Recent Results
in Cancer Research 128

E. Hecker E.G. Jung F. Marks
W. Tilgen (Eds.)

Skin Carcinogenesis in Man and in Experimental Models

With a Foreword by Harald zur Hausen

With 67 Figures and 44 Tables

Springer-Verlag
Berlin Heidelberg New York
London Paris Tokyo
Hong Kong Barcelona
Budapest

Prof. Dr. E. Hecker
Deutsches Krebsforschungszentrum
Division: Mechanisms of Tumorigenesis
Research Program 3: Risk Factors of Cancer
and Cancer Prevention, Im Neuenheimer Feld 280
W-6900 Heidelberg, Germany

Prof. Dr. E.G. Jung
Director, Department of Dermatology
Mannheim Medical School, University of Heidelberg
Postfach 10 80 23, Theodor-Kutzer-Ufer
W-6800 Mannheim, Germany

Prof. Dr. F. Marks
Deutsches Krebsforschungszentrum
Division: Biochemistry of Tissue Specific Regulation
Research Program 2: Tumor Cell Regulation
Im Neuenheimer Feld 280
W-6900 Heidelberg, Germany

Privatdozent Dr. W. Tilgen
Department of Dermatology
University of Heidelberg, Voss-Str. 2
W-6900 Heidelberg, Germany

ISBN-13:978-3-642-84883-4 e-ISBN-13:978-3-642-84881-0
DOI: 10.1007/978-3-642-84881-0

Library of Congress Cataloging-in-Publication Data. Skin carcinogenesis in man and in experimental models / E. Hecker ... [et al.] (ed.). p. cm. – (Recent resuls in cancer research : 128) Includes bibliographical references and index. ISBN-13:978-3-642-84883-4 1. Skin – Cancer – Congresses. 2. Skin – Cancer – Animal models – Congresses. 3. Carcinogenesis – Congresses. 4. Carcinogenesis – Animal models – Congresses. I. Hecker, Erich. II. Series. [DNLM: 1. Disease Models, Animal – congresses. 2. Melanoma – congresses. 3. Neoplasms, Experimental – congresses. 4. Skin Neoplasms – congresses. W1 RE106P v.128 1993 / WR 500 S62828 1993] RC261.R35 no. 128 [RC280.S5] 616.99′4 s – dc20 [616.99′4.77′071] DNLM/DLC

Softcover reprint of the hardcover 1st edition 1993

Typesetting: Best-set Typesetter Ltd., Hong Kong
25/3130/SPS-5 4 3 2 1 0 – Printed on acid-free paper

Secretary General of the Symposium

E. Hecker, Honorary Chairman, Heidelberg

Scientific Program Committee

F. Marks, Chairman experimental aspects, Heidelberg
E. G. Jung/W. Tilgen, Chairmen clinical aspects, Heidelberg
A. Balmain, Glasgow
R. K. Boutwell, Madison
G. Fürstenberger, Heidelberg
N. E. Fusenig, Heidelberg
R. J. M. Fry, Oak Ridge
L. Gissmann, Heidelberg
V. Kinzel, Heidelberg
R. M. Kripke, Houston
J. C. van der Leun, Utrecht
R. M. MacKie, Glasgow
R. Schmidt, Heidelberg
H. W. Thielmann, Heidelberg

Local Organizing Committee

N. E. Fusenig, Chairman, Heidelberg
E. Egenlauf, Heidelberg
J. Hietzker, Heidelberg
E. Mang, Heidelberg
F. Marks, Heidelberg

Foreword

The detection of cancer risk factors and their possible avoidance would most effectively contribute to the fight against cancer. Research in these areas depends to a substantial degree on in vivo experimental animal models and on epidemiologic studies, including data from cancer registries.

When the Deutsches Krebsforschungszentrum was founded in 1964, its division "Mechanisms of Tumorigenesis" and a number of other divisions became engaged in research on chemical carcinogenesis of the skin, mainly using the mouse skin as an experimental model. Their interest originated in part from investigations of the new and at that time controversial pathogenic principle of conditional carcinogens as represented by certain tumor promoters which are *per se* noncarcinogenic. During the past 25 years, conditional carcinogens in terms of tumor promoters were established as a new, nonclassical category of cancer risk factors besides the classical solitary carcinogens.

In the course of this exciting period, scientists of our center started cooperative programs with clinical dermatologists of the University of Heidelberg at the Clinics of Dermatology in Heidelberg and Mannheim, to extend the scope of their investigations into clinical oncology and to contribute by experimental approaches to solving problems in clinical oncology. This led to a gradual shift from mere animal studies to the more direct analyses of human tumors and opened up for us a new phase of research. At this stage it appeared to be most appropriate that the scientists of the Deutsches Krebsforschungszentrum and the clinicians of the University of Heidelberg jointly organize an international symposium on Skin Carcinogenesis in Man and in Experimental Models. It was held on October 29–31, 1991, at the Deutsches Krebsforschungszentrum in Heidelberg.

The inviting institutions were pleased to welcome clinicians and experimentalists active in skin cancer research from all over the world. Intensive discussions during the meeting documented the interest of the scientific community. I am, therefore, pleased that the present volume of *Recent Results in Cancer Research* documents as the proceedings of the symposium the most important areas of current research which were, unanimously, recognized to mark problems deserving particular scientific efforts. It should provide an overview of the current state of the art in experimental and clinical investigations of skin carcinogenesis, a particularly important topic in cancer research and cancer prevention.

I trust these Proceedings will be welcomed by the scientific community.

Heidelberg,
January 1993

Harald zur Hausen
Chairman of the Management Board
Deutsches Krebsforschungszentrum

Preface

The slow, but steady increase in the incidence of skin cancers in human beings urged scientists of the Deutsches Krebsforschungszentrum (DKFZ) and clinicians of the University of Heidelberg to call and invite experts in science and medicine for an international symposium on which this book is based. The increase of skin cancer over the last decades is well documented by epidemiologic evidence. It may have a number of different causes, of which the generation and existence of so-called "holes" in the ozone layer resulting from a depletion of stratospheric ozone—now to be found above both of the earth's poles—causes many headlines in the media and deep general concern as expressed, e.g., by the United Nations Environment Program (UNEP)[1]. Investigations on risk factors for cancer of the skin and on prevention of skin cancer are therefore considered "hot spots" in present-day cancer research. Scientists of the DKFZ have been dealing with etiologies and mechanisms of skin carcinogenesis in experimental models for about 25 years, and continue to do so. As a result, many contacts were developed with the Departments of Dermatology of the University of Heidelberg, one located traditionally in Heidelberg city and the other in the neighboring city of Mannheim. Such a background of traditional, experimental, and clinical engagement in skin cancers made it seem particularly appropriate and timely to invite scientists to an international symposium on Skin Carcinogenesis in Man and in Experimental Models. It was held October 29–31, 1991, at the DKFZ and intended to update, analyze,

[1] See especially the contribution by van der Leun et al. on p. 263.

and discuss the latest facts in the etiology of, and in the mechanisms involved in, the generation of cancer of the skin.

For the first time, a report was presented on the German Melanoma Register which collects in Germany scientific data on the incidence and possible causes of this most aggressive skin cancer. Besides the many other practical aspects, numerous theoretical considerations on the generation of skin cancer were discussed, nourished essentially by experimental models. Thus, a large body of experimental facts on the impact of exogenous (environmental) risk factors on genetic and epigenetic elements of target cells in the skin were presented. Also, the role of genetic predisposition and elimination of crucial genomic damage were themes of the symposium. In this context the role of oncogenes and suppressor genes as sources of endogenous risk factors was accounted for specifically.

The organizers of the symposium—the Secretary General, the international scientific program committee and the local organizing committee—were pleased to welcome in the DKFZ about 250 registered participants, clinicians from many departments of dermatology as well as experimentalists working on skin cancer from Western and Eastern Europe, from the USA, and from the Far East. To take part, some of the visitors had travelled long distances, from as far as Japan, or had come from areas such as Slovenia and Russia. Many of them contributed actively to the symposium—by holding one of the 27 invited lectures, as chairpersons of the scientific sessions, or as presenters of more than 70 posters. The organizers believe that this symposium has generated an overview of the current state of the art in scientific experimental and clinical investigations on the generation and the prevention of cancer of the skin. From the results presented, marked refinements in the assessment of the risk of cancer associated with environmental and endogenous factors, including tumor viruses, will hopefully be stimulated. Moreover, new ideas should emerge for developing specific approaches to explore the mechanistic, i.e., ultimately the molecular-biological, causes of skin cancers and others. In addition, the experimental utilization of oncogenes and of other techniques from molecular biology at all levels of the biology of tissues and cells may open up entirely new facets in research on skin cancer. Detailed knowledge of the mechanistic aspects of skin carcinogenesis may give important hints on how to "tailor-make" and utilize new antitumor agents in the therapy of skin cancer for the benefit of the cancer patient.

This book, as the proceedings of the symposium, covers all 27 invited lectures, arranged according to the three sections of the symposium's scientific program; for the corresponding posters the book of abstracts for the symposium may be consulted (J Cancer Res Clin Oncol 116 (Suppl) S61–S88 (1991)). Many thanks are due from the organizers to Mrs. E. Mang and Dr. B. Sorg for compiling the indices of the book and to the publishers, Springer-Verlag, for their efficient cooperation in the technical editing and production of the proceedings.

Heidelberg,
January 1993

Erich Hecker
Director at the
Deutsches Krebsforschungszentrum,
Head, Division Mechanisms of
Tumorigenesis Research Program 3,
Risk Factors of Cancer and
Cancer Prevention

Contents

*List of Contributors**

* The address of the principal author is given on the first page of each contribution.
[1] Page on which contribution begins.

I. General Aspects

Genetic Determinants in Carcinogenesis

J.C. Barrett

Laboratory of Molecular Carcinogenesis, National Institute of Environmental Health Sciences, National Institutes of Health, P.O. Box 12233, Research Triangle Park, NC 27709, USA

Introduction

There are three types of risk factors that determine whether an individual will develop cancer – environmental exposures, intrinsic susceptibility, and age/time. It is important, therefore, to understand the genetic determinants underlying these risk factors. The critical target genes for environmental factors are, in part, known and include protooncogenes and tumor suppressor genes (Boyd and Barrett 1990; Bishop 1991). These are discussed further by Balmain, Bowden, and others in this volume. The genetic determinants for intrinsic susceptibility to cancer are of two types. On the one hand, genetic variations exist in genes that influence the impact of environmental agents on an individual, such as genes that control carcinogen metabolism or repair of carcinogenic damage (Hanawalt and Sarasin 1986; Lehmann and Dean 1990). On the other hand, individuals may inherit germ line mutations in genes that are directly involved in the neoplastic conversion of normal cells (Malkin et al. 1990). For example, inherited mutations in tumor suppressor genes can increase the risk of specific cancers. The magnitude of this increased risk can vary greatly depending on the number of additional steps required for the genesis of the tumor. For example, mutations in the *rb* gene increase the relative risk for retinoblastoma by 10^5-fold whereas the same mutation, increases the risk for lung cancer by only 10-fold (A. Knudson, personal communication). This is probably because retinoblastomas only require one additional mutation, inactivation of the wild-type allele of the *rb* gene, whereas lung cancers require this mutation plus multiple mutations in other genes. Germ line mutations of other genes also contribute to increased risk of cancer, including the APC (adenopolyposis of the colon) gene, p53 gene, Wilms tumor gene, neurofibromatosis gene, early onset breast cancer susceptibility gene, and possibly others. The proportion of cancers arising as the consequence of germ line mutations in tumor suppressor genes is unknown but

Recent Results in Cancer Research, Vol. 128

may be greater than previously appreciated due to the facts that multiple tumor suppressor genes exist, which affect different types of cancers, and that most of these mutations are de novo germ line mutations (Malkin et al. 1990)

The third risk factor for cancer is time or age. The incidence for common cancers rises exponentially with the fourth, fifth, or higher power of age (Cutler and Semsei 1989). Thus, time or age is the most potent carcinogen known. The critical question is which of these two chronological parameters is important: Is time per se the only risk factor or does the aging process play a role in the development of cancers?

Role of Aging Versus Time in Carcinogenesis

There are arguments to support the hypothesis that time per se is all that is important in the age-dependent incidence curves for cancer as well as evidence to support the concept that the aging and cancer processes are interrelated.

There are two lines of reason that favor the role of time in cancer development. First, the exponential increase in cancer incidence as a function of time is completely predicted on the basis of mathematical models that describe the development of cancer as a multihit process (Peto et al. 1975; Kaldor and Day 1987), which is now supported by molecular studies of cancer genetics (Bishop 1991; Boyd and Barrett 1990). If one assumes that a cancer arises as the consequence of multiple independent mutations that occur in a stochastic manner, then an age/time-dependent occurrence of different cancers is predicted and the slope of the curve is determined by the number of mutations required for a given cancer (Kaldor and Day 1987).

This model generates time-dependent exponential increases in cancer incidence. However, there is evidence against the hypothesis that the aging process enhances the development of cancers. In general, animals become less susceptible, not more susceptible, to carcinogenesis as they age. For example, older animals are generally less susceptible to carcinogen-induced tumorigenesis (Anisimov and Turusov 1981; Peto et al. 1975), and tumor transplantation studies reveal that tumors grow less well in older animals, indicating that physiological functions, such as declining immunological responses, do not facilitate growth of tumors in older animals (Ershler 1986; Ershler et al. 1984; Volk and Ershler 1991).

These observations fail to support the concept that the aging process contributes to the development of cancers. However, there is other evidence that suggests an interrelationship between aging and cancer. One way to test the hypothesis that these two processes are related would be to examine animals that have mutations in genes affecting lifespan and ask whether genetic effects on lifespan affect cancer development. If cancer and aging were unrelated, then mutants with accelerated aging would not be expected to develop cancers at a faster rate. Fortunately, nature has provided some interesting examples of such genetic experiments. In humans, there are genetic variants that exhibit premature aging. One example is Werner syndrome, which is characterized by premature aging in midlife (Salk et al. 1985). The onset of this disease is typically between 21 and 58 years of age (mean 38.7 years) and the individuals die in the fourth or fifth decade of life (Goldstein et al. 1990). The causes of death are similar to those of the general population – arteriosclerosis and cancer. Interestingly, Werner syndrome patients with accelerated aging have an earlier appearance of certain cancers, which suggests an association between the gene or genes causing aging and cancer.

A more striking example of decreased lifespan and accelerated cancer formation is provided by comparisons of evolutionarily divergent species, such as rodents and humans. Rats, for example, have approximately the same spontaneous incidence of cancer (≈30%) at 2 years as humans at 80 years (Cutler and Semsei 1989). Similar exponential increases in the incidence of cancer as a function of age occur in rodents and humans, except that common tumors arise within 1–2 years in rodents and only after decades in humans. If the same processes are involved in the development of cancer in rodents and humans, why do rats get cancer? They should die of "old age" before getting cancer. Since rats do get cancer at a similar (and sometimes higher) incidence than humans, there must be some relationship between the genetic determinants for aging and cancer. Aging does not cause cancer, but genes involved in controlling lifespan and aging may also affect cancer development. A further understanding of the genes controlling aging should increase our understanding of the cancer process and vice versa.

Why Do Rodents Get Cancer?

While there appears to be an interrelationship between lifespan and cancer development, the nature of this relationship is unknown. Therefore, it is a fundamental problem in cancer biology to understand why tumors arise more rapidly in rodents than in humans. Elucidation of the molecular basis for cancer development in different species may provide some insight into this question.

Given that cancer is a multistep process involving multiple genetic changes (and there is ample evidence to support this conclusion in rodents and humans), the difference in time of occurrence of human versus rodent cancers suggests either that: (a) fewer steps (genetic events) are required in the evolution of rodent tumors, or (b) the rates of transition between the steps are slower in humans. A combination of these two differences may also contribute to accelerated tumor development in rodents (or in its delayed development in humans).

It is very difficult to address these possibilities in vivo. However, one approach to the elucidation of differences in neoplastic development between humans and rodents is to dissect the carcinogenic process in vitro using cells from each species. Extensive studies by multiple laboratories over many years have used such an approach, and a number of similarities have emerged in the neoplastic process of cells from different mammalian species. Neoplastic conversion of both human and rodent cells in culture is a multistep process involving both activation of protooncogenes and inactivation of tumor suppressor genes (Barrett and Fletcher 1987; Bishop 1991). Cooperation between oncogenes (e.g., *ras* plus *myc*) increases the neoplastic progression of both human and rodent cells (Hurlin et al. 1989; Rhim et al. 1985), and inactivation of multiple tumor suppressor genes has been shown in human and rodent tumors (Bishop 1991; Boyd and Barrett 1990). Despite these similarities, one major species difference is clear from studies of cell transformation; the ability of rodent cells in culture to escape cellular senescence spontaneously or following carcinogen treatment is significantly greater than that of human cells (Barrett and Fletcher 1987; McCormick and Maher 1988).

Both human and rodent cells in culture can be grown for only a limited number of cell divisions, after which they exhibit morphological changes and cease proliferation, a process termed cellular senescence or cellular aging (Hayflick 1976). Thirty years ago, Hayflick and Moorhead (1961) reported that normal human fibroblasts are able to undergo a limited, fixed number of cell divisions, after which they cease proliferation. For example, embryonic human fibroblasts can be grown for 50–60 population doublings before senescence. The failure of the cells to grow beyond this limit is an inherent property of the cells that cannot be explained simply by inadequate media components (Hayflick 1976). The key determinant in the lifespan of cells in culture is the number of cell doublings, not the length of time in culture (Hayflick 1976). Normal cells transplanted serially in vivo also exhibit a finite lifespan, suggesting that cellular senescence is not a cell culture artifact (Daniel et al. 1986).

Three lines of evidence suggest that the aging of cells in culture may be related to the aging of the organism (Hayflick 1976):

1. The doubling potential of cells in culture is inversely proportional to the age of the donor. Cells from embryonic tissue exhibit the longest lifespan (50–60 cell doublings). Cells from adult tissue can be grown for only 14–29 doublings, and there is a general decrease in the lifespan of cells in culture with increasing age of the donor tissue.
2. Cells derived from individuals who exhibit premature aging have a decreased lifespan in culture. Patients with progeria (Hutchinson–Gilford syndrome) manifest signs of aging at the end of their first decade of life that are typical of normal individuals in the seventh decade of life. Werner syndrome individuals also have accelerated aging but in later

years – the mean age of death is 47. The main causes of death in these individuals are cancer and cardiovascular disease, similar to the causes in normal individuals. Fibroblasts derived from individuals with the premature aging characteristics senesce prematurely in culture, after only 2–10 population doublings.

3. The lifespan of cells in culture is correlated in general with the maximun lifespan of the species, although the variability in this experimental data is great. Cells from humans (maximum lifespan 100–120 years) can be grown for 50–60 population doublings, whereas cells from rodents (3–5-year lifespan) can be grown for only 20–40 population doublings. Cells from the Galapagos tortoise, which has a lifespan of 175–200 years, undergo a greater number of population doublings (90–125) in culture than human cells.

These lines of evidence, although not conclusive, provide provocative support for the hypothesis that aging of cells is related to the aging process of the organism.

Escape from cellular senescence is an important step in neoplastic progression of human and rodent cancers (Barrett and Fletcher 1987). Many, but not all, tumor cells can be grown indefinitely in culture and therefore have escaped senescence and are termed immortal. It is not clear whether the failure of some tumor cells to grow in culture is a technical artifact or an indication that escape from senescence is not required for these cancers. Many of these tumors cannot be maintained in vivo in nude mice, suggesting that only a small growth fraction of cells exists in the tumor. Improvements in cell culture techniques have led to the establishment of many cell lines from most tumor types, suggesting that it is possible to obtain immortal cell lines if the culture conditions are optimal. Since no property of cancer cells is universal, it is not necessary to demonstrate that escape from senescence has occurred in every cancer. However, in those cancers where this change is evident, it is probably a critical change, based on the following addtional lines of evidence (Barrett and Fletcher 1987).

The observation that treatment of normal cells with diverse carcinogenic agents, including chemical carcinogens, viruses, and oncogenes, allows cells to escape senescence indicates that this change is important in cancer induction. While immortality is not sufficient for neoplastic transformation, most immortal cells have an increased propensity for spontaneous, carcinogen-induced, or oncogene-induced neoplastic progression (Barrett and Fletcher 1987). Therefore, escape from senescence is a preneoplastic change that predisposes a cell to neoplastic conversion. It is clear that immortal cells are further along the multistep pathway to neoplasia than normal cells.

Cellular senescence may be one of the mechanisms by which tumor suppression occurs (Sager 1986; Barrett and Fletcher 1987). Tumor suppression is controlled by a family of normal cellular genes that must be inactivated, lost, or mutated in cancer cells. Since cellular senescence limits the growth of cells, it is reasonable that senescence might be one mechanism by which tumor suppressor genes operate.

Two major theories of cellular senescence have been proposed for many years (Macieira-Coelho 1988). One is the error catastrophe or damage model, which proposes that random accumulation of damage or mutations in DNA, RNA, or protein leads to the loss of proliferative capacity. The experimental evidence supporting the error accumulation hypothesis has been criticized (Macieira-Coelho 1988). A second hypothesis is that senescence is a genetically programmed process, and recent support for a genetic basis for senescence was provided by experiments of Pereira-Smith and Smith (1988) and by Sugawara et al. (1990).

It is possible to fuse cells of different origins and then to select for the hybrid cells using biochemical markers for drug sensitivity or resistance that differ in the parental cells. When cells with a finite lifespan are fused to immortal cells with an indefinite lifespan, the majority of these hybrids senesce, indicating that senescence is dominant over immortality (Koi and Barrett 1986; Pereira-Smith and Smith 1988). Even hybridization of two different immortal human cell lines with each other can result in senescence, indicating that different complementation groups exist for the senescence function lost in these cells. Four complementation groups have been established, suggesting that loss or inactivation of one of multiple genes might allow escape from senescence (Pereira-Smith and Smith 1988). If this hypothesis is correct, it should be possible to map the genes involved in cellular senescence. Recent findings with hamster and human interspecies hybrids have mapped putative senescence genes to specific human chromosomes (Sugawara et al. 1990).

When we fused normal human lung fibroblasts (MRC-5), which have a finite lifespan, to immortal hamster cells, the hybrids that formed exhibited a finite lifespan characteristic of the normal human cells (Sugawara et al. 1990). At the end of this lifespan, the cells displayed signs of cellular senescence characteristic of the parental human cells at the end of their lifespan. When MRC-5 cells, which have a lifespan of 60 population doublings, were used at a population doubling level of 40, the human–hamster hybrids grew for approximately 20 population doublings, i.e., the remaining lifespan of the parental human cells. Since the cell hybrids grew extensively before dying, the cessation of growth was not due to a toxic effect of the fusion protocol or some other trivial reason. Furthermore, when earlier passage MRC-5 cells were used (population doubling level 30), the hybrids grew longer, for up to 30 population doublings, again achieving the lifespan of the parental cells. Therefore, the senescence of the hybrids is an active process dictated by the senescence program of the normal human cells. The limited lifespan of the hybrids indicates that cellular senescence is dominant in these hamster–human hybrids. A similar conclusion was drawn from studies of intraspecies hybrids, i.e., human–human and hamster–hamster (Koi and Barrett 1986; Pereira-Smith and Smith 1988).

Although the majority of the hamster–human hybrids senesced, some of the hybrids ultimately escaped senescence. Senescent cells appeared in all of the hybrid clones after two to three passages. In some of the clones a few nonsenescent cells continued to proliferate, achieving 100 population doublings with high labeling indices and colony forming efficiencies (Sugawara et al. 1990). This was an indication that these hybrid clones had escaped senescence. Because human chromosomes are usually lost in interspecies hybrids, the possibility that escape from senescence is due to loss of an essential chromosome or chromosomes was examined by karyotypic analysis of the hybrids after escape from senescence (approximately 40 population doublings). It is possible to distinguish human and hamster chromosomes; therefore, the simple question was asked whether escape from senescence involved the loss of any specific human chromosome. Without exception, all of the human–hamster hybrid clones that escaped senescence had lost both copies of human chromosome 1. All other human chromosomes were present in one or two copies in at least one of the immortal hybrids (Sugawara et al. 1990).

In order to determine whether the loss of chromosome 1 in nonsenescent hybrids was the fortuitous consequence of human chromosome loss in the hybrid or an indication that a gene on this chromosome influenced the senescence process, two additional approaches were undertaken. One involved interspecies cell hybrids with human cells carrying X; autosomal chromosome translocations. These experiments showed that applying selective pressure for the long arm of chromosome 1 increased the percentage of senescent hybrids. The second approach involved microcell hybrids containing individual human chromosomes by which we could introduce only chromosome 1 to show induction of cellular senescence. The data strongly implicated a gene or genes on human chromosome 1 being involved in cellular senescence.

Recently, in collaboration with Dr. Max Costa and coworkers, we have mapped another senescence gene to chromosome X (Klein et al. 1991). In addition, Pereira-Smith and Smith (1988) and Ning et al. (1991) have mapped a senescence gene for HeLa cells to chromosome 4. Thus, three senescence genes have now been mapped (Table 1).

These results have led us to propose the following hypothesis: Cellular senescence is controlled by genes that are activated or whose functions become manifested at the end of the lifespan of the cell. Defects in the function of these gene products can allow cells to escape the program of senescence and become immortal. Immortalization relieves one constraint on tumor cell growth, allowing malignant progression. Current efforts are focused on the cloning of these genes and on understanding how they operate to arrest cell growth.

Table 1. Mapping of putative senescence genes

Chromosome localization of *sen*$^+$ gene	Cell line(s)	Reference
Chromosome 1	Syrian hamster 10W	Sugawara et al. (1990)
	Human endometrium	Yamada et al. (1990)
Chromosome 4	Cervical carcinoma (HeLa)	Ning et al. (1991)
Chromosome X	Chinese hamster (Ni-2)	Klein et al. (1991)

Possible Role of Cell Cycle Controls in Cellular Senescence

The retinoblastoma susceptibility gene encodes a nuclear phosphoprotein of 110 kDa (H.-H. Lee et al. 1987; Zu et al. 1989). Inactivation of both alleles of this gene leads to the development of retinoblastoma and has been implicated in several malignancies including osteosarcoma, soft tissue sarcomas, lung carcinoma, and breast carcinoma (Friend et al. 1987; Harbour et al. 1988; E.Y.-H.P. Lee et al. 1988; Stratton et al. 1989; T'Ang et al. 1988; Weichselbaum et al. 1988). Recent work has shown that the RB protein is differentially phosphorylated during the cell cycle (Buchkovich et al. 1989; Chen et al. 1989; DeCaprio et al. 1989; Furukawa et al. 1990; Mihara et al. 1989). It was found that the RB protein is unphosphorylated in the G_1/G_0 compartment of the cell cycle and is phosphorylated as cells enter into S phase. The protein is increasingly phosphorylated as the cells progress through G_2 and M, and is again primarily in the unphosphorylated form as cells reenter G_1. Also, the RB protein was found to be unphosphorylated in cells induced to differentiate (Buchkovich et al. 1989; Chen et al. 1989; Furukawa et al. 1990; Mihara et al. 1989). These data suggest that the unphosphorylated form of the protein is growth inhibitory and that the tumor suppressor function of the RB protein may be linked to cell cycle control and differentiation. Therefore, we examined whether the product of the retinoblastoma tumor suppressor gene may be a key regulator of cellular senescence (Futreal and Barrett 1991).

Examination of RB protein expression levels in senescent Syrian hamster embryo (SHE) cells was accomplished by SDS-PAGE separation of cellular lysates, followed by the western blotting procedure and immunochemical detection using monoclonal antibodies to the human retinoblastoma protein (Futreal and Barrett 1991). This antibody detected bands of approximately 110–116 kDa by western blot in the hamster cells, which is similar to the reported sizes of both human and mouse RB proteins (Furukawa et al. 1990; Futreal and Barrett 1991; Zu et al. 1989). Senescent SHE cell cultures expressed comparable levels of RB protein to young cells; however, only the unphosphorylated form of RB was observed.

We examined whether the senescent cells could be stimulated to phosphorylate the RB protein in response to growth stimulatory signals (Futreal and Barrett 1991). When cultures of young or senescent cells were maintained for 48 h in media containing 0.5% serum, both young and senescent cells exhibited only the unphosphorylated form of the RB protein as determined by western blot analysis. When the cells were stimulated with medium containing 10% serum, the phosphorylated form of the RB protein was observed in the young cells by 10 h after serum stimulation, peaking at 20 h, which corresponds to the time course for stimulation of DNA synthesis under similar conditions. In the senescent cells, the RB protein remained unphosphorylated at all time points examined (up to 120 h). This result indicates that senescent cells are blocked in their ability to phosphorylate the RB protein in response to normal growth stimuli (Fig. 1).

Studies by Stein et al. (1990) also found that the RB protein was not phosphorylated in senescent human cells, which further substantiates the possible growth regulatory role of the unphosphorylated RB protein in cellular senescence of cells from different species. We have shown that senescent cells no longer possess the capability to phosphorylate the RB protein in response to growth stimulation (Futreal and Barrett 1991). This finding implicates upstream modifiers of RB phosphorylation as possible crucial regulatory elements in mediating cellular senescence, with the end result being a block to proliferation caused by the presence of unphosphorylated RB protein acting on its own or through other effector molecules. Downregulation of a RB kinase activity in senescent cells and/or upregulated activity of a RB phosphatase are possible mechanisms for the alterations of RB phosphorylation in senescent cells. Recent studies indicate that the p34 cdc2 kinase, which is a candidate RB kinase, is downregulated in senescent human and hamster cells (Richter et al. 1991).

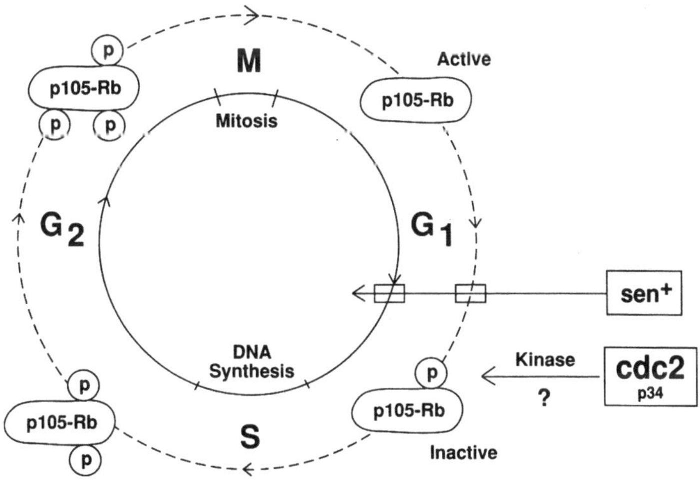

Fig. 1. The block to DNA synthesis in senescent cells appears to be in late G_1 prior to the phosphorylation of the RB protein

In conclusion, an important difference between the neoplastic transformation in human and rodent cells is the propensity of rodent cells to escape cellular senescence. Cellular senescence has been shown to be controlled by a family of genes and defects in these genes allow cells to become immortal. Senescence genes have been mapped to three chromosomes (1, 4, and X), and these genes are active in both human and rodent cells. Therefore, the difference in immortalization (escape from senescence) of these different cells cannot be explained on the basis of a different genetic mechanism for human versus rodent cells. It is possible, however, that the difference between human and rodent cells is the number of genes (or gene defects) required for immortalization. Immortalization is a multistep process for both human and rodent cells, but the number of steps involved for any cell type is not clearly established (Barrett and Fletcher 1987; Bols et al. 1991). An alternative possibility is that the rates at which changes occur differ between cells of different species. In support of this hypothesis, we have shown that induction of aneuploidy correlates with chemically induced immortalization of SHE cells (Barrett 1987) and that the rates of aneuploidy induction in human cells are approximately tenfold lower than in hamster cells (Tsutsui et al. 1990). However, the difference in induction of aneuploidy is less than the difference in immortalization between these species (Barrett 1987). Further explanation of the differences between human and rodent cell immortalization must therefore await cloning of the genes involved in senescence and elucidation of how the growth arrest process occurs in senescent cells.

References

Anisimov VN, Turusov VS (1981) Modifying effect of aging on chemical carcinogenesis. A review. Mech Ageing Dev 15:399–414

Barrett JC (1987) Relationship between mutagenesis and carcinogenesis. In: Barrett JC (ed) Mechanisms of environmental carcinogenesis, vol I. CRC, Boca Raton, pp 129–142

Barrett JC, Fletcher WF (1987) Cellular and molecular mechanisms of multistep carcinogenesis in cell culture models. In: Barrett JC (ed) Mechanisms of environmental carcinogenesis: multistep models of carcinogenesis, vol II. CRC, Boca Raton, pp 73–116

Bishop JM (1991) Molecular themes in oncogenesis. Cell 64:235–248

Bols BL, Naaktgeboren JM, Simons JW (1991) Immortalization of Syrian hamster embryo cells is in itself a multistep event. Cancer Res 51:1177–1184

Boyd J, Barrett JC (1990) Tumor suppressor genes: possible functions in the negative regulation of cell proliferation. Mol Carcinog 3:325–329

Buchkovich K, Duffy LA, Harlow E (1989) The retinoblastoma protein is phosphorylated during specific phases of the cell cycle. Cell 58:1097–1105

Chen P-L, Scully P, Shew J-Y, Wang JYJ, Lee W-H (1989) Phosphorylation of the retinoblastoma gene product is modulated during the cell cycle and cellular differentiation. Cell 58:1193–1198

Cutler RG, Semsei I (1989) Development, cancer and aging: possible common mechanisms of action and regulation. J Gerontol 44:25–34

Daniel CW, DeOme KB, Young JT, Blair PB, Faulkin LJ Jr (1968) The in vivo span of normal and preneoplastic mouse mammary glands: a serial transplantation study. Proc Natl Acad Sci USA 61:53–60
DeCaprio JA, Ludlow JW, Lynch D, Furukawa Y, Griffin J, PiwnicaWorms H, Huang C-M, Livingston DM (1989) The product of the retinoblastoma susceptibility gene has properties of a cell cycle regulatory element. Cell 58:1085–1095
Ershler WB (1986) Why tumors grow more slowly in old people. J Natl Cancer Inst 77:837–839
Ershler WB, Stewart JA, Hacker MP, Moore AL, Tindle BH (1984) B16 murine melanoma and aging: slower growth and longer survival in old mice. J Natl Cancer Inst 72:161–164
Friend SH, Horowitz JM, Gerber MR, Wang X-F, Bogenmann E, Li FP, Weinberg RA (1987) Deletions of a DNA sequence in retinoblastomas and mesenchymal tumors: organization of the sequence and its encoded protein. Proc Natl Acad Sci USA 84:9059–9063
Furukawa Y, DeCaprio JA, Freedman A, Kanakura Y, Makamura M, Ernst TJ, Livingston DM, Griffin JD (1990) Expression and state of phosphorylation of the retinoblastoma susceptibility gene product in cycling and noncycling human hematopoietic cells. Proc Natl Acad Sci USA 87:2770–2774
Futreal PA, Barrett JC (1991) Failure of senescent cells to phosphorylate the RB protein. Oncogene 6:1109–1113
Goldstein S, Murano S, Reis RJS (1990) Werner syndrome: a molecular genetic hypothesis. J Gerontol 45:B3–B8
Hanawalt PC, Sarasin A (1986) Cancer-prone hereditary diseases with DNA processing abnormalities. Trends Genet 2:124–129
Harbour JW, Lai S-L, Whang-Peng J, Gazdar AF, Minna JD, Haye FJ (1988) Abnormalities in structure and expression of the human retinoblastoma gene in SCLC. Science 241:353–357
Hayflick L (1976) The cell biology of human aging. N Engl J Med 295:1302–1308
Hayflick L, Moorhead PS (1961) The serial cultivation of human diploid cell strains. Exp Cell Res 25:585–621
Hurlin PJ, Maher VM, McCormick JJ (1989) Malignant transformation of human fibroblasts caused by expression of a transfected T24 HRAS oncogene. Proc Natl Acad Sci USA 86:187–191
Kaldor JM, Day NE (1987) Interpretation of epidemiological studies on the context of the multistage model of carcinogenesis. In: Barrett JC (ed) Mechanisms of environmental carcinogenesis, vol II. CRC, Boca Raton, pp 21–57
Klein CB, Conway K, Wang XW, Bhamra RK, Lin X, Cohen MD, Annab L, Barrett JC, Costa M (1991) Senescence of nickel-transformed cells by a mammalian X chromosome: possible epigenetic control. Science 251:796–799
Koi M, Barrett JC (1986) Loss of tumor-suppressive function during chemically induced neoplastic progression of Syrian hamster embryo cells. Proc Natl Acad Sci USA 83:5992–5996
Lee EY-HP, To H, Shew Y-Y, Bookstein R, Scully P, Lee W-H (1988) Inactivation of the retinoblastoma susceptibility gene in human breast cancers. Science 241:218–221
Lee H-H, Shew J-Y, Hong FD, Shery TW, Domoso LA, Young L-J, Bookstein R, Lee ER-H (1987) The retinoblastoma susceptibility gene encodes a nuclear phosphoprotein associated with DNA binding activity. Nature 329:642–646
Lehmann AR, Dean SW (1990) Cancer-prone human disorders with defects in DNA repair. In: Cooper CS, Grover PL (eds) Chemical carcinogenesis and mutagenesis II. Springer, Berlin Heidelberg New York, pp 71–101 (Handbook of experimental pharmacology, vol 94)

Macieira-Coelho A (1988) Biology of normal proliferating cells in vitro. Relevance for in vivo aging. In: von Hang HP (ed) Interdisciplinary topics in gerontology, vol 23. Karger, Basel

Malkin D, Li FP, Strong LC, Fraumeni JF Jr, Nelson CE, Kim DH, Kassel J, Gryka MA, Bischoff FZ, Tainsky MA, Friend SH (1990) Germ line p53 mutations in a familial syndrome of breast cancer, sarcomas, and other neoplasms. Science 250:1233–1238

McCormick JJ, Maher VM (1988) Towards an understanding of the malignant transformation of diploid human fibroblasts. Mutat Res 199:273–291

Mihara K, Cao X-R, Yen A, Chandler S, Driscoll B, Murphree AL, T'Ang A, Fung Y-KY (1989) Cell cycle-dependent regulation of phosphorylation of the human retinoblastoma gene product. Science 246:1300–1303

Ning Y, Weber JL, Killary AM, Ledbetter DH, Smith JR, Pereira-Smith OM (1991) Genetic analysis of indefinite division in human cells: evidence for a cell senescence-related gene(s) on human chromosome 4. Proc Natl Acad Sci USA 88:5635–5639

Pereira-Smith OM, Smith JR (1988) Genetic analysis of indefinite division in human cells: identification of four complementation groups. Proc Natl Acad Sci USA 85:6043–6046

Peto R, Roe FJC, Lee PN, Levy L, Clack J (1975) Cancer and ageing in mice and men. Br J Cancer 32:411–426

Rhim JS, Jay G, Arnstein P, Price FM, Sanford KK, Aaronson SA (1985) Neoplastic transformation of human epidermal keratinocytes by AD12-SV40 and Kirsten sarcoma viruses. Science 227:1250–1252

Richter KH, Afshari CA, Annab LA, Burkhart BA, Owen RD, Boyd J, Barrett JC (1991) Downregulation of cdc2 in senescent human and hamster cells. Cancer Res 51:6010–6013

Sager R (1986) Genetic suppression of tumor formation: A new frontier in cancer research. Cancer Res 46:1573–1580

Salk D, Fujiwara Y, Martin GM (1985) Werner's symdrome and human aging. Plenum, New York (Advances in experimental medicine and biology, vol 190)

Stein GH, Beeson M, Gordon L (1990) Failure to phosphorylate the retinoblastoma gene product in senescent human fibroblasts. Science 249:666–669

Stratton MR, Williams S, Fisher C, Ball A, Westbury G, Gusterson BA, Fletcher CDM, Knight JC, Fung Y-K, Reeves BR, Cooper CS (1989) Structural alterations in the RB1 gene in human soft tissue tumours. Br J Cancer 60:202–205

Sugawara O, Oshimura M, Koi M, Annab L, Barrett JC (1990) Induction of cellular senescence in immortalized cells by human chromosome 1. Science 247:707–710

T'Ang A, Varley JM, Chakraborty S, Murphree AL, Fung Y-KT (1988) Structural rearrangement of the retinoblastoma gene in human breast carcinoma. Science 242:263–266

Tsutsui T, Suzuki N, Maizumi H, Barrett JC (1990) Aneuploidy induction in human fibroblasts: comparison with results in Syrian hamster fibroblasts. Mutat Res 240:241–249

Volk MK, Ershler WB (1991) The influence of immunosenescence on tumor growth and spread; lesions from animal models. Cancer Cells 3:13–18

Weichselbaum RR, Beckett M, Diamond A (1988) Some retinoblastomas, osteosarcomas, and soft tissue sarcomas may share a common etiology. Proc Natl Acad Sci USA 85:2106–2109

Yamada H, Wake N, Fujimoto S, Barrett JC, Oshimura M (1990) Multiple chromosomes carrying tumor suppressor activity for a uterine endometrial

carcinoma cell line identified by microcell mediated chromosome transfer. Oncogene 5:1141–1147
Zu H-J, Hu-S-X, Hashimoto T, Takahashi R, Benedict WF (1989) The retinoblastoma susceptibility gene product: a characteristic pattern in normal and abnormal expression in malignant cells. Oncogene 4:807–812

Transforming Growth Factor Regulation of Keratinocyte Growth

L. Dagnino[1], J.A. Pietenpol[1,2], E.Y. Yang[1], and H.L. Moses[1]

[1] Department of Cell Biology, Vanderbilt University School of Medicine, Nashville, TN 37232, USA
[2] Present address: Johns Hopkins Oncology Center, 424 North Bond Street, Baltimore, MD 21231, USA

Introduction

Transforming growth factors (TGF) were originally defined by their ability to induce morphologic transformation in monolayer culture and stimulate soft agar growth of rodent fibroblast cell lines (DeLarco and Todaro 1978; Moses et al. 1981; Roberts et al. 1981). Early studies with TGF indicated that they may play a role in neoplastic transformation and led to the purification and cloning of two very important growth regulatory molecules, TGF-α and TGF-β.

TGF-α is a 50-amino-acid molecule structurally and functionally similar to epidermal growth factor (EGF) (Marquardt et al. 1984). TGF-α appears to exert its biological effects by binding and activating the EGF transmembrane tyrosine kinase receptor; the biological effects of TGF-α are virtually identical to those of EGF (for review, see Derynck et al. 1989). TGF-α was originally thought to be an embryonic molecule inappropriately expressed in some cancer cells. It was in conjunction with the discovery of TGF-α that the autocrine hypothesis was first published as an explanation for the excessive growth that occurs in neoplastic cells (Sporn and Todaro 1980). TGF-α is now known to be produced by many normal epithelial cells both in culture and in vivo (Coffey et al. 1987; Derynck et al. 1989), and thus may normally function as an autocrine factor. Recent data indicate that autocrine stimulation by TGF-α does occur in carcinoma cells (Sizeland and Burgess 1991).

While negative regulators of cell proliferation had been hypothesized to be important, this field did not gain respectability until the demonstration that TGF-β_1 is a potent inhibitor of cell growth (Tucker et al. 1984). Although TGF-β_1 remains the prototypic diffusible negative regulator of cell proliferation, it has an extraordinary diversity of biological effects (reviewed in Moses 1990). TGF-β_1 belongs to a very large family of related molecules with a wide range of regulatory activities during embryonic development

Recent Results in Cancer Research, Vol. 128

and in the adult state. Of the numerous TGF-β-like molecules, the mammalian TGF-β_1, TGF-β_2, and TGF-β_3 proteins are potent inhibitors of cell growth (Graycar et al. 1989). Recent studies (Pietenpol et al. 1990a,b, 1991; Moses et al. 1990; Murphy et al. 1992) have indicated that antioncogenes, or tumor suppressor genes, may be involved in the negative regulation of cell proliferation by TGF-β_1. This review will discuss the growth inhibitory effects of TGF-β_1 in one in vivo model system, as well as evidence for oncogene and tumor suppressor gene involvement in the growth inhibitory pathway for TGF-β_1.

TGF-β Regulation of Cell Proliferation In Vitro

Although originally described as a factor that stimulated soft agar growth of rodent fibroblasts (Roberts et al. 1981; Moses et al. 1981), it is unlikely that TGF-β_1, or any of the TGF-βs, are direct mitogens for any cell type. They are indirect mitogens for certain mesenchymal cells by inducing endogenous growth factor expression, which stimulates cell proliferation in an autocrine manner (Leof et al. 1986; Battegay et al. 1990). TGF-β_1 was first demonstrated to be a growth inhibitor in studies comparing the biological activities of the growth inhibitor from African green monkey (BSC-1) cells originally described by Holley et al. (Holley et al. 1978) and human platelet-derived TGF-β_1 (Tucker et al. 1984). The growth inhibitor produced by BSC-1 cells has been identified as TGF-β_2 (Hanks et al. 1988). Subsequent studies have demonstrated that TGF-β_1 and TGF-β_2 are the most potent growth inhibitory polypeptides known for a wide variety of cultured cells, including those originating from epithelial, lymphoid, endothelial, and myeloid tissues (for review, see Moses 1990). TGF-β_3 has also been shown to be growth inhibitory for epithelial cells in culture (Graycar et al. 1989). In general, the inhibitory effects of the TGF-βs are reversible. The TGF-βs cause growth arrest in the G_1 phase of the cell cycle (Shipley et al. 1986).

TGF-β Regulation of Cell Proliferation In Vivo

TGF-β_1 and TGF-β_2 also inhibit cell proliferation in vivo. Silberstein and Daniel (1987) reported that TGF-β_1 administered in semisolid pellets reversibly inhibited mammary epithelial cell proliferation in mice. Russell et al. (1988) found that intravenously administered TGF-β_1 and TGF-β_2 inhibited the early phase of liver regeneration following partial hepatectomy. Inhibition of hematopoietic cell proliferation has been demonstrated by Goey et al. (1989) following intraarterial administration of TGF-β_1. TGF-β_1 administration also resulted in suppression of the immune response to immunogenic tumors and of cytotoxic T lymphocyte production in vivo (Torre-Amione et al. 1990; Fontana et al. 1989).

Additional in vivo studies have demonstrated that TGF-β_1 has remarkable effects on the chicken chorioallantoic membrane (CAM) (Yang and Moses 1990). When TGF-β_1 was focally applied to the CAM, gross angiogenesis was induced. Furthermore, a central hypercellular lesion was observed, and was characterized by increases in fibroblast, epithelial, and endothelial cell densities. The formation of this lesion was quite rapid, and fibroblasts and epithelial cells accumulated at the point of treatment within 4 h of exposure to TGF-β_1. This area of increased cell density should have the highest concentration of TGF-β_1. These density changes were not mediated by increases in proliferation, since fibroblasts, endothelial cells, and epithelial cells were markedly growth inhibited in the central area of TGF-β_1 application. Thus, fibroblast and epithelial cell accumulation must have been due to stimulated cell migration from regions peripheral to the site of TGF-β_1 treatment.

These observations are reminiscent of in vitro studies which demonstrated that the chemotactic effects of TGF-β_1 occur at a much lower (subpicomolar) concentration than that required for other TGF-β_1 effects (Postlethwaite et al. 1987). At picomolar concentrations, TGF-β_1 is no longer chemotactic and other biological effects are induced, including growth inhibition and stimulation of extracellular matrix production. The

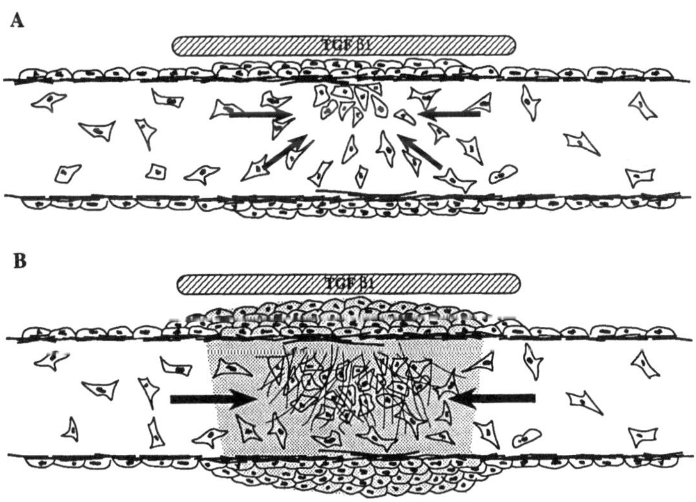

Fig. 1A,B. In Vivo effects of TGF-β_1 on the chicken CAM. When TGF-β_1 is focally applied to the CAM in the form of a methylcellulose disk (*cross-hatched ovals*), TGF-β_1 likely diffuses into the CAM and forms a concentration gradient. **A** Within 4 h, fibroblasts and epithelial cells accumulate centrally through chemotaxis (*arrows*). **B** Beyond 8 h, when more TGF-β_1 has diffused into the CAM, centrally accumulated cells form a zone of growth inhibition (*stippled area*), and chemotaxis probably occurs from more peripheral regions (*arrows*). Angiogenesis then occurs by 16 h (Yang and Moses 1990)

effects of TGF-β_1 on the CAM suggest that similar concentration-dependent mechanisms may specify different zones of cellular function in vivo (Fig. 1). With initial TGF-β_1 administration, rapid inward chemotaxis of cells is observed (Fig. 1A), but with continued administration and increased diffusion of TGF-β_1 into the CAM, the region of chemotactic stimulation moves outward peripherally (Fig. 1B). As cells migrate centrally and accumulate where TGF-β_1 concentrations are higher, they no longer proliferate. However, they perform differentiated functions such as deposition of extracellular matrix by fibroblasts, and formation of capillary tubes and secretion of basement membrane materials by endothelial cells. Thus, TGF-β_1-induced growth inhibition is an integral, and perhaps necessary, component of the mesenchymal reorganization stimulated in the CAM. Similar functions may be stimulated by TGF-β_1 in the physiologic contexts of wound healing and embryogenesis, as well as in the pathologic process of neoplasia. Many cancer cells have lost the growth inhibitory response to TGF-β (Shipley et al. 1986; Masui et al. 1986; Moses et al. 1985) and produce increased quantities of TGF-β_1 (Derynck et al. 1985). The latter could play a role in tumor stroma formation and angiogenesis, as illustrated by the CAM studies (Yang and Moses 1990). TGF-β produced by tumors could also enhance tumor growth by suppression of immune surveillance (Torre-Amione et al. 1990).

TGF-β Effects on Early Growth Factor-Induced Events

In studying the mechanisms of TGF-β growth inhibition, we have utilized secondary cultures of human skin keratinocytes grown in low-calcium, serum-free medium (Moses et al. 1985; Shipley et al. 1986) and a continuous line of mouse keratinocytes cultured in low-calcium, serum-containing medium (Coffey et al. 1988a,b). Both cell types require EGF/TGF-α for proliferation. TGF-β_1, TGF-β_2 and TGF-β_3 are potent inhibitors of keratinocyte proliferation (Coffey et al. 1988a; Graycar et al. 1989). The majority of keratinocytes cultured in the presence of TGF-βs arrest in the G_1 phase of the cell cycle (Shipley et al. 1986; Coffey et al. 1988b). This effect is not due to cytotoxicity since growth inhibition is reversible (Shipley et al. 1986; Coffey et al. 1988b). Induction of terminal differentiation, although reported for bronchial epithelial cells (Masui et al. 1986), does not appear to be a general phenomenon, and does not occur in either the human foreskin keratinocytes or the mouse keratinocyte cell line (Shipley et al. 1986; Coffey et al. 1988b). It is possible that prior growth inhibition of keratinocytes by the TGF-βs may render them more susceptible to induction of differentiation by physiologic inducers such as calcium. TGF-β_1 does not appear to interfere with growth factor–receptor interactions or with many of the early events induced by growth stimulatory factors, including some signal transduction events (Chambard and Pouyssegur 1988; Coffey et al.

1988a). For example, EGF induction of c-*fos* in mouse keratinocytes is not affected by TGF-β_1, even though EGF stimulation of DNA synthesis is inhibited (Coffey et al. 1988a).

Perhaps the best evidence that TGF-β does not interfere with early growth factor-induced events is provided by data demonstrating that TGF-β_1 can prevent EGF-stimulated DNA synthesis in epithelial cells even when added late in G_1, long after early events induced by EGF have occurred (Pietenpol et al. 1990b; Howe et al. 1991; Laiho et al. 1990). Following EGF addition to mouse keratinocytes that have been growth arrested by depletion of EGF, there is a 12-h delay prior to entry of the cells into the S phase of the cell cycle (Coffey et al. 1988b). TGF-β_1 was shown to inhibit subsequent entry into the S phase if added at any time up to the G_1/S boundary (Pietenpol et al. 1990b). Thus, in considering mechanisms of TGF-β growth inhibition, events other than those induced early by growth factors must be examined.

The Role of c-*myc* in Growth Inhibition by TGF-β

The protooncogene c-*myc* has been shown to be necessary for the proliferation of a number of cell types (for review, see Murphy et al. 1992). Decreased proliferation by TGF-β is associated with inhibition of c-*myc* expression in endothelial cells (Takehara et al. 1987) and lymphocytes (Ruegemer et al. 1990), as well as in breast carcinoma (Fernandez-Pol et al. 1987) and colon carcinoma cell lines (Mulder et al. 1988; Mulder 1991). However, negative regulation of cell growth by TGF-β does not appear to require c-*myc* downregulation in all cell types, as evidenced by the lack of suppression of c-*myc* expression in some fibroblasts sensitive to the growth inhibitory effects of TGF-β (Sorrentino and Bandyopadhyay 1989; Chambard and Pouyssegur 1988). In exponentially proliferating human and mouse keratinocytes, the presence of TGF-β_1 resulted in a rapid decrease of c-*myc* mRNA and protein (Coffey et al. 1988a). Half-maximal reduction in c-*myc* mRNA levels following TGF-β addition occurred in approximately 30 min. Since the half-life of c-*myc* mRNA following addition of actinomycin D is approximately 20 min, the suppression of c-*myc* expression by TGF-β must occur quite rapidly, although protein synthesis appears to be required for this effect (Coffey et al. 1988a). In addition, the presence of antisense c-*myc* oligonucleotides in mouse keratinocyte cultures reduced c-*myc* protein levels and cell proliferation as effectively as TGF-β_1 (Pietenpol et al. 1990b), suggesting that c-*myc* is necessary for mouse keratinocyte growth.

Like other immediate-early genes, c-*myc* is induced rapidly by the addition of EGF to quiescent cells of many types, including skin keratinocytes (Coffey et al. 1988a). However, unlike other immediate-early genes, c-*myc* expression remains elevated throughout the G_1 and S phases (Coffey et al. 1988a; Münger et al. 1992). Thus, c-*myc* expression could be a target of TGF-β_1 effects, even in late G_1. Expression of c-*myc* mRNA and protein were shown to be rapidly inhibited by TGF-β_1 addition throughout the G_1 and S phases of the cell cycle (Coffey et al. 1988a; Münger et al. 1992). Use of antisense c-*myc* oligonucleotides that inhibit *myc* protein synthesis inhibited progression through the cell cycle in a pattern very similar to that observed with TGF-β_1 (Münger et al. 1992). Antisense oligonucleotides inhibited progression into S phase when added at any point in G_1, but had no inhibitory effect when added during S phase. This indicates that in keratinocytes the c-*myc* protein may be required for initiation, but not for progression of the S phase. Thus, the phase of the cell cycle in which TGF-β_1 inhibits proliferation appears to overlap with the period in which c-*myc* is needed. In addition, these observations are consistent with the concept that TGF-β suppression of c-*myc* may be a critical component in the pathway for TGF-β_1-induced growth inhibition. However, certain studies have presented data against c-*myc* suppression being a critical component in the TGF-β pathway for growth inhibition. Transfection of *myc* into breast epithelial cells (Telang et al. 1990; Sarubbi et al. 1990) or skin keratinocytes (Reiss et al. 1989) did not result in resistance to TGF-β. One problem with these studies is that they did not show overexpression of *myc* protein or lack of TGF-β regulation of *myc* protein expression in the transfected cells.

The mechanism of TGF-β suppression of c-*myc* has been investigated. Nuclear run-on assays using single-stranded, exon- and intron-specific probes demonstrated that the inhibition of c-*myc* expression by TGF-β_1 occurred at the level of transcriptional initiation (Pietenpol et al. 1990b). Studies with a series of 5′ deletion c-*myc*/chloramphenicol acetyltransferase (CAT) constructs indicated that a region between positions −100 and +71 relative to the P1 transcription start site is necessary for TGF-β_1 suppression. Based on these data, it was proposed that TGF-β_1 may induce the interaction of a factor(s) with a specific *cis* element in the c-*myc* gene promoter, resulting in inhibition of transcriptional initiation of this gene (Pietenpol et al. 1990a,b).

Requirement for p^{RB} in TGF-β_1 Suppression of c-*myc* Transcription

In considering other proteins that may be involved in TGF-β_1 regulation of c-*myc* transcription, the protein product of the retinoblastoma gene, p^{RB}, seemed a likely candidate. p^{RB} has properties of a cell cycle regulatory factor (DeCaprio et al. 1989). It is a differentially phosphorylated 105-kDa nuclear protein that has been postulated to contribute to growth suppression, directly or indirectly (Friend et al. 1986). Evidence of tumor suppressor activity by p^{RB} is provided by the observations that loss or inactivation of the *rb* gene has been found in a variety of malignant cell types including retinoblastomas, osteosarcomas, small cell carcinoma of the lung, and carcinomas of the breast, bladder, and prostate. Furthermore, introduction of a cloned *rb* gene into cells results in marked changes in morphology, decreased growth rates, and reduced tumorigenic potential in neoplastic cells (Huang et al. 1988; Takahashi et al. 1991). It has been demonstrated that p^{RB} associates with the transforming proteins of the DNA tumor virus SV40 (DeCaprio et al. 1988), adenovirus (Whyte et al. 1988), and human papilloma virus 16 (HPV-16) (Dyson et al. 1989b). The specific transforming proteins are large T antigen (TAg), E1A, and E7, respectively. Furthermore, mutant forms of these virus proteins incapable of binding p^{RB} are also transformation defective. It has been hypothesized that binding of p^{RB} by DNA viral transforming proteins may block the growth suppressive activity of p^{RB}, resulting in some of the aberrations of growth control associated with transformation by these viruses (DeCaprio et al. 1988; Whyte et al. 1988; Dyson et al. 1989a,b).

Keratinocytes transformed by the DNA tumor viruses SV40 and HPV-16 or HPV-18 are resistant to the growth inhibitory effects of TGF-β_1 (Pietenpol et al. 1990a,b). TGF-β_1 is also unable to decrease c-*myc* mRNA levels in these DNA tumor virus-transformed cells. Subsequent studies tested whether blocking of TGF-β_1 suppression of c-*myc* expression is mediated through the p^{RB}-binding domain of the DNA tumor virus-transforming proteins. Transient expression in nontransformed keratinocytes of the DNA tumor virus proteins that bind p^{RB}, including HPV-16 E7, adenovirus E1A, and SV40 TAg, prevented TGF-β_1 suppression of c-*myc* expression. Mutants of E1A and TAg with impaired association to p^{RB} failed to block the TGF-β_1 suppression of c-*myc* (Pietenpol et al. 1990b). These data indicate that a cellular protein that interacts with the conserved domain of the DNA viral oncoproteins is necessary for TGF-β_1 suppression of c-*myc* transcription. However, proteins other than p^{RB} bind to the p^{RB} binding domain of the DNA virus-transforming proteins (Dyson et al. 1989a,b, McCormick et al. 1981; Whyte et al. 1988, 1989), and their involvement in this cannot be excluded. To further examine the possible involvement of p^{RB} in the TGF-β_1 pathway for suppression of c-*myc* transcription, the effect of p^{RB} on c-*myc* expression was investigated (Pietenpol et al. 1991). Transient expression of p^{RB} in skin keratinocytes repressed transcription of the human c-*myc* promoter as effectively as TGF-β_1 treatment. The same c-*myc* promoter region was required for regulation by both TGF-β_1 and p^{RB}. This sequence, termed the *T*GF-β *c*ontrol *e*lement (TCE), lies between 86 and 63 bp upstream from the P1 transcription start site. The demonstration that transient expression of p^{RB} inhibits *myc* transcription like TGF-β_1, and that such inhibition requires the same promoter element as TGF-β_1 supports the concept that p^{RB} may be a component in the TGF-β_1 pathway targeted by DNA tumor virus oncoproteins.

Kerr et al. (1990) have presented results indicating that TGF-β_1 suppression of transin/stromelysin gene transcription is mediated through binding of a *fos*-containing protein complex to a promoter sequence termed the TGF-β_1 inhibitory element (TIE). Robbins et al. (1990) have reported that expression of p^{RB} in mouse fibroblasts suppresses transcription of c-*fos*, and have indentified an element in the c-*fos* promoter (retinoblastoma control element, RCE) necessary for this suppression. The TIE and RCE show some similarity to the TCE. Sequences homologous to the RCE have been identified in the TGF-β_1, -β_2, and -β_3 promoters by Kim et al. (1991). Cotransfection with an RB expression plasmid was shown to regulate expression from TGF-β_1 promoter/CAT constructs positively or negatively depending on the cell type. In contrast to the effects observed in keratinocytes, RB overexpression in mink lung (Mv1Lu) cells enhanced c-*myc* expression, even though these cells are very sensitive to the growth inhibitory effect of TGF-β (Kim et al. 1991). TGF-β treatment of p^{RB}-defective DU-145 prostate carcinoma cells was reported to decrease c-*myc* mRNA levels without any effect on cell proliferation (Zentella et al. 1991); however, another study showed that TGF-β did not affect either proliferation or c-*myc* transcription in these cells (Murphy et al. 1992).

We have examined the effect of TGF-β_1 treatment or overexpression of p^{RB} on c-*myc* expression in the Mv1Lu cells. TGF-β_1 suppressed transcription, whereas RB had little or no effect (C.S. Murphy, J.A. Pietenpol, and H.L. Moses, unpublished observations). Since p^{RB} did not suppress transcription of c-*myc* in the Mv1Lu cells, it was suspected that another tumor suppressor gene that encodes a DNA-binding protein, such as p53, might be involved. Expression of wild-type p53 was found to regulate transcription of c-*myc* in transient assays in these cells. Whereas wild-type p53 markedly suppressed transcription, four different mutant p53 clones caused transactivation. Preliminary data indicate that the TCE is not required for wild-type p53 suppression or mutant p53 transactivation of c-*myc*. This indicates that cell type differences may exist in the tumor suppressor genes involved in the response pathway for suppression of c-*myc* expression and growth inhibition. The possibility that p53 may be involved in the response pathway for growth inhibition by TGF-β_1 in the Mv1Lu cells in a manner analogous to p^{RB} in the keratinocytes is currently being investigated.

TCE Binding to Cellular Proteins

Evidence for keratinocyte protein binding to the TCE was obtained in both mobility shift assays (Pietenpol et al. 1991) and southwestern blots (Murphy et al. 1992). By gel shift, oligonucleotide probes containing TCE sequences formed three complexes, whereas southwestern blots showed TCE binding predominantly to a 106-kDa polypeptide termed p106. Which, if any, of the complexes identified in the gel shift assay corresponds to p106 is not known.

Because p^{RB} is a nuclear phosphoprotein of 105–110 kDa capable of binding DNA (Lee et al. 1987), and because p^{RB} appears to be involved in the suppression of c-*myc* transcription in response to TGF-β_1 treatment, the

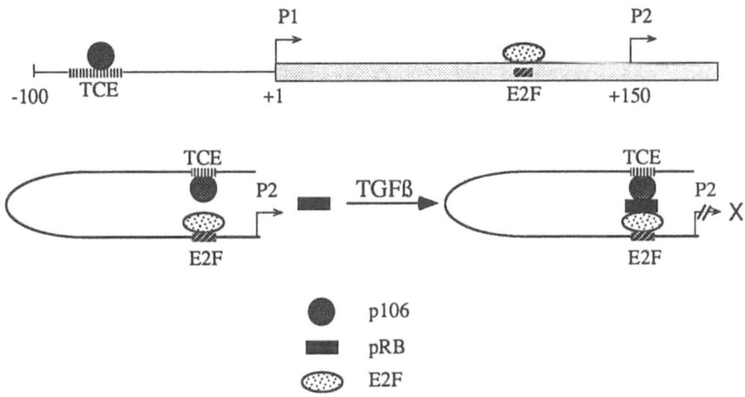

Fig. 2. Schematic model of TGF-β_1 inhibitory action on keratinocyte cell growth. This model represents possible modes of action for TGF-β_1 inhibition of c-*myc* expression and, subsequently, cell growth (see text)

possibility of TCE binding directly to p^{RB} was examined. No binding of the TCE oligonucleotide was obtained with cellular proteins coprecipitated with antibodies to DNA tumor viral oncoproteins (Pietenpol et al. 1991; Murphy et al. 1992). Additional evidence that p106 is distinct from p^{RB} is provided by experiments on extracts from retinoblastoma cell lines (WERI and Y-79) lacking the *rb* gene and a human prostatic adenocarcinoma cell line (DU-145) that produces a functionally defective RB protein (Pietenpol et al. 1991; Murphy et al. 1992). TCE binding to the shifted complexes and to p106 was observed in extracts from these cell lines, similar to that observed with normal human foreskin keratinocyte extracts.

Recent experiments have shown that p^{RB} can form complexes with several cellular proteins, including the transcription factor E2F (Chellappan et al. 1991; Bagchi et al. 1991; Bandara et al. 1991). E2F was originally characterized as a factor important in the activation of adenovirus E2 genes (reviewed in Nevins 1991), and was subsequently shown to *trans*-activate c-*myc* transcription (Hiebert et al. 1989). Thus, it is possible that the inhibition of c-*myc* transcription by TGF-β involves the formation of a complex containing p^{RB}, E2F and p106, as illustrated in Fig. 2. The interaction of E2F with p^{RB} and p106 may preclude activation of c-*myc* transcription.

Effect of TGF-β_1 Treatment on p^{RB} Phosphorylation State

Following growth factor stimulation of quiescent keratinocytes, TGF-β_1 can inhibit progression into the S phase at any point prior to the G_1/S transition but does not inhibit progression through the S phase of the cell cycle (Pietenpol et al. 1990b). Since p^{RB} is underphosphorylated during G_1 and hyperphosphorylated during S and G_2 (DeCaprio et al. 1989), the G_1/S specific phosphorylation of p^{RB} becomes an attractive target for the growth inhibitory activities of TGF-β_1 (Laiho et al. 1990). However, in TGF-β_1-treated primary human keratinocytes and a series of HPV- and SV40-transformed human keratinocyte cell lines, the phosphorylation status of p^{RB} strictly correlated with cell growth (Münger et al. 1992). Treatment of rapidly growing nontransformed keratinocytes with TGF-β_1 caused a decrease in p^{RB} phosphorylation over a period of several hours that correlated with growth arrest of the cells. In addition, placement of keratinocytes in amino acid-deficient or growth factor-depleted medium, growth conditions that cause a G_1 arrest similar to TGF-β_1 treatment, also caused a slow decrease in the phosphorylation state of p^{RB}. In the transformed keratinocytes that are resistant to the growth inhibitory effect of TGF-β, treatment with TGF-β_1 had no effect on p^{RB} phosphorylation. Thus, no evidence was found for a direct effect of TGF-β_1 on the phosphorylation status of these cells, indicating that the p^{RB}-dependent suppression of c-*myc* transcription by TGF-β_1 in keratinocytes is not mediated through an alteration in the phosphorylation state of p^{RB}.

Conclusions

Control of keratinocyte proliferation involves both positive and negative polypeptide regulators that bind to cell surface membrane receptors. Keratinocytes produce peptides such as TGF-α and TGF-β, which have, respectively, stimulatory and inhibitory effects on proliferation (Coffey et al. 1987) (Fig. 3). TGF-β is secreted in a latent form that could be activated in

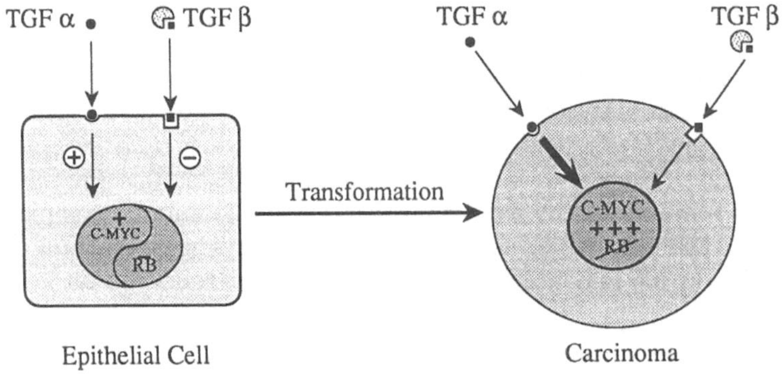

Fig. 3. Model for positive and negative growth factor regulation of keratinocyte proliferation. TGF-β_1 suppresses transcription of c-*myc*, a protooncogene required for cell proliferation, utilizing a pathway that requires the protein product of the retinoblastoma susceptibility gene (p^{RB}) (see text). This predicts that one mechanism for loss of the growth inhibitory response in carcinoma cells is mutational inactivation of the *rb* gene

the medium or at the cell membrane by proteolytic action, resulting in a negative effect on cell proliferation. Autocrine regulation by both stimulators and inhibitors of proliferation is likely an important physiologic mechanism of regulation of keratinocyte growth. The presence of opposing regulatory pathways should allow for a more precise control of cell proliferation than would an on/off stimulatory pathway provided by the growth factors. The growth inhibitory polypeptides probably play as important a role in the control of cell proliferation as the growth stimulatory factors. Data summarized here indicate that the mechanism of TGF-β_1 growth inhibition in skin keratinocytes involves suppression of transcription of the protooncogene *c-myc*, the expression of which is required for cell proliferation. The data further indicate that the tumor suppressor gene product p^{RB} is a critical component in this pathway. This would predict that one mechanism for loss of the growth inhibitory response to TGF-β_1 in carcinoma cells could be mutational inactivation of the *rb* gene (Fig. 3).

Acknowledgment. Lina Dagnino is recipient of a Centennial Fellowship of the Medical Research Council of Canada.

References

Bagchi S, Weinmann R, Raychaudhuri P (1991) The retinoblastoma protein copurifies with E2F-I, an E1A-regulated inhibitor of the transcription factor E2F. Cell 65:1063–1072

Bandara LR, Adamszewski JP, Hunt T, La Thangue NB (1991) Cyclin A and the retinoblastoma gene product complex with a common transcription factor. Nature 352:249–251

Battegay EJ, Raines EW, Seifert RA, Bowen-Pope DF, Ross R (1990) TGF-β induces bimodal proliferation of connective tissue cells via complex control of an autocrine PDGF loop. Cell 63:515–524

Chambard J-C, Pouyssegur J (1988) TGF-β inhibits growth factor-induced DNA synthesis in hamster fibroblasts without affecting the early mitogenic events. J Cell Physiol 135:101–107

Chellappan SP, Hiebert S, Mudryj M, Horowitz JM, Nevins JR (1991) The E2F transcription factor is a cellular target for the RB protein. Cell 65:1053–1061

Coffeyy RJ Jr, Derynck R, Wilcox JN, Bringman TS, Goustin AS, Moses HL, Pittelkow MR (1987) Production and auto-induction of transforming growth factor-α in human keratinocytes. Nature 328:817–820

Coffey RJ Jr, Bascom CC, Sipes NJ, Graves-Deal R, Weissman BE, Moses HL (1988a) Selective inhibition of growth-related gene expression in murine keratinocytes by transforming growth factor β. Mol Cell Biol 8:3088–3093

Coffey RJ Jr, Sipes NJ, Bascom CC, Graves-Deal R, Pennington CY, Weissman BE, Moses HL (1988b) Growth modulation of mouse keratinocytes by transforming growth factors. Cancer Res 48:1596–1602

DeCaprio JA, Ludlow JW, Figge J, Shew J-Y, Huang C-M, Lee W-H, Marsilio E, Paucha E, Livingston DM (1988) SV40 large tumor antigen forms a specific complex with the product of the retinoblastoma susceptibility gene. Cell 54:275–283

DeCaprio JA, Ludlow JW, Lynch D, Furukawa Y, Griffin J, Piwnica-Worms H, Huang C-M, Livingston DM (1989) The product of the retinoblastoma susceptibility gene has properties of a cell cycle regulatory element. Cell 58:1085–1095

DeLarco JE, Todaro GJ (1978) Growth factors from murine sarcoma virus-transformed cells. Proc Natl Acad Sci USA 75:4001–4005

Derynck R, Jarrett JA, Chen EY, Eaton DH, Bell JR, Assoian RK, Roberts AB, Sporn MB, Goeddel DV (1985) Human transforming growth factor-β complementary DNA sequence and expression in normal and transformed cells. Nature 316:701–705

Derynck R, Lindquist PB, Bringman TS, Wilcox JN, Elder JT, Fisher GL, Vorhees JJ, Moses HL, Pittelkow MR, Coffey RJ Jr (1989) Expression of the transforming growth factor-α gene in tumor cells and normal tissue. Cancer Cells 7:297–301

Dyson N, Buchkovich K, Whyte P, Harlow E (1989a) The cellular 107 K protein that binds to adenovirus E1A also associates with the large T antigens of SV40 and JC virus. Cell 58:249–255

Dyson N, Howley PM, Münger K, Harlow E (1989b) The human papilloma virus-16 E7 oncoprotein is able to bind to the retinoblastoma gene product. Science 243:934–937

Fernandez-Pol JA, Talked VD, Klos DJ, Hamilton PD (1987) Suppression of the EGF-dependent induction of c-*myc* proto-oncogene expression by transforming growth factor-β in a human breast carcinoma cell line. Biochem Biophys Res Commun 144:1197–1205

Fontana A, Frei K, Bodmer S, Hofer E, Schreier MH, Palladino MA Jr, Zinkernagel RM (1989) Transforming growth factor-β inhibits the generation of cytotoxic T cells in virus-infected mice. J Immunol 143:3230–3234

Friend SH, Bernards R, Rogelj S, Weinberg RA, Rapaport JM, Albert DM, Dryja TP (1986) A human DNA segment with properties of the gene that predisposes to retinoblastoma and osteosarcoma. Nature 323:643–646

Goey H, Keller JR, Back T, Longo DL, Ruscetti FW, Wiltrout RH (1989) Inhibition of early murine hemopoietic progenitor cell proliferation after in vivo locoregional administration of transforming growth factor-β1. J Immunol 143:877–880

Graycar JL, Miller DA, Arrick BA, Lyons RM, Moses HL, Derynck R (1989) Human transforming growth factor-β3: recombinant expression, purification, and biological activities in comparison with transforming growth factors-β1 and -β2. Mol Endocrinol 3:1977–1986

Hanks SK, Armour R, Baldwin JH, Maldonado F, Spiess J, Holley RW (1988) Amino acid sequence of the BSC-1 cell growth inhibitor (polyergin) deduced from the nucleotide sequence of the cDNA. Proc Natl Acad Sci USA 85:79–82

Hiebert SW, Lipp M, Nevins JR (1989) E1A-dependent trans-activation of the human MYC promoter is mediated by the E2F factor. Proc Natl Acad Sci USA 86:3594–3598

Holley RW, Armour R, Baldwin JH (1978) Density-dependent regulation of growth of BSC-1 cells in cell culture: growth inhibitors formed by the cells. Proc Natl Acad Sci USA 75:1864–1866

Howe PH, Draetta G, Leof EB (1991) Transforming growth factor β1 inhibition of p34cdc2 phosphorylation and histone H1 kinase activity is associated with G1S-phase growth arrest. Mol Cell Biol 11:1185–1194

Huang H-JS, Yee J-K, Shew J-Y, Chen P-L, Bookstein R, Friedmann T, Lee EY-HP, Lee W-H (1988) Suppression of the neoplastic phenotype by replacement of the RB gene in human cancer cells. Science 242:1563–1566

Kerr LD, Miller DB, Matrisian LM (1990) TGF-β1 inhibition of transin-stromelysin gene expression is mediated through a fos binding sequence. Cell 61:267–278

Kim SJ, Lee HD, Robbins PD, Busam K, Sporn MB, Roberts AB (1991) Regulation of transforming growth factor β1 gene expression by the product of the retinoblastoma-susceptibility gene. Proc Natl Acad Sci USA 88:3052–3056

Laiho M, DeCaprio JA, Ludlow JW, Livingston DM, Massague J (1990) Growth inhibition by TGF-β linked to suppression of retinoblastoma protein phosphorylation. Cell 62:175–185

Lee W-H, Shew JY, Hong FD, Sery TW, Donosco LA, Young L-J, Bookstein R, Lee EY-HP (1987) The retinoblastoma susceptibility gene encodes a nuclear phosphoprotein associated with DNA binding activity. Nature 329:642–644

Leof EB, Proper JA, Goustin AS, Shipley GD, DiCorleto PE, Moses HL (1986) Induction of c-*sis* mRNA and activity similar to platelet-derived growth factor by transforming growth factor-β: a proposed model for indirect mitogenesis involving autocrine activity. Proc Natl Acad Sci USA 83:2453–2457

Marquardt H, Hunkapiller MW, Hood LE, Todaro GJ (1984) Rat transforming growth factor type 1: structure and relation to epidermal growth factor. Science 223:1079–1082

Masui T, Wakefield LM, Lechner JF, LaVeck MA, Sporn MB, Harris CC (1986) Type β transforming growth factor is the primary differentiation-inducing serum factor for normal human bronchial epithelial cells. Proc Natl Acad Sci USA 83:2438–2442

McCormick F, Clark R, Harlow E, Tjian R (1981) SV40 T antigen binds specifically to a cellular 53 K protein in vitro. Nature 292:63–65

Moses HL (1990) The biological actions of transforming growth factor β. In: Sara V, Hall K, Low H (eds) Growth factors from genes to clinical application. Raven, New York, pp 141–155

Moses HL, Branum EB, Proper JA, Robinson RA (1981) Transforming growth factor production by chemically transformed cells. Cancer Res 41:2842–2848

Moses HL, Tucker RF, Leof EB, Coffey RJ Jr, Halper J, Shipley, GD (1985) Type β transforming growth factor is a growth stimulator and a growth inhibitor. Cancer Cells 3:65–71

Moses HL, Yang EY, Pietenpol JA (1990) TGF-β stimulation and inhibition of cell proliferation: new mechanistic insights. Cell 63:245–247

Mulder KM (1991) Differential regulation of c-*myc* and transforming growth factor-α messenger RNA expression in poorly differentiated and well-differentiated colon carcinoma cells during the establishment of a quiescent state. Cancer Res 51:2256–2262

Mulder KM, Levine AE, Hernandez X, McKnight MK, Brattain DE, Brattain MG (1988) Modulation of c-*myc* by transforming growth factor-β in human colon carcinoma cells. Biochem Biophys Res Commun 150:711–716

Münger K, Pietenpol JA, Pittelkow MR, Holt JT, Moses HL (1992) TGF-β regulation of c-*myc* expression, p^{RB} phosphorylation, and cell cycle progression in keratinocytes (submitted)

Murphy CS, Pietenpol JA, Münger K, Howley PM, Moses HL (1992) c-*myc* and p^{RB}: role in TGF-β1 inhibition of keratinocyte proliferation. Cold Spring Harbor Symp Quant Biol (in press)

Nevins JR (1991) Utilization of cellular transcription factors for adenovirus-induced transcription. Virus Res 20:1–10

Pietenpol JA, Holt JT, Stein RW, Moses HL (1990a) Transforming growth factor β-1 suppression of c-*myc* gene transcription: role in inhibition of keratinocyte proliferation. Proc Natl Acad Sci USA 87:3758–3762

Pietenpol JA, Stein RW, Moran E, Yaciuk P, Schlegel R, Lyons RM, Pittelkow MR, Münger K, Howley PM, Moses HL (1990b) TGF-β1 inhibition of c-*myc* transcription and growth in keratinocytes is abrogated by viral transforming proteins with p^{RB} binding domains. Cell 61:777–785

Pietenpol JA, Münger K, Howley PM, Stein RW, Moses HL (1991) Factor-binding element in the human c-*myc* promoter involved in transcriptional regulation by transforming growth factor β1 and by the retinoblastoma gene product. Proc Natl Acad Sci USA 88:10227–10231
Postlethwaite AE, Keski-Oja J, Moses HL, Kang AH (1987) Stimulation of the chemitactic migration of human fibroblasts by transforming growth factor β. J Exp Med 165:251–256
Reiss M, Dibble CL, Narayanan R (1989) Transcriptional activation of the c-*myc* proto-oncogene in murine keratinocytes enhances the response to epidermal growth factor. J Invest Dermatol 93:136–141
Robbins PD, Horowitz JM, Mulligan RC (1990) Negative regulation of human c-fos expression by the retinoblastoma gene product. Nature 346:668–671
Roberts AB, Anzano MA, Lamb LC, Smith JM, Sporn MB (1981) New class of transforming growth factors potentiated by epidermal growth factor: Isolation from non-neoplastic tissues. Proc Natl Acad Sci USA 78:5339–5343
Ruegemer JJ, Ho SN, Augustine JA, Schlager JW, Bell MP, McKean DJ, Abraham RT (1990) Regulatory effects of transforming growth factor-β on IL-2- and IL-4-dependent T cell cycle progression. J Immunol 144:1767–1776
Russell WE, Coffey RJ Jr, Ouellette AJ, Moses HL (1988) Type β transforming growth factor reversibly inhibits the early proliferative response to partial hepatectomy in the rat. Proc Natl Acad Sci USA 85:5126–5130
Sarubbi DJ, Narayanan R, Telang NT, Newman MJ (1990) Evaluation of the role of extracellular matrix proteins, polyunsaturated fatty acids and c-*myc* expression in the inhibition of the serum-free growth of epithelial cells by TGF-β1. In Vitro Cell Dev Biol 26:1195–1201
Shipley GD, Pittelkow MR, Wille JJ Jr, Scott RE, Moses HL (1986) Reversible inhibition of normal human prokeratinocyte proliferation by type β transforming growth factor-growth inhibitor in serum-free medium. Cancer Res 46:2068–2071
Silberstein GB, Daniel CW (1987) Reversible inhibition of mammary gland growth by transforming growth factor-β. Science 237:291–293
Sizeland AM, Burgess AW (1991) The proliferative and morphologic responses of a colon carcinoma cell line (LIM 1215) require the production of two autocrine factors. Mol Cell Biol 11:4005–4014
Sorrentino V, Bandyopadhyay S (1989) TGF-β inhibits Go/S-phase transition in primary fibroblasts. Loss of response to the antigrowth effect of TGF-β is observed after immortalization. Oncogene 4:569–574
Sporn MB, Todaro GJ (1980) Autocrine secretion and malignant transformation of cells. N Engl J Med 303:878–880
Takahashi R, Hashimoto T, Xu H-J, Hu S-X, Matsui T, Miki T, Bigo-Marshall H, Aaronson SA, Benedict WF (1991) The retinoblastoma gene functions as a growth and tumor suppressor in human bladder carcinoma cells. Proc Natl Acad Sci USA (in press)
Takehara K, LeRoy EC, Grotendorst GR (1987) TGF-β inhibition of endothelial cell proliferation: Alteration of EGF binding and EGF-induced growth-regulatory (competence) gene expression. Cell 49:415–422
Telang NT, Osborne MP, Sweterlitsch LA, Narayanan R (1990) Neoplastic transformation of mouse mammary epithelial cells by deregulated *myc* expression. Cell Regul 1:863–872
Torre-Amione G, Beauchamp RD, Koeppen H, Park BH, Schreiber H, Moses HL, Rowley DA (1990) A highly immunogenic tumor transfected with a murine transforming growth factor type β1 cDNA escapes immune surveillance. Proc Natl Acad Sci USA 87:1486–1490
Tucker RF, Shipley GD, Moses HL, Holley RW (1984) Growth inhibitor from BSC-1 cells closely related to the platelet type β transforming growth factor. Science 226:705–707

Whyte P, Buchkovich KJ, Horowitz JM, Friend SH, Raybuck M, Weinberg RA, Harlow E (1988) Association between an oncogene and an anti-oncogene: the adenovirus E1A proteins bind to the retinoblastoma gene product. Nature 334:124–129

Whyte P, Williamson NM, Harlow E (1989) Cellular targets for transformation by the adenovirus E1A proteins. Cell 56:67–75

Yang EY, Moses HL (1990) Transforming growth factor β1-induced changes in cell migration, proliferation, and angiogenesis in the chicken chorioallantoic membrane. J Cell Biol 111:731–741

Zentella A, Weis FMB, Ralph DA, Laiho M, Massagué J (1991) Early gene responses to transforming growth factor-β in cells lacking growth-suppressive RB function. Mol Cell Biol 11:4952–4958

Epithelial Stem Cells, Hair Follicles, and Tumor Formation

R.M. Lavker[1], S.J. Miller[1], and T.-T. Sun[2]

[1] Departments of Dermatology, University of Pennsylvania School of Medicine, Philadelphia, PA 19014, USA
[2] Ronald O. Perleman Department of Dermatology and Pharmacology, New York University School of Medicine, New York, NY 10016, USA

Introduction

The hair follicle is a remarkable structure that undergoes a phase of sustained growth (anagen), followed by a period of cellular degeneration and rearrangement (catagen), and succeeded by an interval of rest (telogen) (Dry 1926; Chase et al. 1951; Chase 1954; Kligman 1959). This cycle can be repeated many times during the life of a hair follicle. In humans, individual hair follicles cycle independently. However, in many mammals, especially those used in experimental carcinogenesis (e.g., mouse, rat, and rabbit), hair follicles cycle in synchrony (Johnson 1958). The equilibrium that exists between new cell formation and epithelial cell loss due to terminal differentiation are prime examples of a self-renewing or "steady-state" tissue. By definition, the growth and regeneration of all self-renewing tissues (e.g., epidermis, hair follicle, intestinal epithelium, and hematopoietic system) are governed by stem cells. These cells are believed to be long-lived; they have great potential for cell division; and they are ultimately responsible for homeostasis of continuously renewing tissues (Potten et al. 1979; Wright and Alison 1984; Potten and Morris 1988). It is also generally accepted that a subpopulation of cells having stem cell characteristics are the target cells that interact with carcinogens and eventually become transformed (Boutwell 1964; Stenbach et al. 1981; Van Duuren et al. 1975; Argyris 1985; Morris et al. 1986).

Previous evidence has indicated that the hair follicle plays a central role in mouse skin tumorigenesis. In early studies on chemical skin carcinogenesis it has been shown that the phase of the hair cycle (growing vs resting) dramatically influences the yield of chemically induced mouse skin tumors (Whiteley 1957; Andreasen and Engelbreth-Holm 1953; Borum 1954; Berenblum et al. 1958). Furthermore, it has been suggested that target cells for epithelial skin carcinogenesis may exist in the hair follicle (Argyris and Slaga 1981; De Young et al. 1978; Klein-Szanto et al. 1983; Cotsarelis

Recent Results in Cancer Research, Vol. 128

et al. 1990). Thus, a knowledge of the location and properties of hair follicle stem cells would ultimately contribute to our understanding of follicular involvement of carcinogenesis. Therefore, we will discuss in the following sections: (a) properties of epithelial stem cells; (b) the location of the putative hair follicle stem cells and its relationship to the control of the hair cycle; and (c) the role of the hair follicle in the development of non-melanoma skin cancer.

Epithelial Stem Cells

Investigations on stem cells of the hemopoietic system, and of several stratified squamous and simple epithelia, have revealed that stem cells possess many of the following properties: (a) they are relatively primitive, both biochemically and ultrastructurally; (b) they have great proliferative potential and are responsible for the long-term maintenance and regeneration of the tissue; (c) they are normally slow-cycling; (d) they can be induced to proliferate in response to wounding and certain growth stimuli; (e) when they undergo cell division, they give rise to more rapidly cycling "transient or transit amplifying" (TA) cells, which have a limited capacity for division, before they become postmitotic or terminally differentiated in the scheme of "stem cell → TA cell → postmitotic cell; and finally, (f) stem cells are often found in well-protected, highly vascularized and innervated areas (Gilbert and Lajtha 1965; Potten et al. 1979; Leblond 1981; Lavker and Sun 1982, 1983; Buick and Pollak 1984; Wright and Alison 1984; Schermer et al. 1986; Potten and Morris 1988; Cotsarelis et al. 1989, 1990). A comparison of the stem cell location in several stratified squamous epithelia is presented in Fig. 1.

We have shown that in palmar epidermis, the "nonserrated" basal keratinocytes at the bottom of the *deep* rete ridges did not incorporate tritiated thymidine (^{3}H-TdR) after a single exposure (pulse), but they could be recruited into the proliferative pool in response to wounding, implying that these nonserrated cells are normally slow-cycling (Lavker and Sun 1982, 1983). In addition, these cells were ultrastructurally "primitive," containing copious amounts of ribosomes and melanosomes but relatively few keratin filament bundles. In contrast, the ("serrated") basal keratinocytes located at the bottom of the *shallow* rete ridges had a cytoplasm filled with keratin filaments, resulting in a more differentiated appearance. These cells incorporated ^{3}H-TdR after a single pulse, like cells located immediately above the nonserrated cells, indicating that they were more rapidly cycling. Based on these findings, we postulated that the nonserrated basal cells of deep rete ridges were putative stem cells, whereas their suprabasal cells as well as the basal serrated cells of the shallow rete ridges were TA cells (Lavker and Sun 1982, 1983; Fig. 1b).

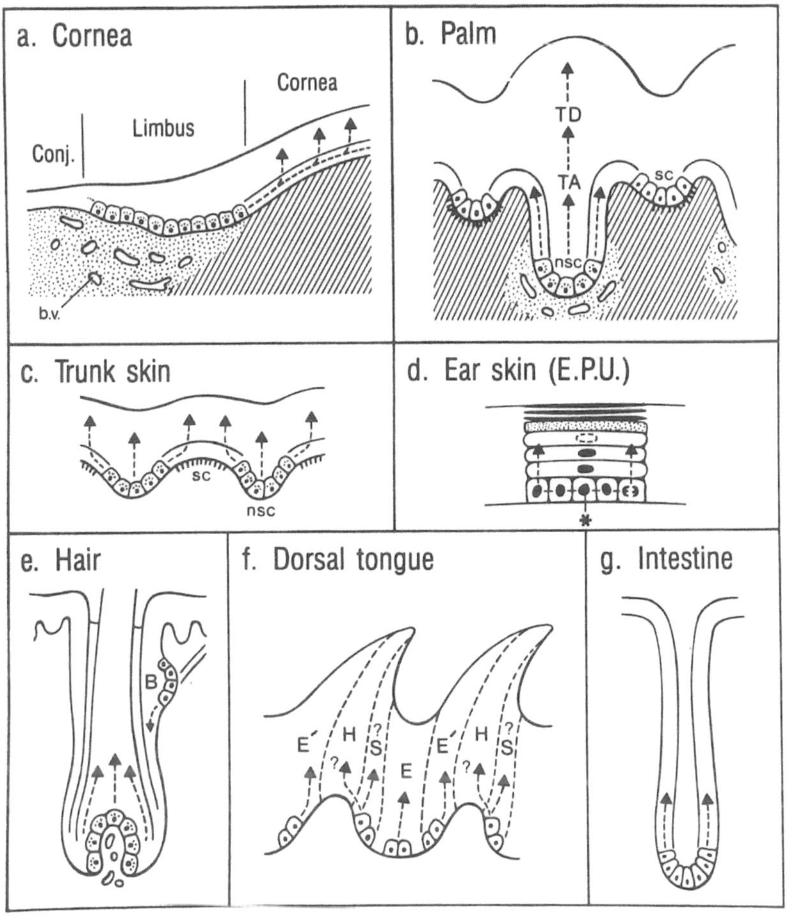

Fig. 1a–g. Localization of epithelial stem cells in cornea (**a**), palm (**b**), trunk skin (**c**), ear skin (**d**), hair follicle (**e**), dorsal tongue epithelium (**f**), and small intestinal epithelium (**g**). The stem cells of the corneal epithelium are found to be limited to the basal layer of the limbal region. The putative stem cells of the palm and trunk epidermis are the nonserrated basal cells (*nsc*) located at the bottom of the deep rete ridges. Stem cells give rise to transient amplifying (*TA*) cells, which differentiate into terminally differentiated (*TD*) cells. In the ear epidermis, it has been postulated (Potten and Morris 1988) that stem cells are located in the center of the basal layer in the so-called "epidermal proliferative unit" (*E.P.U.*). In the hair follicle, stem cells are now thought to be present in the bulge (*B*) area. Dorsal tongue epithelium may contain separate stem cell populations which give rise to cells which express different major keratin polypeptides that are characteristic of hair-type (*H*), esophageal-type (*E*, *E'*), and skin-type (*S*) differentiation. Intestinal epithelium, a simple epithelium, has its stem cells located at the bottom of the crypt. A comparison of the location and properties of the stem cells of these epithelial systems has revealed that they all share a common set of characteristics (Cotsarelis et al. 1989) *sc*, serrated cells; *bv*, blood vessels

In our studies on corneal epithelium, we identified a population of slow-cycling basal epithelial cells in the limbus, a region at the edge of the corneal epithelium (Cotsarelis et al. 1989). To accomplish this, we continuously administered to mice ^{3}H-TdR for 2 weeks, a protocol that labeled all cycling cells. After the label was discontinued, only slow-cycling cells retained their labeled thymidine after a 4-week "chase" period, and were detected by autoradiography as "label-retaining cells" (LRCs; Bickenbach 1981; Morris et al. 1985). LRCs were only observed among basal keratinocytes in limbal epithelium; no such cells were detected within central corneal epithelium. In addition to being slow-cycling, these limbal basal cells had other features supporting their stem cell nature. Limbal epithelium could be preferentially stimulated to proliferate in response to either wounding or topical application of a tumor promotor, 12-*O*-tetradecanoylphorbol-13-acetate (TPA), indicating that it has a greater proliferative potential than corneal epithelium (Cotsarelis et al. 1989). Moreover, using a monoclonal antibody to a major 64-kD basic corneal epithelial keratin, K3, Schermer et al. (1986) showed that this keratin was a molecular marker for an advanced stage of corneal epithelial differentiation. This keratin was expressed by both basal and suprabasal cells in central corneal epithelium, but only suprabasally in limbal epithelium, indicating that limbal basal cells were less differentiated or more primitive than corneal basal cells. Taken together, these findings strongly support the hypothesis that corneal epithelial stem cells are primarily located in limbal epithelium (Fig. 1a).

Hair Follicle Stem Cells

The bulbar or lowermost portion of the hair follicle contains a group of relatively undifferentiated epithelial cells, known as the matrix cells. During the growing phase, the matrix cells proliferate extremely rapidly, giving rise to cells that migrate upwards and undergo terminal differentiation forming several specialized hair cell types (Van Scott et al. 1963; Hashimoto and Shibazaki 1976). Although epithelial cells comprise the bulk of the bulb, a group of specialized mesenchymal cells, called follicular papilla cells[1], is known to interact with the matrix cells in regulating hair growth (Moffat 1968; Pierard and de la Brassinne 1975). Thus, it has been generally assumed that the germinative center of the hair follicle was in the bulbar region, and that the follicular stem cells were located in the matrix (Kligman 1959; Van Scott et al. 1963).

---

[1] Although this group of cells are customarily known as dermal papilla cells, it may be more precise to call them follicular papilla to distinguish them from the "dermal papilla" which are the pegs of connective tissue that interdigitate with the epidermal rete ridges forming the dermal/epidermal junction (A. Bernard Ackerman, personnal communication).

Based on our studies of epidermal and corneal epithelial stem cells, we have learned that one of the most diagnostic criteria for identifying keratinocyte stem cells is their slow-cycling nature. When we evaluated the distribution of slow cycling cells (detected as LRCs) within the hair follicle, we were unable to find any LRCs in the matrix. Unexpectedly, however, we found a population of LRCs in the outer root sheath of the upper follicle in a specific area called the bulge (Fig. 2; Cotsarelis et al. 1990). The bulge area, first described by Unna (1876) and Storre (1903), is the portion of the outer root sheath to which the arrector pili muscle attaches. Cells of the bulge area possess the following features: (1) It marks the lower end of the permanent hair follicle. Keratinocytes below the bulge degenerate during catagen and are therefore "dispensable." (2) These cells are ultrastructurally primitive, having a cytoplasm primarily filled with ribosomes and devoid of aggregated keratin filaments. (3) Although these cells are normally slow-cycling, they undergo transient proliferation during early anagen, and can be stimulated to proliferate by hair plucking, retinoic acid and TPA. (4) These cells are located in a physically well protected and highly vascularized area. Based on these findings, we have postulated that

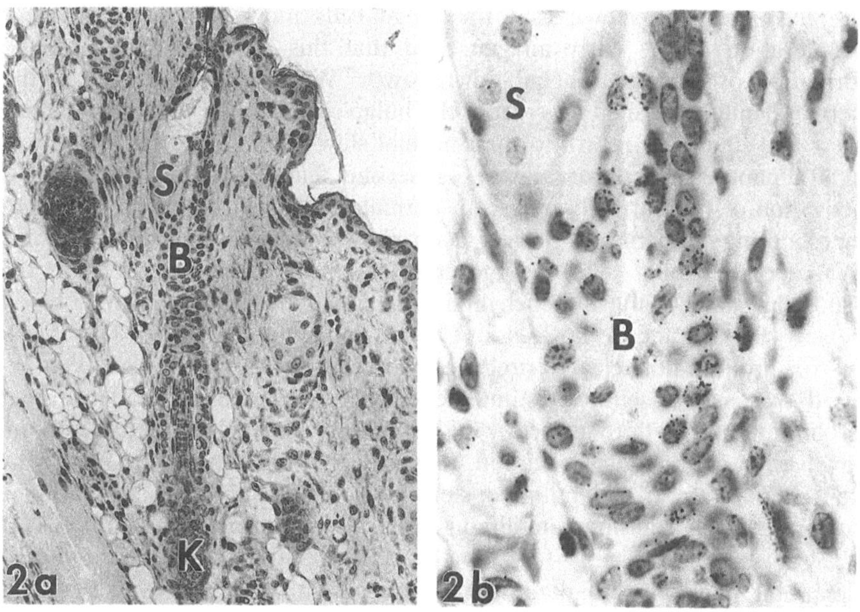

Fig. 2a,b. After 14 days of continuous ^{3}H-thymidine labeling, followed by a 4-week chase period, slow-cycling cells were detected as "label-retaining cells" (LRCs) by autoradiography in the bulge area (*B*) of mouse pelage hair follicles. **a** Low-magnification view showing that LRCs are confined to the bulge (*B*) regions of the follicles. **b** A higher magnification view. LRCs are not detected in matrix keratinocytes (*K*) of the bulge region or in sebaceous glands (*S*)

follicular stem cells reside in the bulge, instead of the matrix (Cotsarelis et al. 1990; Sun et al. 1991; Lavker et al. 1991). Additional support for this conclusion can be obtained from a reevaluation of some previous experiments whose biological significance was unclear. For example, Oliver (1966, 1967a,b) surgically removed the lower follicle (below the bulge region) of rat vibrissae and found that, as long as a new dermal papilla was supplied, the follicle could regenerate. This indicates that the keratinocytes of the lower follicle are "dispensable" and in retrospect, strongly supports our notion that the stem cells are located in the upper half of the follicle. Similarly, surgical removal of the lower portion of human axillary hair follicles, up to a level below the bulge, did not impede the restoration of new hair follicles (Inaba et al. 1979).

Identification of the putative hair follicle stem cells in the bulge region rather than the matrix has enabled us to develop a "bulge-activation hypothesis" (Fig. 3) which provides for the first time a unifying concept that explains many of the puzzling properties of the hair follicle (Cotsarelis et al. 1990; Sun et al. 1991; Lavker et al. 1991). We hypothesized that during the later stages of the resting phase or early portion of the growing phase, the normally slow-cycling stem cells of the bulge area would be activated by the dermal papilla cells which lie in close proximity to the bulge at this time. We have recently shown that the bulge cells indeed undergo transient proliferation during early anagen, and that this activation leads to the formation of a new epithelial downgrowth. We also showed that as the dermal papilla is pushed away from the bulge cells by this epithelial column, the bulge stem cells return to their normal slow-cycling state (R.M. Lavker et al., unpublished observations). A second feature of the hypothesis is activation of the normally quiescent dermal papilla by the matrix keratinocytes during mid-anagen. It has been shown that, during anagen (stage IV), dermal papilla cells undergo transient proliferation, resulting in the "loosening up" of the mesenchymal cells and the formation of new blood vessels (Pierard and de la Brassinne 1975; Sholley and Cotran 1976). Since matrix proliferation clearly precedes papillary proliferation, we hypothesized that matrix cells can stimulate dermal papilla to undergo transient proliferation. The third aspect of the hypothesis is that since matrix cells are involved in continuous replication, they are most likely transient amplifying cells derived from the putative stem cells residing in the distant bulge region. As the transient amplifying cells in the scheme of stem cells → transient amplifying cell → terminally differentiated cells, these cells, by definition, have only a limited proliferative potential. After they exhaust this potential, the bulb region of the hair follicle can no longer grow, hence they undergo terminal differentiation and enter a degenerative or apoptotic phase (catagen). The fourth feature of the hypothesis is that the upward movement of the follicular papilla is critical for subsequent activation of bulge cells. Even though during early catagen, the follicular papilla is distant from the degenerating matrix, these two groups of cells are still connected

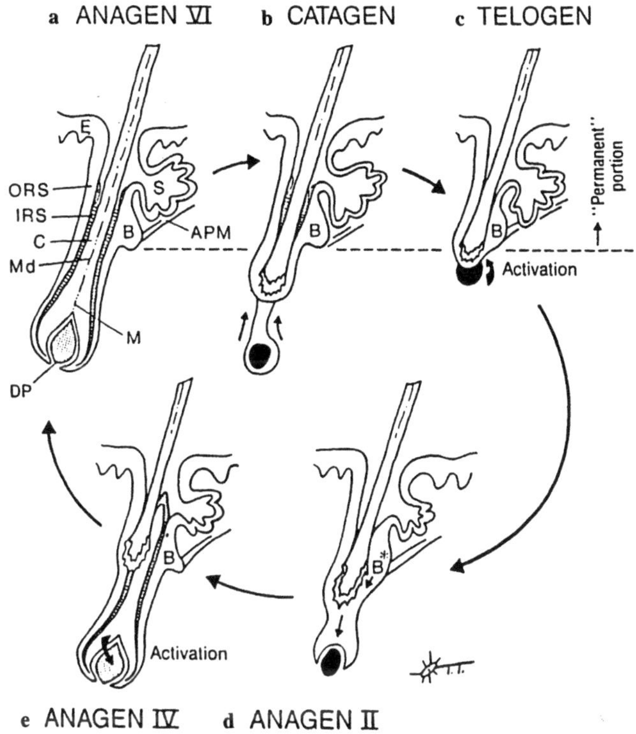

Fig. 3a–e. Hair cycle: the bulge activation hypothesis. The quiescent (*B*) and activated (*B**) states of the bulge cells are indicated. The structures above the *dashed line* represent the permanent portion of the follicle; keratinocytes below the bulge degenerate during catagen and thus can be considered as "dispensable." The four major elements of this hypothesis are: the activation of the bulge by dermal papilla during telogen (**c**), the activation of the dermal papilla by the matrix keratinocytes during anagen IV (**e**), the finite proliferative capability of matrix cells as transient-amplifying cells during late anagen (**a**), and the upward migration of the dermal papilla during catagen (**b**). *Abbreviations*: *APM*, arrector pili muscle; *B*, bulge; *C*, cortex; *DP*, dermal papilla; *E*, epidermis; *IRS*, inner root sheath; *M*, matrix; *MD*, medulla; *ORS*, outer root sheath; *S*, sebaceous gland. (Reprinted with permission from Cotsarelis et al. 1990)

by a "connective tissue sheath/outer root sheath cells." This sheath later contracts to pull the follicular papilla upward. Failure of an upward movement of the follicular papilla will result in no subsequent hair growth. Evidence for this is seen in the *hr/hr* mouse mutant, which has a defect in the connective tissue sheath. This animal has a normal first hair cycle, but the second growth phase never commences, presumably because the bulge cells cannot become activated by the follicular papilla, which remains separated from the permanent portion of the hair follicle (Montagna et al. 1952; Chase 1954).

Hair Follicles and Skin Carcinogenesis

Several lines of evidence indicate a strong relationship between skin carcinogenesis and hair follicle formation. Giovanella et al. (1970) compared tumorigenesis in strains of hairless (*bb/cc hr/hr*) versus haired (Swiss) mice. In this study all newborn mice developed papillomas using a two-stage protocol consisting of dimethylbezanthracene (DMBA) initiation followed by croton oil promotion. However, only a few adult "hairless" mice formed papillomas following the identical two-stage protocol. Based on these results, Giovanella et al. (1970) suggested that hairless mice were refractory to chemical carcinogenesis. Iversen and Iversen (1976) later challenged this notion, as they reported that carcinomas could be induced in adult hairless mouse skin of the Oslo *hr/hr* strain using a complete carcinogenesis protocol of a single application of methylcholanthrene (MCA) in benzene. However, this apparent controversy could be explained by several factors: (1) different strains of the so-called "hairless" mice were employed which might have had different abnormalities in their hair follicles and might have very different intrinsic sensitivities to chemical carcinogens; (2) Giovanella et al. (1970) employed a two-stage protocol, whereas Iversen and Iversen (1976) used a one-stage protocol; (3) Giovanella et al. (1970) used acetone as a vehicle, whereas Iversen and Iversen used benzene, which is itself a mild carcinogen; and finally (4) different aged animals were employed by these two groups. This last point is significant because newborn "hairless" (*hr/hr*) mice actually contain normal follicles during the first hair cycle. Detailed histological evaluations of chemically induced skin tumors from several species implicated the follicle as their possible site of origin. Early work by Zackheim (1964) revealed that chemically induced basal cell carcinomas in rats arose from follicular structures, while squamous cell carcinomas arose primarily from interfollicular epidermis. In an extensive survey of benign rabbit epidermal tumors, Ghadially (1961) reported that the bud-shaped keratoacanthoma (type I), which was the most common tumor produced in rabbit skin, actually arose as a result of enlargement and fusion of the superficial part of the hair follicle. Similar observations were made in mice treated topically with MCA, or MCA followed by TPA. Carcinomas formed were found to originate from the outer root sheath cells of hair follicles (Bhisey et al. 1982). In another study, DMBA was administered intravenously, rather than topically, to 70 Sprague-Dawley rats. This resulted in the production of 257 tumors (Bennington et al. 1976); of these, 250 were mammary tumors and, interestingly, the other seven involved the pilosebaceous unit. No epidermal tumors were observed. Of the pilosebaceous tumors, five displayed morphologic and histochemical evidence of differentiation resembling the lower portion of the hair follicle.

The importance of hair follicles in chemical carcinogenesis was further strengthened by the observation that the hair growth cycle influenced the process of tumor formation. In a series of experiments utilizing rabbits, multiple application of a complete carcinogen resulted in the production of 598 papillomas in regions where hair was in anagen, compared with 296 keratoacanthoma-like lesions in regions where hair was resting (Whitley 1957). This suggested that hair cycle affected not only tumor development, but also tumor type. This phenomenon was more extensively studied in mice, where it was demonstrated that a single application of a complete carcinogen during different phases of the hair cycle (growing vs resting) led to differences in tumor yield (Andreasen and Englebreth-Holm 1953; Borum 1954; Berenblum et al. 1958). The results of these experiments, summarized in Table 1, show that when a single application of 0.5% DMBA in benzene was used as a complete carcinogen, mice treated during the growing phase of the hair cycle produced few, if any, tumors; whereas mice treated during the resting phase of the hair cycle developed many papillomas. Conversely, when a hair cycle-specific study was conducted utilizing a two-stage carcinogenesis protocol (Berenblum et al. 1958), only relatively minor differences in tumor development were seen. This suggests that while complete carcinogen protocols are hair-cycle dependent, two-stage carcinogenesis protocols may not be.

In addition to the above clinical observations, histological studies of the effects of carcinogen application at different times of the hair cycle indicated that a single application of carcinogen caused considerable changes in skin of mice in the resting phase of the cycle, but not in the growing phase. Application of MCA to mouse skin when hairs were in telogen resulted in more follicular alterations and more prolonged sebaceous gland regrowth as opposed to similar treatment when hairs were in the growing phase (Liang and Cowdry 1954). Similarly, a single application of DMBA to mouse skin with hair follicles in the actively growing phase (anagen V or VI) resulted in mild epidermal and follicular hyperplasia. This was contrasted by ulceration, severe hyperplasia of the epidermis and surrounding hair follicles, and loss of sebaceous glands after similar treatment of skin with hair follicles in the resting phase (Andreasen and Borum 1959). Although it is clear that more destruction occurs in the resting phase, it is not apparent why "anagen skin" is less reactive than "telogen skin" to carcinogens.

A possible role of the hair cycle in tumor formation and degree of tissue destruction was also observed in studies where ionizing radiation was used

Table 1. Hair cycle and one-stage[a] mouse skin chemical carcinogenesis

	Strain	Weeks	Anagen	Telogen
Andreasen (1953)	St/Eh	10	6/56	37/64[b]
Borum (1954)	St/Eh	12	0/55	40/53[b]
Berenblum (1958)	Swiss (inbred)	10	0/34	17/24[b]

[a] 0.5% DMBA in benzene.
[b] Ulceration.

as a carcinogen. Albert and coworkers (1967a,b) observed in male albino CD rats that acute injury did not effect tumor production until the radiation penetrated to a depth of 0.36–1.40 mm. At depths above 0.36 mm only the epidermis was damaged, whereas at the lower depths there was extensive hair follicle damage and atrophy. Permanent follicle injury was less severe when growing hairs were irradiated (Albert 1967b). Under a wide range of doses and types of ionizing radiations (alpha instead of electron irradiation), a strong relationship was found between the degree of hair follicle damage and tumor formation, leading Albert et al. (1969) to conclude that hair follicle damage is directly related to tumor formation in rats.

Future Directions

The data that we have summarized here clearly indicate that the hair follicle plays an important role in skin carcinogenesis. Interestingly, in spite of the early observation that tumor formation following two-stage carcinogenesis protocols was not hair cycle-dependent, a central tenet in the field of mouse skin carcinogenesis has emerged that chemical initiation should be done during the resting phase of the hair cycle (Boutwell 1964; Van Duuren et al. 1975; Stenbeck et al. 1981). However, there are many unresolved issues centering around the observations that tumor yield is related to the phase of the hair cycle. For example, in the initial studies mice treated with a complete carcinogen were followed for only 10 weeks, and two-stage treated mice were observed for only 20 weeks (Andreasen and Engelbreth-Holm 1953; Borum 1954; Berenblum et al. 1958). However, current practice utilizes a 40–50-week observation period, which provides information not only on papilloma formation but also on progression of papillomas into carcinomas (Yuspa 1986). Thus, the question arises as to whether tumors progress and behave differently from animals initiated with a single application of a complete carcinogen in the growing versus resting phase of the hair cycle. Similarly, what are the nature of anagen- vs telogen-initiated tumors using a two-stage chemical carcinogenesis protocol? Strains of mice which have been bred for sensitivity to DMBA-initiated/croton oil-promoted skin carcinogenesis (e.g., STS, SENCAR), are now routinely used instead of Swiss and Eh/St albino mice (Hennings and Yuspa 1985). Therefore, does the strain of mice influence the tumor yield when animals are initiated at different times during the hair cycle? Finally, DMBA was applied in benzene in some early studies, while acetone is now routinely used as the carcinogen vehicle. Benzene is, in itself, a mild carcinogen; it is also an extremely strong skin irritant. At the present time, it is not known what confounding effects benzene might have had on the early observations. However, it is well appreciated that production of skin ulceration or erosion can complicate the experimental outcome of tumorigenesis experiments, in that skin healing after ulceration has sufficient promoting action to cause some papillomas to arise without further external promotion (Stenback et al. 1981; Argyris and Slaga 1981; Argyris 1985). In view of these extensive protocol changes and the new understanding of hair follicle stem cells, it is imperative that the relationship between hair cycle and skin tumor formation be reexamined systematically and critically.

Acknowledgments. This work was supported by NIH grants AR39674 and EY06769 (R.M.L.), and AR34511, AR39749, and EY4722 (T.-T.S.), and by the National Alopecia Areata Foundation (R.M.L. and T.-T.S.).

References

Albert RE, Burns FJ, Heimbach RD (1967a) The effect of penetration depth of electron radiation on skin tumor formation in the rat. Radiat Res 30:515–524
Albert RE, Burns FJ, Heimbach RD (1967b) The association between chronic radiation damage of the hair follicles and tumor formation in the rat. Radiat Res 30:590–599
Albert RE, Phillips ME, Bennett P, Burns F, Heimbach R (1969) The morphology and growth characteristics of radiation-induced epithelial skin tumors in the rat. Cancer Res 29:658–668
Andreasen E, Borum K (1959) Histology of early reactions following a single application of 9,10-dimethyl-1,2-benzanthracene to mouse skin in two different stages of hair formation. Acta Pathol Microbiol Scand 46:59–71
Andreasen E, Engelbreth-Holm J (1953) On the significance of the mouse hair cycle in experimental carcinogenesis. Acta Pathol Microbiol Scand 32:165–169
Argyris TS (1985) Promotion of epidermal carcinogenesis by repeated damage to mouse skin. Am J Indust Med 8:329–337
Argyris TS, Slaga TJ (1981) Promotion of carcinomas by repeated abrasion in initiated skin of mice. Cancer Res 41:5193–5195
Bennington JL, Holmes EJ, Combs JW (1976) Tumors of the pilosebaceous unit induced in the rat by the intravenous administration of 7,12-dimethylbenz[a]anthracene. J Invest Dermatol 66:183–187
Berenblum I, Haran-Ghera N, Trainin N (1958) An experimental analysis of the "hair cycle effect" in mouse skin carcinogenesis. Br J Cancer 12:402–413
Bhisey RA, Iyengar B, Sirsat SM (1982) Effects of the active tumor promotor, TPA, on hair follicle growth and development of hair anlage tumors in the mouse skin: a comparison with human adnexal lesions. J Cancer Res Clin Oncol 102:245–252
Bickenbach JR (1981) Identification and behavior of label-retaining cells in oral mucosa and skin. J Dent Res 60:1611–1620
Borum K (1954) The role of the mouse hair cycle in epidermal carcinogenesis. Acta Pathol Microbiol Scand 34:542–553
Boutwell RK (1964) Some biological aspects of skin carcinogenesis. Prog Exp Tumor Res 4:207–250
Buick RN, Pollak MN (1984) Perspectives on clonogenic tumor cells, stem cells and oncogenes. Cancer Res 44:4909–4918
Chase HB (1954) Growth of the hair. Physiol Rev 34:113–126
Chase HB, Rauch H, Smith VW (1951) Critical stages of hair development and pigmentation in the mouse. Physiol Zool 24:1–8
Cotsarelis G, Cheng S-Z, Dong G, Sun T-T, Lavker RM (1989) Existence of slow-cycling limbal epithelial basal cells that can be preferentially stimulated to proliferate: implications on epithelial stem cells. Cell 57:201–209

Cotsarelis G, Sun T-T, Lavker RM (1990) Label-retaining cells reside in the bulge area of pilosebaceous unit: Implications for follicular stem cells, hair cycle and skin carcinogenesis. Cell 61:1329–1337

De Young LM, Richards WL, Bonzelet W, Tsai LL, Boutwell RK (1978) Localization and significance of gammaglutamyltanspeptidase in normal and neoplastic mouse skin. Cancer Res 38:3697–3701

Dry FW (1926) The coat of the mouse (Mus musculus). J Genet 16:287–340

Ghadially FN (1961) The role of the hair follicle in the origin and evolution of some cutaneous neoplasms of man and experimental animals. Cancer 14:801–816

Gilbert CW, Lajtha LG (1965) The importance of cell population kinetics in determining response to irradiation of normal and malignant tissue. In: Cellular and radiation biology. Williams and Wilkins, Baltimore, pp 474

Giovanella BC, Liegel J, Heidelberger C (1970) The refractoriness of the skin of hairless mice to chemical carcinogenesis. Cancer Res 30:2590–2597

Hashimoto K, Shibazaki S (1976) Ultrastructural study on differentiation and function of hair. In: Toda K, Ishibashi Y, Hori Y, Morikawa F (eds) Biology and disease of the hair. University of Tokyo Press, Tokyo, pp 23–57

Hennings H, Yuspa SH (1985) Two-stage tumor promotion in mouse skin: an alternative interpretation. J Natl Cancer Res 74:735–740

Inaba M, Anthony J, McKinstry C (1979) Histologic study of the regeneration of axillary hair after removal with subcutaneous tissue shaver. J Invest Dermatol 72:224–231

Iversen U, Iversen OH (1976) The sensitivity of the skin of hairless mice to chemical carcinogenesis. Cancer Res 36:1238–1241

Johnson E (1958) Quantitative studies of hair growth in the albino rat: I. Normal males and females. J Endocrinol 16:337–350

Klein-Szanto AJ, Nelson KG, Shah Y, Slaga TJ (1983) Simultaneous appearance of keratin modifications and gammaglutamyltransferase activity as indicators of tumor progression in mouse skin papillomas. J Natl Cancer Inst 70:161–168

Kligman AM (1959) The human hair cycle. J Invest Dermatol 33:307–316

Lavker RM, Sun T-T (1982) Heterogeneity in epidermal basal keratinocytes: morphological and functional correlations. Science 215:1239–1241

Lavker RM, Sun T-T (1983) Epidermal stem cells. J Invest Dermatol [Suppl] 81:121s–127s

Lavker RM, Cotsarelis G, Wei Z-G, Sun T-T (1991) Stem cells of pelage, vibrissae and eyelash follicles: the hair cycle and tumor formation. Ann NY Acad Sci 642:214–225

Leblond CP (1981) The life history of cells in renewing systems. Am J Anat 160:114–157

Liang H, Cowdry EV (1954) Changes of hair follicular cells after a single painting of methylcholanthrene in mice. Cancer Res 4:340–345

Moffat GH (1968) The growth of hair follicles and its relation to the adjacent dermal structures. J Anat 102:527–540

Montagna W, Chase HB, Melaragno HP (1952) Skin of hairless mice: I. Formation of cysts and the distribution of lipids. J Invest Dermatol 19:83–94

Morris R, Fischer SM, Slaga TJ (1985) Evidence that the centrally and peripherally located cells in the murine epidermal proliferative unit are two distinct cell populations. J Invest Dermatol 84:277–281

Morris R, Fischer SM, Slaga TJ (1986) Evidence that a slowly cycling subpopulation of adult murine epidermal cells retains carcinogen. Cancer Res 46:3061–3066

Oliver RF (1966) Whisker growth after removal of the dermal papilla and lengths of follicle in the hooded rat. J Embryol Exp Morphol 15:331–347

Oliver RF (1967a) Ectopic regeneration of whisker in the hooded rat from implanted length of vibrissa follicle wall. J Embryol Exp Morphol 17:27–34

Oliver RF (1967b) The experimental induction of whisker growth in the hooded rat by implantation of dermal papillae. J Embryol Exp Morphol 18:43–51
Pierard GE, de la Brassinne M (1975) modulation of dermal cell activity during hair growth in the rat. J Cutan Pathol 2:35–41
Potten CS, Morris RJ (1988) Epithelial stem cells in vivo. J Cell Sci Suppl 10:45–62
Potten CS, Schofield R, Lajtha LG (1979) A comparison of cell replacement in bone marrow, testis and three regions of surface epithelium. Biochim Biophys Acta 560:281–299
Schermer A, Galvin S, Sun T-T (1986) Differentiation-related expression of a major 64K corneal keratin in vivo and in culture suggests limbal location of corneal epithelial stem cells. J Cell Biol 103:49–62
Sholley MM, Cotran RS (1976) Endothelial DNA synthesis in the microvasculature of rat skin during the hair growth cycle. Am J Anat 147:243–254
Slaga TJ, Klein-Szanto AJP (1983) Initiation-promotion versus complete carcinogenesis in mice: importance of dark basal keratinocytes (stem cells). Cancer Invest 1:425–436
Stenbeck F, Peto R, Shubick P (1981) Initiation and promotion at different stages and doses in 2200 mice: I. Methods and the apparent persistence of initiated cells. Br J Cancer 44:1–14
Stohr P (1903–1904) Entwicklungsgeschichte des menschlichen Wollhaares. Anat Hefte Abt 1/23:1–66
Sun T-T, Cotsarelis G, Lavker RM (1991) Hair follicular stem cells: the bulge-activation hypothesis. J Invest Dermatol 96:77–78s
Unna PG (1876) Beitrage zur Histologie und Entwicklungsgeschichte der menschlichen Oberhaut und ihrer Anhangsgebilde. Arch Microskop Anat Entwicklungsmech 12:665–741
Van Duuren BL, Sivak A, Katz C, Seidman I, Melchionne S (1975) The effect of aging and interval between primary and secondary treatment in two-stage carcinogenesis on mouse skin. Cancer Res 35:502–505
Van Scott EJ, Ekel TM, Auerbach R (1963) Determinants of rate and kinetics of cell division in scalp hair. J Invest Dermatol 41:269–273
Whitely HJ (1957) The effect of the hair growth cycle on experimental skin carcinogenesis in the rabbit. Br J Cancer 11:196–205
Wright N, Alison M (1984) The biology of epithelial cell populations, vol 1. Clarendon, Oxford
Yuspa SH (1986) Cutaneous chemical carcinogenesis. J Am Acad Dermatol 15:1031–1044
Zackheim HS (1964) Evolution of squamous cell carcinoma in the rat. J Invest Dermatol 77:434–444

The Skin: Initiation and Target Site of Immune Responses

G. Stingl

Division of Cutaneous Immunobiology, Department of Dermatology I, University of Vienna Medical School, Alser Strasse 4, 1090 Vienna, Austria

Introduction

During the past 15 years, increasing evidence has accumulated that the skin, in addition to its target role in immune reactions, contains the cellular elements which are needed for the initiation and expression of the immune response.

In this review, the immunological functions of various resident and passenger cells of the skin will be summarized briefly. Based on this information, a hypothetical model of the molecular and cellular pathways operative in immune responses originating and terminating in the skin will be constructed.

Immune Functions of Skin Cells

Langerhans Cells

Langerhans cells (LC) are dendritic cells of bone marrow derivation that reside mainly within stratified squamous epithelia but have also been shown to occur in mesenchymal tissues such as the dermis and lymph nodes. In the epidermis, they usually are located at a suprabasal level and constitute approximately 2% to 4% of all epidermal cells. LC visualization at the light microscopic level requires the use of appropriate histochemical and/or immunolabeling techniques. Ultrastructurally, LC exhibit unique trilaminar cytoplasmic organelles (Birbeck granules) that allow their identification (Stingl et al. 1989).

Phenotypic Features of Langerhans Cells. In the past few years, it has become clear that the phenotype of LC is determined by the quality and quantity of mediators present in their microenvironment. Resident as well as

Recent Results in Cancer Research, Vol. 128

freshly isolated LC display nonspecific esterase and adenosinetriphosphatase (ATPase) activity, and are the only cells within the normal epidermis to express Fc IgG receptors type II (FcγRII/CD32) (Romani et al. 1989b; Schmitt et al. 1990), Fc IgE receptors type I (FcεRI) (Bieber et al. 1992; Wang et al. 1992), C3bi receptors (CD11b-CD18), and major histocompatibility complex (MHC)-encoded class II antigens (Stingl et al. 1989).

In epidermal cell cultures, LC acquire a pronounced dendritic configuration, and undergo profound changes in their marker repertoire: while the expression of certain markers (FcγRII, ATPase activity, Birbeck granules) continuously decreases, the surface density of other molecules greatly increases in culture (MHC class I and class II antigens, RFDI, CD25, CD40, CD54, CD58) (Schuler and Steinman 1985; Witmer-Pack et al. 1988; Romani et al. 1989b; Stingl et al. 1989; Teunissen et al. 1990). Thus, cultured LC are essentially indistinguishable from certain MHC class II-bearing dendritic cells (DC) of lymphoid tissues which are potent stimulators of primary and secondary T cell responses (Metlay et al. 1989). It is now clear that the cytokines granulocyte/macrophage colony-stimulating factor (GM-CSF) and interleukin (IL)-1 are responsible for the phenotypic changes LC undergo in epidermal cell cultures (Heufler et al. 1988).

Functional Capacities of Langerhans Cells. Several groups of investigators have demonstrated over the years that LC-containing epidermal cells can induce primary and secondary T cell responses towards alloantigens, haptens, and soluble protein antigens including microbial antigens (Stingl et al. 1989; Stingl and Shevach 1991; Will et al. 1992).

The availability of techniques for the purification of the various epidermal cell subpopulations made it possible to assess the functional capacities of LC per se (i.e., in the absence of other epidermal cells) and to comparatively evaluate the immunological functions of freshly isolated vs cultured LC. Results obtained showed that freshly isolated, but not cultured LC are able of processing large protein antigens (Romani et al. 1989a). On the other hand, it appears that while both freshly isolated and cultured LC are potent antigen-presenting cells for primed cells, cultured LC are far superior to freshly isolated LC in their capacity to stimulate naive, resting T cells (Inaba et al. 1986). The mechanisms underlying these functional differences between freshly isolated and cultured LC are not entirely understood. Recent evidence indicates that the antigen-processing capacity of LC correlates with the level of biosynthesis of MHC class II molecules and with the expression of invariant chain (Puré et al. 1990) and is dependent upon the presence of certain acidic organelles such as endosomes and Birbeck granules (Girolomoni et al. 1990; Stössel et al. 1990).

Ample evidence indicates that these in vitro findings are of relevance for the in vivo situation. Larsen et al. (1990) documented that a few hours after skin transplantation LC begin to enlarge and exhibit increased amounts of surface-bound MHC class II molecules. Subsequently, a marked reduction in the number of epidermal LC occurs concomitantly with the appearance of strongly Ia^+ cells in the dermis of the transplants. In keeping with this finding, Aiba and Katz (1990) found that 24 h after application of a contact sensitizer LC appear larger than normal, exhibit more intense anti-Ia staining, and are several-fold more potent in their T cell stimulatory capacity than LC from nontreated or vehicle-treated animals. Furthermore, it was possible to identify antigen-bearing LC/DC in draining lymph nodes after the application of contact sensitizers (Silberberg-Sinakin et al. 1976; Macatonia et al. 1987; Kripke et al. 1990) and to demonstrate antigen-specific T cell activation by these cells (Macatonia et al. 1987). On the basis of these findings, it appears likely that LC function involves two components: (1) antigens are picked up in the skin and processed by LC; and (2) LC acquire the capacity to leave the skin and trigger resting T cells in the lymphoid organs.

One can therefore assume that the major in vivo function of LC is to provide a sensitizing signal in the induction of an immune response against antigens introduced into the skin (e.g., contactants, microorganisms) or newly generated in the skin (e.g., tumor antigens). The validity of this assumption is supported by several in vivo experiments: (1) While the application of a contact sensitizer to a skin area with high LC density leads to the induction of contact hypersensitivity (CHS), the application of the same contactant to a skin area deficient in LC results in antigen-specific unresponsiveness (Toews et al. 1980; Elmets et al. 1983). (2) Antigen-bearing LC induce sensitization even when administered via routes (e.g., intravenously) that favor the induction of tolerance (Ptak et al. 1980; Sullivan et al. 1986). (3) CD4-bearing T cells that had been sensitized in vitro with hapten-modified LC act as effector cells of CHS (Hauser 1990). (4) Compared to transplants with high LC density (body skin), transplants devoid of LC (central portion of cornea) or subtotally depleted of LC (tape-stripped skin) enjoy a prolonged survival on MHC class II-disparate recipients (Streilein et al. 1979; Streilein et al. 1982). (5) GM-CSF-activated LC-containing epidermal cells, but not LC-depleted epidermal cells are capable of presenting tumor antigens for the generation of protective antitumor immunity in vivo (Grabbe et al. 1991).

Dermal Dendrocytes

In the past few years, several investigators have described a population of dendritic cells in the human dermis which are primarily located in perivascular areas (Cerio et al. 1989; Sontheimer et al. 1989). Morphologically, these so-called dermal dendrocytes (DD) have a folded nucleus and a highly ruffled, irregular surface. Their cytoplasm is relatively dark and contains the organelles needed for an active cellular metabolism, but is devoid of Birbeck granules (Sontheimer et al. 1989). Phenotypic features of DD include

ATPase and nonspecific esterase activity as well as the expression of CD45, CD11b, CD11c, MHC class II antigens, and the subunit A of the clotting proenzyme factor XIII. In contrast, they fail to display CD1, CD14, and CD15 molecules and do not react with antibodies against von Willebrand factor (Cerio et al. 1989; Sontheimer et al. 1989). Thus, they do not qualify as endothelial cells and are also clearly distinct from typical CD1-bearing LC which are also regularly present around the dermal microvasculature. Functional studies with DD purified on the basis of a thorough phenotypic analysis are needed to understand their biological role as well as their relationship to the various leukocyte lineages.

Keratinocytes

Keratinocytes are capable of producing and secreting various mediators of the inflammatory reaction and of the immune response such as eicosanoids (Kragballe et al. 1990) and cytokines (Kupper 1988; Luger and Schwarz 1991). Keratinocyte-derived cytokines include IL-1, IL-6, IL-7, IL-8, and other intercrines, GM-CSF, and tumor necrosis factor α (TNF-α), as well as some of the factors regulating the growth of certain epithelial and/or mesenchymal cells, e.g., transforming growth factors (TGF) α and β, platelet-derived growth factor (PDGF), and basic fibroblast growth factor (bFGF) (Luger and Schwarz 1991). It should be kept in mind that – with the notable exceptions of IL-1, IL-7 and TGF-β – most of these mediators are not constitutively produced by keratinocytes, but only after the delivery of certain noxious stimuli (hypoxia, trauma, ultraviolet radiation, certain chemicals, etc.) (Enk and Katz 1992; O. Kilgus, E. Payer, S. Schreiber, A. Elbe, R. Strohal, and G. Stingl, submitted for publication). Application of contact allergens, for example, leads to an upregulation in the transcription of various cytokine genes in keratinocytes including those (IL-1, GM-CSF, TNF-α) which affect LC phenotype and function. One may therefore speculate that the induction of CHS does not only require the allergen uptake by LC, but also the hapten-induced alteration of cytokine production by keratinocytes. According to this concept, the latter event would be responsible for the in vivo activation of LC.

Evidence is accumulating that keratinocytes, in addition to their secretory capacities, can functionally interact with lymphocytes in an antigen-specific fashion. The observation that keratinocytes can be effectively lysed by $CD8^+$ cytotoxic T cells in an MHC class I-restricted fashion (Symington and Santos 1990) may be of pathogenetic significance in herpes simplex virus infections, graft-versus-host disease, and other skin disorders with a lichenoid infiltrate and keratinocyte necrosis.

While keratinocytes in culture and in normal skin do not constitutively express MHC class II molecules, the expression of these moieties may be induced by interferon-γ (IFN-γ) both in vitro (Basham et al. 1984; Volc-

Platzer et al. 1985) and in vivo (Nathan et al. 1986). It has been amply documented that keratinocytes synthesize and express MHC class II antigens in many skin disorders with prominent lymphocytic infiltration (Volc-Platzer et al. 1984; Auböck et al. 1986). This phenomenon has been attributed to IFN-γ production by infiltrating T cells. Functionally, class II-bearing keratinocytes are capable of inducing proliferation in allogeneic $CD4^+$ cell lines, but not in resting T cells (Niederwieser et al. 1988; Gaspari and Katz 1988). Although unable to process exogenously added protein antigen, keratinocytes present processing-independent peptide to a T cell hybridoma. This indicates that keratinocytes can express functional peptide/class II complexes, but lack the capacity to process exogenous protein antigen (Gaspari and Katz, 1988). In T helper 1 cell (Th1) clones, class II^+ keratinocytes induce nonresponsiveness (tolerance) to subsequent antigen-specific stimulation (Gaspari and Katz 1988; Bal et al. 1990). Because the same phenomenon has been shown to occur in models using antigen-presenting cells which cannot provide the so-called "second signal" necessary for T cell activation, one can assume that keratinocytes are unable to deliver auxiliary stimuli critical to this event. The in vivo importance of the tolerizing potential of class II^+ keratinocytes has been demonstrated by the finding that injection of hapten-modified, class II^+ keratinocytes into naive mice leads to a transient specific hyporesponsiveness to subsequent sensitization by hapten (Gaspari and Katz 1991).

Lymphocytes

The lymphocytes of mammalian skin belong almost exclusively to the T cell lineage as defined by the surface expression of CD3-associated T cell antigen receptors (TCR). To date, two major species of TCR have been identified: TCR α/β heterodimers are expressed on most peripheral T cells and recognize the nominal antigen in conjunction with MHC-encoded antigens (Allison and Lanier 1987). The more recently identified TCR γ/δ heterodimers are present on early fetal thymocytes, on a minor fraction of adult thymocytes and peripheral T cells, and, at least in the mouse system, on a varying percentage of lymphocytes populating epithelial tissues (Raulet 1989). Although the occurrence of signal transduction via CD3-TCR γ/δ has been demonstrated under several experimental conditions, the physiological ligand of this type of TCR has yet to be identified. Some evidence exists that TCR γ/δ may be receptors for first-line defense (e.g., enterotoxins, heat shock proteins); that they function as adhesion molecules (homing receptors); that they recognize MHC or MHC-like molecules (MHC class I and class II, Qa and TL in mouse, CD1 in humans); that they recognize antigen in conjunction with MHC or MHC-like structures; and that they behave as anti-self receptors, thereby regulating ontogeny and response of TCR α/β-bearing cells (Ferrick et al. 1989).

The mouse epidermis harbors a population of basally located cells that are $CD45^+$, Thy-1^+, asialo-$GM1^+$, $CD5^-$, $CD4^-$, $CD8^-$, MHC class II^-, and uniformly dendritic in shape. Thus, they were originally referred to as Thy-1^+ dendritic epidermal cells (Tschachler et al. 1983; Bergstresser et al. 1983). They have been renamed dendritic epidermal T cells (DETC) because of their uniform expression of surface-bound, CD3-associated 35-kDa/45-kDa TCR γ/δ heterodimers (Steiner et al. 1988). The TCR repertoire of DETC is very limited (preferential, if not exclusive usage of Vγ3 and Vδ1 determinants) and most closely resembles that of early fetal thymocytes (Havran and Allison 1988; Havran et al. 1989).

Based on these observations, Havran and Allison (1988) proposed that Vγ3-bearing early fetal thymocytes leave the thymus during the last days of gestation, migrate to the skin, home into the epidermis and thus become DETC. This hypothesis gained strong support from the observations that: (1) implantation of day 14 fetal thymic lobes from euthymic mice into either syngeneic athymic nude mice or Thy-1-disparate euthymic newborn mice results in the appearance of $V\gamma3^+$ DETC (Havran and Allison 1990); and (2) intravenous injection of fetal thymocytes (containing a TCR Vγ3-expressing subpopulation), but not of adult thymocytes (containing no TCR $V\gamma3^+$ cells) into Thy-1-disparate athymic nude mice results in the appearance of CD3/TCR $V\gamma3^+$ DETC (Payer et al. 1991). In other experiments, Elbe et al. (1992) have obtained evidence that transplantation of day 16 fetal skin onto a Thy-1-disparate recipient results in the appearance of donor-type DETC within the graft. Their further observation that the fetal skin graft contains $CD45^+$, Thy-1^+, $CD3^-$ lymphocytes, but no mature T cells at the time of transplantation, implies that fetal skin can provide stimuli promoting the expression of CD3/TCR genes in immature ($CD3^-$) DETC precursors. Thus, the relative contribution of the thymic vs the cutaneous microenvironment in the physiological maturation of DETC precursors into DETC is not yet clear and remains a subject for further investigations.

Similarly unclear is the functional role of DETC and, closely linked to this question, the functional ligand of their Vγ3/Vδ1-expressing TCR. Very recent evidence exists that keratinocyte extracts can specifically stimulate the proliferation of DETC (Havran et al. 1991), but the molecular nature of the relevant DETC-stimulating peptide has yet to be determined.

Although several investigators have searched for the human equivalent to murine DETC, no comparable T cell population has so far been identified in human skin. Most T cells of human skin are round to polygonal in shape, are found in the dermis rather than in the epidermis, and predominantly express TCR α/β rather than TCR γ/δ (Bos et al. 1990; Foster et al. 1990). Intradermal T cells are clustered preferentially around postcapillary venules and around the appendages and consist of both $CD4^+$ and $CD8^+$ cells (Bos et al. 1987). Most of the intraepidermal T cells exhibit the $CD4^-$, $CD8^+$, $CD2^+$, $CD3^+$/TCR α/β^+ phenotype and are located within the basal layer of the epidermis and the acrosyringial epithelium (Foster et al. 1990). Their highest density is encountered within the plantar epidermis (Foster et al. 1990). The further observation by these authors that the vast majority of T cells of human skin are $CD45RO^+$ suggests that they are memory cells.

The derivation of these intraepidermal memory cells can be explained in two ways. First, they might be generated by LC-mediated antigenic stimulation of naive T cells indigenously residing within the epidermis. Alternatively, they could already enter the skin/epidermis in a sensitized state. Because the ontogenetic development of skin T cells has not yet been carefully studied in man, no meaningful statement can currently be made about the validity of the former concept. In contrast, there exist some experimental data, mainly derived from studies with the monoclonal antibody HECA-452, which support the latter theory. This antibody reacts with 10%–20% of peripheral blood T cells and with 85% of lymphocytes in inflammatory skin lesions (Picker et al. 1990). HECA-452-reactive cells have the $CD45^{low}$, $CD44^{high}$ phenotype and, thus, qualify as memory cells. Cell attachment experiments have shown that memory T cells, but not resting T cells, adhere to endothelial cell lymphocyte adhesion molecule 1 (ELAM-1)$^+$ cells (Shimizu et al. 1991) and that the HECA-452$^+$ T cell subset is the predominant ELAM-1-binding population among circulating lymphocytes (Picker et al. 1991). It has further been observed that ELAM-1 is preferentially expressed on endothelial cells of venules within inflammatory skin lesions and that these venules are associated with a predominantly HECA-452$^+$ T cell infiltrate (Picker et al. 1991). These data strongly suggest that the interaction between HECA-452-reactive molecules (termed CLA, cutaneous leukocyte antigen) and ELAM-1 mediates the adhesion of memory T cells to the endothelial cells of the dermal microvasculature and, thus, promotes the migration of memory T cells into the dermis. The further migration of these cells into the epidermis involves various cytokines, chemotactic factors, and adhesion molecules. Primarily on the basis of in vitro studies, one would assume that members of the IL-8 family (intercrines; Oppenheim et al. 1991) are the most important keratinocyte-derived T cell chemotactic signals. In vitro, IFN-γ and TNF-α are capable of inducing intercrine production by keratinocytes (Barker et al. 1990) and presumably play an important role in T cell recruitment to the epidermis. Additionally, these cytokines trigger the expression of intercellular adhesion molecule 1 (ICAM-1) by keratinocytes (Barker et al. 1990), rendering these cells capable of binding lymphocyte function-associated antigen 1 (LFA-1) (Dustin et al. 1988). These data support the concept that the epidermotropic migration of dermal T cells is initiated by certain keratinocyte-derived cytokines (the production of which can also be induced or enhanced by secretory products of activated T cells themselves, e.g., IFN-γ) and that their attachment to and, finally, their entrance into the epidermis can be mediated by the LFA-1/ICAM-1 interaction.

Thus, it appears likely that human epidermal T cells (or at least the vast majority thereof) are not the descendants of naive, resting T cells indigenously residing in the epidermis, but rather represent the progeny of activated T cells which enter the skin and epidermis in the course of inflammatory reactions.

Skin-Induced Immune Responses: A Hypothesis

The above data clearly show that the skin harbors the cell types needed for the initiation of an immune response, i.e., antigen-presenting cells and lymphocytes. In addition, a variety of other cells reside in this organ (keratinocytes, mast cells, eosinophils, endothelial cells) which, by means of their secretory products, can regulate and modulate the function of immunocompetent cells and, by themselves, can display important effector functions in the immune response.

While the preeminent role of LC as sensitizing cells in cutaneous immune responses is generally accepted, it is not yet clear at which anatomical site the functional interactions between LC and lymphocytes occurs. While it is conceivable that T cells within the skin are the targets of antigen-bearing LC, more evidence exists for the assumption that, at least in the primary immune response, T cell sensitization occurs in the draining lymph node. The finding that patent lymphatics are required for the onset of sensitization (Frey and Wenk 1958), together with the demonstration of increased numbers of antigen-bearing LC in the dermal lymphatics and draining nodes during the sensitization period (Silberberg-Sinakin et al. 1976; Macatonia et al. 1987; Kripke et al. 1990), indicates that, upon antigen exposure, LC migrate from the epidermis to the dermis (to become DD?) and, then, via the dermal lymphatics (as veiled cells?) to the paracortical areas of the draining lymph nodes. At this site, they present (as lymphoid dendritic cells?) the antigen in an immunologically relevant fashion to the surrounding resting T cells. In order to fulfill their task (i.e., to mediate or, at least, to initiate effector mechanisms against the noxious pathogens), T cell blasts thus generated must find their way back to the skin and, ideally, should accumulate at the cutaneous sites harboring the antigen. Evidence exists that this is, in fact, the case. Several investigators have reported that T cell blasts generated in lymph nodes draining the skin preferentially infiltrate cutaneous sites of hapten-induced inflammation, while blast cells obtained from mesenteric lymph nodes accumulate after adoptive transfer in highest number in the gut wall and the mesenteric lymph nodes (Griscelli et al. 1969; Asherson et al. 1973; Rose et al. 1976). Increasing evidence is emerging that tissue-specific homing receptors on lymphocytes and corresponding addressins on endothelial cells are responsible for these preferential homing patterns of lymphocytes (Berg et al. 1989; Shimizu et al. 1991; Picker et al. 1991). Upon arrival in the skin and upon receipt of a renewed antigen stimulus by MHC class II-bearing accessory cells, these sensitized T cells can undergo clonal expansion, resulting in the generation of effector cells/molecules sufficient in magnitude to ensure the elimination of the pathogen.

This hypothesis about the mechanisms and the pathways of immune responses originating in the skin corresponds to the SALT (skin-associated lymphoid tissues) concept originally put forward by Streilein (1983). According to this concept, antigen-presenting Langerhans cells, cytokine-producing keratinocytes, epidermotropic T cells, and draining peripheral lymph nodes collectively form an immunological unit which provides the skin with unique immune surveillance mechanisms, i.e., the capacity to generate protective immune responses against exogenous and endogenous pathogens (Mitchinson and Kinlen 1980). Following this reasoning, an injury of the LC population, for instance by ultraviolet radiation (Toews et al. 1980; Stingl et al. 1981; Cruz et al. 1989) or by the human immunodeficiency virus 1 (HIV-1; Belsito et al. 1984; Tschachler et al. 1987), will lead to a functional impairment of SALT and, thus, to a progressive spread of infections and/or neoplastic processes affecting the skin.

Acknowledgments. I thank Mrs. Marlies Kaufmann for carefully typing this manuscript. This work was supported, in part, by grant no. P8536-MED from the Austrian Science Foundation, Vienna, Austria.

References

Aiba S, Katz SI (1990) Phenotypic and functional characteristics of in vivo-activated Langerhans cells. J Immunol 145:2791–2796

Allison JP, Lanier LL (1987) Structure, function, and serology of the T-cell antigen receptor complex. Annu Rev Immunol 5:503–540

Asherson GL, Allwood GG, Mayhew B (1973) Contact sensitivity in the mouse. XI. Movement of T blasts in the draining lymph nodes to sites of inflammation. Immunology 25:485–494

Auböck J, Romani N, Grubauer G, Fritsch P (1986) HLA-DR expression on keratinocytes is a common feature of diseased skin. Br J Dermatol 114:465–472

Bal V, McIndoe A, Denton G, Hudson D, Lombardi G, Lamb J, Lechler R (1990) Antigen presentation by keratinocytes induces tolerance in human T cells. Eur J Immunol 20:1893–1897

Barker JNWN, Sarma V, Mitra RS, Dixit VM, Nickoloff BJ (1990) Marked synergism between tumor necrosis factor-α and interferon-γ in regulation of keratinocyte-derived adhesion molecules and chemotactic factors. J Clin Invest 85:605–608

Basham TY, Nickoloff BJ, Merigan TC, Morhenn VB (1984) Recombinant gamma interferon induces HLA-DR expression on cultured human keratinocytes. J Invest Dermatol 83:88–90

Belsito DV, Sanchez MR, Baer RL, Valentine F, Thorbecke GJ (1984) Reduced Langerhans' cell Ia antigen and ATPase activity in patients with the acquired immunodeficiency syndrome. N Engl J Med 310:1279–1282

Berg EL, Goldstein LA, Jutila MA, Nakache M, Picker LJ, Streeter PR, Wu NW, Zhou D, Butcher EC (1989) Homing receptors and vascular addressins: cell surface molecules that direct lymphocyte traffic. Immunol Rev 108:5–18

Bergstresser PR, Tigelaar RE, Dees JH, Streilein JW (1983) Thy-1 antigen bearing dendritic cells populate murine epidermis. J Invest Dermatol 81:286–288
Bieber T, de la Salle H, Wollenberg A, Hakimi J, Chizzonite R, Ring J, Hanau D, de la Salle C (1992) Human epidermal Langerhans cells express the high affinity receptor for immunoglobulin E (FcεRI). J Exp Med 175:1285–1290
Bos JD, Zonneveld I, Das PK, Krieg SR, van der Loos CM, Kapsenberg ML (1987) The skin immune system (SIS): Distribution and immunophenotype of lymphocyte subpopulations in normal human skin. J Invest Dermatol 88:569–573
Bos JD, Teunissen MBM, Cairo I, Krieg SR, Kapsenberg ML, Das PK, Borst J (1990) T-cell receptor γδ bearing cells in normal human skin. J Invest Dermatol 94:37–42
Cerio R, Griffiths CEM, Cooper KD, Nickoloff BJ, Headington JT (1989) Characterization of factor XIIIa positive dermal dendritic cells in normal and inflamed skin. Br J Dermatol 121:421–431
Cruz PD, Nixon-Fulton J, Tigelaar RE, Bergstresser PR (1989) Disparate effects of in vitro low-dose UVB irradiation on intravenous immunization with purified epidermal cell subpopulations for the induction of contact hypersensitivity. J Invest Dermatol 92:160–165
Dustin ML, Singer KH, Tuck DT, Springer TA (1988) Adhesion of T lymphoblasts to epidermal keratinocytes is regulated by interferon γ and is mediated by intercellular adhesion molecule 1 (ICAM-1). J Exp Med 167:1323–1340
Elbe A, Kilgus O, Strohal R, Payer E, Schreiber S, Stingl G (1992) Fetal skin – a site of DETC development. J Immunol 149:1694–1701
Elmets CA, Bergstresser PR, Tigelaar RE, Wood PJ (1983) Analysis of the mechanism of unresponsiveness produced by haptens painted on skin exposed to low-dose ultraviolet irradiation. J Exp Med 158:781–794
Enk AH, Katz SI (1992) Early molecular events in the induction phase of contact sensitivity. Proc Natl Acad Sci USA 89:1398–1402
Ferrick DA, Ohashi PS, Wallace V, Schilham M, Mak TW (1989) Thymic ontogeny and selection of αβ and γδ T cells. Immunol Today 10:403–407
Foster CA, Yokozeki H, Rappersberger K, Koning F, Volc-Platzer B, Rieger A, Coligan JE, Wolff K, Stingl G (1990) Human epidermal T cells predominately belong to the lineage expressing α/β T cell receptor. J Exp Med 171:997–1013
Frey JR, Wenk P (1958) Über die Funktion der regionalen Lymphknoten bei der Entstehung des Dinitrochlorbenzol-Kontaktekzems am Meerschweinchen. Dermatologica 116:243–259
Gaspari AA, Katz SI (1988) Induction and functional characterization of class II MHC (Ia) antigens on murine keratinocytes. J Immunol 140:2956–2963
Gaspari AA, Katz SI (1991) Induction of in vivo hyporesponsiveness to contact allergens by hapten-modified Ia^+ keratinocytes. J Immunol 147:4155–4161
Girolomoni G, Cruz PD Jr, Bergstresser PR (1990) Internalization and acidification of surface HLA-DR molecules by epidermal Langerhans cells: a paradigm for antigen processing. J Invest Dermatol 94:753–760
Grabbe S, Bruvers S, Gallo RL, Knisely TL, Nazareno R, Granstein RD (1991) Tumor antigen presentation by murine epidermal cells. J Immunol 146:3656–3661
Griscelli C, Vassalli P, Mc Cluskey RT (1969) The distribution of large dividing lymph node cells in syngeneic recipient rats after intravenous injection. J Exp Med 130:1427–1451
Hauser C (1990) Cultured epidermal Langerhans cells activate effector T cells for contact sensitivity. J Invest Dermatol 95:436–440
Havran WL, Allison JP (1988) Developmentally ordered appearance of thymocytes expressing different T-cell antigen receptors. Nature 335:443–445
Havran WL, Allison JP (1990) Origin of $Thy\text{-}1^+$ dendritic epdidermal cells of adult mice from fetal thymic precursors. Nature 344:68–70

Havran WL, Grell S, Duwe G, Kimura J, Wilson A, Kruisbeek AM, O'Brien RL, Born W, Tigelaar RE, Allison JP (1989) Limited diversity of T-cell receptor γ-chain expression of murine Thy-1$^+$ dendritic epidermal cells revealed by Vγ3-specific monoclonal antibody. Proc Natl Acad Sci USA 86:4185–4189

Havran WL, Chien YH, Allison JP (1991) Recognition of self antigens by skin-derived T cells with invariant $\gamma\delta$ antigen receptors. Science 252:1430–1432

Heufler C, Koch F, Schuler G (1988) Granulocyte/macrophage colony-stimulating factor and interleukin 1 mediate the maturation of murine epidermal Langerhans cells into potent immunostimulatory dendritic cells. J Exp Med 167:700–705

Inaba K, Schuler G, Witmer MD, Valinsky J, Atassi B, Steinman RM (1986) Immunologic properties of purified epidermal Langerhans cells. Distinct requirements for stimulation of unprimed and sensitized T lymphocytes. J Exp Med 164:605–613

Kragballe K, Fisher GJ, Voorhees JJ (1990) Eicosanoids in inflammatory and immunologic skin disorders. In: Bos JD (ed) Skin immune system (SIS). CRC Press, Boca Raton, pp 243–255

Kripke ML, Munn CG, Jeevan A, Tang JM, Bucana C (1990) Evidence that cutaneous antigen-presenting cells migrate to regional lymph nodes during contact sensitization. J Immunol 145:2833–2838

Kupper TS (1988) Interleukin 1 and other human keratinocyte cytokines: molecular and functional characterization. In: Callen, Dahl, Golitz, Schachner, Stegman (eds) Advances in dermatology, vol 3. Year Book, Chicago, pp 293–307

Larsen CP, Steinman RM, Witmer-Pack M, Hankins DF, Morris PJ, Austyn JM (1990) Migration and maturation of Langerhans cells in skin transplants and explants. J Exp Med 172:1483–1493

Luger TA, Schwarz T (1991) Epidermal cell derived secretory regulins. In: Schuler (ed) Epidermal Langerhans cells. CRC Press, Boca Raton, pp 217–251

Macatonia SE, Knight SC, Edwards AJ, Griffiths S, Fryer P (1987) Localization of antigen on lymph node dendritic cells after exposure to the contact sensitizer fluorescein isothiocyanate. Functional and morphological studies. J Exp Med 166:1654–1667

Metlay JP, Puré E, Steinman RM (1989) Control of the immune response at a level of antigen-presenting cells: a comparison of the function of dendritic cells and B lymphocytes. In: Dixon, Austen, Hood, Uhr (eds) Advances in immunology, vol 47. Academic, Orlando, pp 45–116

Mitchinson NA, Kinlen LJ (1980) Present concepts on immune surveillance. Prog Immunol 4:641–645

Nathan CF, Kaplan G, Levis WR, Nusrat A, Witmer MD, Sherwin SA, Job CK, Path FRC, Horowitz CR, Steinman RM, Cohn ZA (1986) Local and systemic effects of intradermal recombinant interferon-γ in patients with lepromatous leprosy. N Engl J Med 315:6–15

Niederwieser D, Auböck J, Troppmair J, Herold M, Schuler G, Boeck G, Lotz J, Fritsch P, Huber C (1988) IFN-mediated induction of MHC antigen expression on human keratinocytes and its influence on in vitro alloimmune responses. J Immunol 140:2556–2564

Oppenheim JJ, Zachariae COC; Mukaida N, Matsushima K (1991) Properties of the novel proinflammatory supergene "intercrine" cytokine family. Annu Rev Immunol 9:617–648

Payer E, Elbe A, Stingl G (1991) Circulating CD3$^+$/TCR Vγ3$^+$ fetal murine thymocytes home to the skin and give rise to proliferating dendritic epidermal T cells. J Immunol 146:2536–2543

Picker LJ, Michie SA, Rott LS, Butcher EC (1990) A unique phenotype of skin-associated lymphocytes in humans. Preferential expression of the HECA-452

epitope by benign and malignant T cells at cutaneous sites. Am J Pathol 136:1053–1068
Picker LJ, Kishimoto TK, Smith CW, Warnock RA, Butcher EC (1991) ELAM-1 is an adhesion molecule for skin-homing T cells. Nature 349:796–799
Ptak W, Ruzycka DW, Askenase PW, Gershon RK (1980) Role of antigen-presenting cells in the development and persistence of contact hypersensitivity. J Exp Med 151:362–375
Puré E, Inaba K, Crowley MT, Tardelli L, Witmer-Pack MD, Ruberti G, Fathman G, Steinman RM (1990) Antigen processing by epidermal Langerhans cells correlates with the level of biosynthesis of major histocompatibility complex class II molecules and expression of invariant chain. J Exp Med 172:1459–1469
Raulet DH (1989) The structure, function, and molecular genetics of the γ/δ T cell receptor. Annu Rev Immunol 7:175–207
Romani N, Koide S, Crowley M, Witmer-Pack M, Livingstone AM, Fathman CG, Inaba K, Steinman RM (1989a) Presentation of exogenous protein antigens by dendritic cells to T cell clones. Intact protein is presented best by immature, epidermal Langerhans cells. J Exp Med 169:1169–1178
Romani N, Lenz A, Glassel H, Stössel H, Stanzl U, Majdic O, Fritsch P, Schuler G (1989b) Cultured human Langerhans cells resemble lymphoid dendritic cells in phenotype and function. J Invest Dermatol 93:600–609
Rose ML, Parrot DMV, Bruce RG (1976) Migration of lymphoblasts to the small intestine. II. Divergent migration of mesenteric and peripheral immunoblasts to sites of inflammation in the mouse. Cell Immunol 27:36–46
Schmitt DA, Hanau D, Bieber T, Dezutter-Dambuyant C, Schmitt D, Fabre M, Pauly G, Cazenave J-P (1990) Human epidermal Langerhans cells express only the 40-kilodalton Fcγ receptor (FcRII). J Immunol 144:4284–4290
Schuler G, Steinman RM (1985) Murine epidermal Langerhans cells mature into potent immunostimulatory dendritic cells in vitro. J Exp Med 161:526–546
Shimizu Y, Shaw S, Graber N, Gopal TV, Horgan KJ, Van Seventer GA, Newman W (1991) Activation-independent binding of human memory T cells to adhesion molecule ELAM-1. Nature 349:799–802
Silberberg-Sinakin I, Thorbecke GJ, Baer RL, Rosenthal SA, Berezowsky V (1976) Antigen-bearing Langerhans cells in skin, dermal lymphatics and in lymph nodes. Cell Immunol 25:137–151
Sontheimer RD, Matsubara T, Seelig LL Jr (1989) A macrophage phenotype for a constitutive, class II antigen-expressing, human dermal perivascular dendritic cell. J Invest Dermatol 93:154–159
Steiner G, Koning F, Elbe A, Tschachler E, Yokoyama WM, Shevach EM, Stingl G, Coligan JE (1988) Characterization of T cell receptors on resident murine dendritic epidermal T cells. Eur J Immunol 18:1323–1328
Stingl G, Shevach EM (1991) Langerhans cells as antigen-presenting cells. In: Schuler (ed) Epidermal Langerhans cells. CRC Press, Boca Raton, pp 159–190
Stingl G, Gazze-Stingl LA, Aberer W, Wolff K (1981) Antigen presentation by murine epidermal Langerhans cells and its alteration by ultraviolet B light. J Immunol 127:1707–1713
Stingl G, Hauser C, Tschachler E, Groh V, Wolff K (1989) The immune functions of epidermal cells. In: Norris (ed) Immune mechanisms in cutaneous disease. Dekker, New York, pp 3–72
Stössel H, Koch F, Kämpgen E, Stöger P, Lenz A, Heufler C, Romani N, Schuler G (1990) Disappearance of certain acidic organelles (endosomes and Langerhans cell granules) accompanies loss of antigen processing capacity upon culture of epidermal Langerhans cells. J Exp Med 172:1471–1482
Streilein JW (1983) Skin-Associated lymphoid tissues (SALT): origins and functions. J Invest Dermatol 80:12s–16s

Streilein JW, Toews GB, Bergstresser PR (1979) Corneal allografts fail to express Ia antigens. Nature 282:326–327
Streilein JW, Lonsberry LW, Bergstresser PR (1982) Depletion of epidermal Langerhans cells and Ia immunogenicity from tapestripped mouse skin. J Exp Med 155:863–871
Sullivan S, Bergstresser PR, Tigelaar RE, Streilein JW (1986) Induction and regulation of contact hypersensitivity by resident bone marrow-derived, dendritic epidermal cells: Langerhans cells and Thy-1$^+$ epidermal cells. J Immunol 137:2460–2467
Symington FW, Santos EB (1990) Recognition of keratinocytes by cytotoxic T cells specific for conventional HLA-class-I alloantigen. J Invest Dermatol 95:224–228
Teunissen MBM, Wormmeester J, Krieg SR, Peters PJ, Vogels IMC, Kapsenberg ML, Bos JD (1990) Human epidermal Langerhans cells undergo profound morphologic und phenotypical changes during in vitro culture. J Invest Dermatol 94:166–173
Toews GB, Bergstresser PR, Streilein JW (1980) Epidermal Langerhans cell density determines whether contact hypersensitivity or unresponsiveness follows skin painting with DNFB. J Immunol 124:445–453
Tschachler E, Schuler G, Hutterer J, Leibl H, Wolff K, Stingl G (1983) Expression of Thy-1 antigen by murine epidermal cells. J Invest Dermatol 81:282–285
Tschachler E, Groh V, Popovic M, Mann DL, Konrad K, Safai B, Eron L, di Marzo Veronese F, Wolff K, Stingl G (1987) Epidermal Langerhans cells – a target for HTLV-III/LAV infection. J Invest Dermatol 88:233–237
Volc-Platzer B, Majdic O, Knapp W, Wolff K, Hinterberger W, Lechner K, Stingl G (1984) Evidence of HLA-DR antigen biosynthesis by human keratinocytes in disease. J Exp Med 159:1784–1789
Volc-Platzer B, Leibl H, Luger T, Zahn G, Stingl G (1985) Human epidermal cells synthesize HLA-DR alloantigens in vitro upon stimulation with γ-interferon. J Invest Dermatol 85:16–19
Wang B, Rieger A, Kilgus O, Ochiai K, Maurer D, Födinger D, Kinet JP, Stingl G (1992) Epidermal Langerhans cells from normal human skin bind monomeric IgE via FcεRI. J Exp Med 175:1353–1365
Will A, Blank C, Röllinghoff M, Moll H (1992) Murine epidermal Langerhans cells are potent stimulators of an antigen-specific T cell response to Leishmania major, the cause of cutaneous leishmaniasis. Eur J Immunol 22:1341–1347
Witmer-Pack MD, Valinsky J, Olivier W, Steinman RM (1988) Quantification of surface antigens on cultured murine epidermal Langerhans cells: rapid and selective increase in the level of surface MHC products. J Invest Dermatol 90:387–394

II. Melanocyte Carcinogenesis

Melanocyte Carcinogenesis: Facts and Fancies

W. Tilgen

Universitäts-Hautklinik, Voss-Str. 2, W-6900 Heidelberg, Fed. Rep. of Germany

Introduction

On reviewing the literature on malignant melanoma it is evident that little has been added to the basic concept of etiology, although our understanding of the biology of melanoma has improved considerably (Bagnara et al. 1985; Balch et al. 1985; Cascinelli et al. 1990; Ferrone 1990; Gallagher 1986; Lynch and Fusaro 1991; MacKie 1983; Veronesi et al. 1987). Our knowledge of pathogenesis concerning inducing agents and predisposing conditions is increasing. The basic mechanism, however, by which normal melanocytes develop into melanoma cells is not known. Thus, an introduction to melanocyte carcinogenesis consists more of questions than of answers. Melanocyte carcinogenesis seems to be a complex event which covers the disposition and exposure of an individual; both may be interacting and regulated by additional factors. As long as reliable animal models are lacking, most data must be based on epidemiological studies and in vitro investigations. There is only circumstantial evidence for the causal role of the various factors; a direct correlation is only possible for a small percentage of melanomas. Research has focused on endogenous as well as exogenous key processes (Table 1) such as genetic, endocrine, and immunologic factors, as well as on ultraviolet radiation (UVR) and chemical carcinogens. Factors modulating the individual susceptibility for melanoma development as determined by ethnic origin and skin complexion include, for example, antigen phenotype and the interaction between the pigmentary system and UV light.

This review focuses on only some of these cofactors for melanoma development.

Recent Results in Cancer Research, Vol. 128

Table 1. Etiology and pathogenesis of melanoma: "Melanomagenesis" hypotheses

Endogenous factors	Exogenous factors
Genetic factors	*Ultraviolet light exposure*
Ethnic origin: Caucasian race	Sunlight
Pigmentary traits: melanin synthesis	Occupational
Family history	Recreational
Melanoma susceptibility gene	Vacation
HLA phenotype (oncogenes/suppressor genes)	Artificial sources
Endocrine factors	Sunbeds and -lamps
Hormonal influences	Fluorescent light
Reproductive factors (endogenous estrogen/androgen)	*Oncogenic viruses*
Oral contraceptives	*Dietary factors*
Growth factors	*Chemical carcinogens*
Immunological factors	*Miscellaneous*
Antigen phenotypes	X-ray therapy
Differentiation antigens	Chronic scars
Progression antigens	Injury
Immunosuppression	
(*Precursor lesions*)	

Endogenous Factors

The implication for *genetic factors* is based on known ethnic influences on the incidence of melanoma. In the last century the occurrence and mortality rates for malignant melanoma have increased substantially in Caucasians but not in black and oriental individuals. The different incidences of melanomas in the various ethnic groups leave no doubt that individuals with fair skin complexion, red hair, numerous freckles, and a tendency to sunburn are at greatest risk. Epidemiological studies suggest that exposure to sunlight is the main causal factor. This is evidenced by higher incidence and mortality rates among Caucasians living at lower latitudes with more intense sun exposure than among persons with similar complexions who live in temperate climates.

Moreover, a failure in the pigmentary trait may possibly be related to melanocyte carcinogenesis. There are two types of melanin in everyone's skin and hair, regardless of race: the black or brown pigment eumelanin and the yellow-red pheomelanin. While Caucasians have more pheomelanin, those with black or brown skin have more eumelanin. One function of melanin is to protect the skin from sunlight and those chemical carcinogens that cause the formation of oxygen radicals in the skin as a major source for damage. Eumelanin can eliminate toxic intermediates and thus seems to be protective. Pheomelanin, however, is supposed to contribute to the generation of mutagenic photoproducts after exposure to UVR. Histochemical studies with monoclonal antibodies against melanosomal proteins led to the suggestion that an altered melanosome and melanin synthesis is a step in the neoplastic transformation of melanocytes. Recently, increased pheomelanin in malignant melanoma and dyplastic melanocytic nevi, but not in normal skin and common melanocytic nevi, has been described (Jimbow et al. 1991). There is an inverse relationship between the melanoma incidence and the skin pigmentation of various populations: the darker the race, the lower melanoma incidence. One may conclude that the impaired "self-defense" of Caucasian melanocytes lacking UVR-absorbing melanin leads to melanoma: "Having black skin is an equivalent to wearing a sunscreen all the time" (Kopf et al. 1984).

A family history of melanoma is reported by 4%–12% of patients (Lynch and Fusaro 1991). In the majority of cases pedigree analysis indicated an autosomal dominant trait, although polygenic inheritance was also discussed. It is not known, however, whether familial and sporadic melanomas represent the same biological entity. The occurrence of the dysplastic nevus syndrome in melanoma-prone families argued for hereditary factors. However, both common and dysplastic nevi are also associated with sporadic melanomas.

Cytogenetic studies in primary tumors, metastases, and cell lines of melanoma have identified a large variety of nonrandom chromosomal changes which are believed to play an important role in the neoplastic disease. Some of them were particularly observed in melanomas and may be considered primary changes, possibly responsible for tumor initiation; others are shared by many tumor types and may play a role in tumor progression. Earlier studies performed on cell lines, but also more recent ones on biopsy material or early passage cultures, showed the frequent involvement of chromosomes 1, 6, 7, and 10. Altered chromosomes were also identified from dysplastic nevi of patients with a dysplastic nevus syndrome, while congenital and common acquired nevi showed no karyotype abnormality. A melanoma susceptibility gene has been suggested for chromosome 6, as it is frequently involved in aberrations in melanoma cells. This melanoma susceptibility gene might be linked to HLA in men. Recently, a more closely defined chromosome region, 1p36, was identified by a multipoint linkage analysis of six families with predisposition to melanoma. The chromosome region 10q seems to be involved in an early stage of melanocytic transformation. However, it must be stressed that the significance of most chromosomal changes for melanoma development remains unknown (Della Porta et al. 1990; Trent et al. 1990).

Recent progress in molecular biology has allowed the possible role of oncogenes in melanoma development to be studied (Della Porta et al. 1990). So far it has been difficult to detect a consistent abnormality or association of any oncogene in melanomas. In most cases the activated genes were members of the *ras* family. Of the cultured melanomas, 24% contained activated *ras* genes, with N-*ras* being activated 10 times more often than Harvey (Ha)-*ras*. The frequency of N-*ras* mutations in noncultured metastatic melanomas, however, was only 6%, and 5% in primary melanomas. No *ras* mutations were detected in any specimen of common or dysplastic nevi. All the melanomas with an activated *ras* gene had a number of phenotypic characteristics in common, suggesting that they were derived from a similar stage of differentiation in the melanocyte lineage. Moreover, *ras* mutations were often found in primary tumors located on sun-exposed body sites, suggesting that activation occurred by UV-induced mutation (Van't Veer et al. 1989). According to Elder (1990) the question is: "c-Ha-*ras* and UV photocarcinogenesis: do rays raise ras?" The general conclusion was that activation of *ras* genes does not appear to be involved in the initiation, maintenance, or progression of *most* melanomas. Normal diploid melanocytes infected with a retrovirus containing the viral Ha-*ras* and the c-*myc* oncogene undergo complete transformation and acquire all characteristics of melanoma cells (Albino et al. 1989); an isochromosome 6p was the only structural chromosomal abnormality of these transformed melanocytes.

The influence of *endocrine factors*, especially sex hormones, on the incidence and prognosis of melanoma was discussed controversially for the last 50 years (MacKie 1983; Walker 1988). There was no relationship to changes in steroid hormone secretion. The literature on melanoma and pregnancy is confusing and mainly consists of case reports. As a consequence, there is no common agreement on the advice for family planning, pregnancy, or oral contraceptives to be given to melanoma patients. A prospective study on 289 women with clinical stage I cutaneous melanoma showed that prior use of estrogen and oral contraceptives had no deleterious effect (Ledermann et al. 1985). A number of recent studies have searched for estrogen receptors in malignant melanomas to identify patients who might respond to hormone therapy. The proportion of tumors expressing receptors varied from 0 to 80%, but most reports failed to characterize the hormone receptor. Results of studies using a receptor-specific antibody suggest that the apparent estrogen-binding capacity of human melanoma tissues represents unspecific interactions, e.g., with tyrosinase (Flowers et al. 1987). On the other hand, it has also been suggested that melanoma could be an androgen-dependent tumor (Rampen and Mulder 1980), since a receptor for androgen was found in 10%–25% of melanoma specimens. The idea that melanoma could be an estrogen- or androgen-dependent tumor resulted in the use of major hormone-depriving surgical procedures such as orchiectomy, oophorectomy, or hypophysectomy, but without providing substantial benefit for the patients. In a number of studies, melanoma patients were treated with estrogens or antiestrogen, with poor response rates which were independent of the receptor status tested.

Due to the availability of normal melanocytes as well as melanoma cells in culture, derived from different tumor stages, tumor-associated changes in growth regulation could be studied by the determination and isolation of growth factors (Halaban 1990; Herlyn et al. 1988; Rodeck et al. 1991). One clear-cut difference in growth regulation in vitro between normal and malignant melanocytes is documented by a progressive decrease in the requirement for exogenous growth factors, up to growth factor independence of advanced melanoma cells, indicating that these factors may contribute to a transformation mechanism of melanocytes to melanoma cells.

Clinical and histopathological observations suggest *immunological mechanisms* in the pathopysiology of melanoma. In this context, the idea of tumorigenesis as the stepwise development of a malignant tumor from the normal cell through precursor lesions prompted many efforts to characterize these intermediate steps. One approach has been to search for monoclonal antibodies against different cell surface- and melanosome-associated antigens of melanocytes and melanoma cells. Due to the pioneer work on differentiation- and progression-associated melanoma antigens it is possible to distinguish between (1) antigens common to all melanocytes, (2) antigens which discriminate between benign and malignant melanocytic lesions, and (3) antigen patterns which correlate with tumor progression (Houghton et al. 1987; Ruiter et al. 1990). The function of tumor-associated cellular infiltrates is not fully understood. It is still an open question whether melanoma progresses in spite of or because of inflammation (Bröcker et al. 1990).

The significance of *precursor lesions* (congenital melanocytic nevi, dysplastic nevi, acquired nevi) for malignant transformation is still under debate. Since the true risk of various types of nevi progressing into melanoma is not known, the therapeutic recommendations for nevi are likewise controversial.

Exogenous Factors

Ultraviolet radiation exposure seems to be the most important factor in melanoma pathogenesis. This hypothesis is based on large epidemiological studies from Australia, the USA, the United Kingdom, Denmark, and Germany (Elder 1989; Gallagher 1986; Garbe and Orfanos 1989; Holman et al. 1986; Kopf et al. 1984; Osterlind 1991; Sober 1987). Melanoma-susceptible phenotypes with a fair complexion, who tan poorly, and sunburn easily have been identified. The risk of UVR exposure for development of melanoma of the skin may be estimated in two ways (Jung 1988): (1) Cumulative total lifetime exposure to sunlight may be responsible for lentigo maligna melanoma only, because generally the melanoma patient is not an elderly individual with a high total lifetime sun exposure. (2) Intense intermittent sun exposure in early life seems to be an important factor in the development of nodular and superficial spreading melanoma and in the dysplastic nevus syndrome. Thus, sunlight damage should be avoided no matter where or how it occurs.

Some general principles are:

1. On approaching the equator, melanoma rates raise, indicating increasing incidences in sunbelt areas where UVR is more intense.
2. Immigrants from Europe coming to Israel or Australia as children have a higher incidence of malignant melanoma than Europeans who emigrated as adults, pointing to higher risk of intense exposure to sunlight early in life.
3. Various occupational groups, especially outdoor workers, also have an increased risk. Interestingly, US Navy personnel with indoor occupations had a higher age-adjusted incidence rate of melanoma than the US civilian population. Persons in occupations requiring both indoor and outdoor work had the lowest rate (Garland et al. 1990).
4. A significant increase in risk with increasing sun exposure through recreational activities was documented.
5. Migration data and case control studies emphasized the importance of painful blistering sunburn in childhood; but, pigmentation type and skin reaction to sun are more closely related to melanoma risk than are sunburn histories.
6. Melanoma tends to occur in locations more heavily exposed to the sun. The US Navy study, however, suggested a protective role of brief regular sun exposure. Sunburn appears even to be protective for nodular melanoma (Holman et al. 1986).
7. The effects of artificial UV sources like sunlamps and sunbeds, and fluorescent light are controversial (Swerdlow et al. 1988).
8. An increased risk for development of nevi with sun exposure has been described.

Obviously, additional coincidences are required between different risk factors for melanoma to arise, e.g., the individual predisposition and exposure: ethnic origin, the special pigmentary trait of Caucasians, and high sun sensitivity together with residency closer to the equator or excessive UVR exposure accompanied by sunburns early in life. Also, some intrinsic events may be modulated or regulated by UVR exposure (Elder 1990; Kripke 1986).

A lot of unsolved questions remain, showing the gaps in our knowledge of the etiology of cutaneous malignant melanoma: Laboratory models studying the effect of UVR on the induction of melanoma gave no hints as to the precise mechanism by which sunlight is involved in melanocyte carcinogenesis (Dore and Anders 1990; van Weelden et al. 1990). Also unsolved is how sun exposure is related to the cause of plantar melanomas (39%) in Japan (Takematsu et al. 1985). Most patients do not precisely fit the postulated susceptible phenotype. The spectrum of UVR which is in fact responsible for the increased risk has still to be determined. UVR, especially UVB, possibly acts as a dose-dependent carcinogen (= initiator) for skin, perhaps also inducing lentigo maligna melanoma and malignant melanoma in the autosomal recessively inherited disorder xeroderma pigmentosum. In other melanomas, UVR may be a later event in pathogenesis, acting as a cocarcinogen or promotor, since it promotes the development of melanoma in animals that were previously exposed to carcinogens.

Conclusions

"Further work has to be done", as shown by most studies and the interpretation of published data. Epidemiological studies have demonstrated an antihypothesis for every hypothesis. Technological advances in molecular biology and immunology have opened important new tools to study basic processes in tumor biology. Our knowledge, however, still lags far behind our technical possibilities. Nevertheless, epidemiological data have clearly demonstrated that the development of most melanomas is intertwined with the environmental factor UVR exposure, which could be changed, and with a variety of genetic factors that cannot be modified. Future research and, hopefully, this volume may help to clarify what is causal and what is casual in melanocyte carcinogenesis.

References

Albino AP, Nanus DM, Mentle IR et al. (1989) Analysis of ras oncogenes in malignant melanoma and precursor lesions: correlation of point mutations with differentiation phenotype. Oncogene 4:1363–1374

Bagnara J, Klaus SN, Paul E, Schartl M (eds) (1985) Pigment cell 1985. Biological, molecular and clinical aspects of pigmentation. University of Tokyo Press, Tokyo

Balch CM, Soong S-J, Shaw HM, Milton GW (1985) An analysis of prognostic factors in 4000 patients with cutaneous melanoma. In: Balch CM, Milton GW, Shaw HM, Soong S (eds) Cutaneous melanoma. Clinical management and treatment results worldwide. Lippincott, Philadelphia, pp 321–352

Bröcker EB, Macher E, Sorg C (1990) Changes in the tumor-associated inflamatory infiltrates in the course of local and systemic progression of cutaneous melanoma In: Ferrone S (ed) Human melanoma. From basic research to clinical application. Springer, Berlin Heidelberg New York, pp 278–293

Cascinelli N, Santinami M, Veronesi U (eds) (1990) Cutaneous melanoma biology and management. Masson, Milan

Della Porta G, Ghidoni A, Pierotti MA (1990) Cytogenetics and molecular biology of human malignant melanomas. In: Cascinelli N, Santinami M, Veronesi U (eds) Cutaneous melanoma biology and management. Masson, Milan, pp 45–54

Dore J-F, Anders F (1990) Contribution of experimental models to understanding of human melanoma. In: Cascinelli N, Santinami M, Veronesi U (eds) Cutaneous melanoma biology and management. Masson, Milan, pp 63–74

Elder DE (1989) Human melanocytic neoplasms and their etiologic relationship with sunlight. J Invest Dermatol 92 [Suppl]:297s–303s

Elder JT (1990) c-Ha-ras and UV photocarcinogenesis: do rays raise ras? Arch Dermatol 126:379–382

Ferrone S (ed) (1990) Human melanoma. From basic research to clinical application. Springer, Berlin Heidelberg New York
Flowers JL, Seigler HF, McCarty KS Sr, Konrath J, McCarty KS Jr (1987) Absence of estrogen receptor in human melanoma as evaluated by a monoclonal antiestrogen receptor antibody. Arch Dermatol 123:764–765
Gallagher RP (ed) (1986) Epidemiology of malignant melanoma. Springer, Berlin Heidelberg New York (Recent results in cancer research, vol 102)
Garbe C, Orfanos CE (1989) Epidemiologie des malignen Melanoms in der Bundesrepublik Deutschland im internationalen Vergleich. Onkologie 12:253–262
Garland FC, White MR, Garland CF, Shaw E, Gorham ED (1990) Occupational sunlight exposure and melanoma in the U.S. Navy. Arch Environ Health 45:261–267
Halaban R (1990) Growth regulation in normal and malignant melanocytes. In: Ferrone S (ed) Human melanoma. From basic research to clinical application. Springer, Berlin Heidelberg New York, pp 3–14
Herlyn M, Mancianti ML, Jambrosic J, Bolen JB, Koprowski H (1988) Regulatory factors that determine growth and phenotype of normal human melanocytes. Exp Cell Res 179:322–331
Holman CDJ, Armstrong BK, Heenan PJ (1986) Relationship of cutaneous malignant melanoma to individual sunlight-exposure habits. J Natl Cancer Inst 76:403–414
Houghton AN, Real FY, Davis LJ, Cordon-Cardo C, Old LJ (1987) Phenotypic heterogeneity of melanoma; relation to the differentiation program of melanoma cells. J Exp Med 164:812–829
Jimbow K, Salopek TG, Dixon WT, Searles GE, Yamada K (1991) The epidermal melanin unit in the pathophysiology of malignant melanoma. Am J Dermatopathol 13:179–188
Jung EG (1988) Ist das Melanom-Risiko kalkulierbar? Z Hautkr 63:559–562
Kopf AW, Kripke ML, Stern RS (1984) Sun and malignant melanoma. J Am Acad Dermatol 11:674–684
Kripke ML (1986) Immunology and photocarcinogenesis. New light on an old problem. J Am Acad Dermatol 14:149–155
Lederman JS, Lew RA, Koh HK, Sober AJ (1985) Influence of estrogen administration on tumor characteristics and survival in women with cutaneous melanoma. J Natl Cancer Inst 74:981–985
Lynch HT, Fusaro RM (1991) Hereditary malignant melanoma. CRC Press, Boca Raton
MacKie RM (ed) (1983) Malignant melanoma. Advances of a decade. Karger, Basel (Pigment cell, vol 6)
Osterlind A (1991) Etiology and epidemiology of melanoma and skin neoplasms. Curr Opin Oncol 3:355–359
Rampen FHJ, Mulder JH (1980) Malignant melanoma: an androgen-dependent tumor? Lancet 1:562–564
Rodeck U, Melber K, Kath R, Menssen H-D, Varello M, Atkinson B, Herlyn M (1991) Constitutive expression of multiple growth factor genes by melanoma cells but not normal melanocytes. J Invest Dermatol 97:20–26
Ruiter DJ, Van Muijen GNP, van Nouhuys H, Ferrone S (1990) Immunopathology of melanoma with monoclonal antibodies. In: Ferrone S (ed) Human melanoma. From basic research to clinical application. Springer, Berlin Heidelberg New York, pp 253–277
Sober AJ (1987) Solar exposure in the etiology of cutaneous melanoma. Photodermatology 4:23–31

Swerdlow AJ, English JSC, MacKie RM, O'Doherty CJ, Hunter JAA, Clark J, Hole DJ (1988) Fluorescent lights, ultraviolct lamps, and risk of cutaneous melanoma. BMJ 297:647–650

Takematsu H, Tomita Y, Kato T, Takahashi M, Abe R, Seiji M (1985) Melanoma in Japan: experience at Tohoku University Hospital Sendai. In: Balch CM, Milton GW, Shaw HM, Soong S (eds) Cutaneous melanoma. Clinical management and treatment results worldwide. Lippincott, Philadelphia, pp 499–506

Trent JM, Meyskens FL, Salmon SE, Ryschon K, Leong SPL, Davis JR, McGee DL (1990) Relation of cytogenetic abnormalities and clinical outcome in metastatic melanoma. N Engl J Med 322:1508–1511

Van't Veer LJ, Burgering BMTh, Versteeg R, Boot AJM, Ruiter DJ, Osanto S, Schrier PI, Boos JL (1989) N-ras mutations in human cutaneous melanoma correlated with sun exposure. Mol Cell Biol 9:3114–3116

van Weelden H, van der Putte SC, Toonstra J, van der Leun JC (1990) Ultraviolet B-induced tumors in pigmented hairless mice, with an unsuccessful attempt to induce cutaneous melanoma. Photodermatol Photoimmunol Photomed 7:68–72

Veronesi U, Cascinelli N, Santinami M (eds) (1987) Cutaneous melanoma. Status of knowledge and future perspective. Academic, London

Walker MJ (1988) Role of hormones and growth factors in melanomas. Semin Oncol 15:512–523

The German Melanoma Registry and Environmental Risk Factors Implied

C. Garbe[1], J. Weiß[3], S. Krüger[1], E. Garbe[1], P. Büttner[2], J. Bertz[4], H. Hoffmeister[4], I. Guggenmoos-Holzmann[2], E.G. Jung[3], and C.E. Orfanos[1]

[1] Department of Dermatology, University Medical Center Steglitz, Free University of Berlin, W-1000 Berlin 45, Fed. Rep. of Germany
[2] Institute for Statistics, University Medical Center Steglitz, Free University of Berlin, W-1000 Berlin 45, Fed. Rep. of Germany
[3] Department of Dermatology Mannheim, University of Heidelberg, W-6800 Mannheim, Fed. Rep. of Germany
[4] Institute for Epidemiology, Federal Health Office, Berlin, Fed. Rep. of Germany

Introduction

There is no nationwide, population-based cancer registry in the Federal Republic of Germany (FRG). Only the cancer registry of the federal state of Saarland, a region with about 1 000 000 inhabitants bordering on France, has reliably documented the incidence of malignant melanoma in western Germany. The annual incidence of melanoma registered for this region in the mid-1980s was 6/100 000 inhabitants for both sexes (age-adjusted for the European standard population) (Garbe et al. 1986). The increase in the incidence of melanoma in the 1970s documented by the Saarland cancer registry suggested that the incidence would double every 15 years (Garbe et al. 1986). This rate of increase is in good agreement with data from the two internationally longest existing cancer registries in Denmark and Connecticut (USA) (Houghton et al. 1980). However, the question arises whether the data from the Saarland cancer registry and the melanoma incidence derived from this more rural area are representative for the entire FRG. Another drawback of the Saarland cancer registry is that only the diagnoses were registered, without detailed information on histologic subtypes and other histologic or prognostic parameters and without documentation of possible risk factors for developing melanoma.

In view of this situation, the German Dermatological Society decided in 1983 to establish the Central Malignant Melanoma Registry (CMMR) under the guidence of the society. The dermatology departments were asked to cooperate in this initiative, and by 1986 22 had joined the project (Garbe et al. 1987). The data registered included patient characteristics such as age, sex, and nationality as well as detailed information on histology, tumor stage, and therapy (Garbe et al. 1989a). Complete registration for population-based incidence calculations was achieved in some regions (Garbe et al. 1991). Routine registration also included data on profession, work performed longest, drug intake, and sun exposure. Additionally, detailed case control studies were performed to identify risk factors for developing melanoma (Garbe et al. 1989b; Weiß et al. 1990).

It is the aim of this report to present basic data on the melanoma cases documented by the CMMR of the German Dermatological Society and then give a detailed survey of the results obtained by the CMMR studies investigating potential environmental risk factors for the development of malignant melanoma.

Material and Methods

Data Sources. The data stored in the CMMR of the German Dermatological Society between July 1983 and February 1990 were collected by 30 German departments as well as dermatology clinics in Graz (Austria) and Zurich (Switzerland) (Fig. 1). Patient data were documented by the attending physicians using a questionnaire suitable for computerized evaluation. The new questionnaire used from 1989 onwards no longer registered data on potential risk factors, e.g., occupation, sun exposure. The postal code was entered to register the patient's place of residence. A special computer program to transfer postal codes into district codes was used to relate the patients to specific geographic areas. These data were then used to calculate crude incidence rates for the different regions in Germany on the basis of population statistics. The crude incidence rates serve as a basis for assessing the completeness of registration in the different regions by the hospital-based melanoma registry.

Comparative analysis of professional data was done using a classification of professions of the Federal Employment Office (Federal Bureau of Statistics Wiesbaden 1975). The analysis was based on data on the work performed longest. Patients without employment (housewives, students, pensioners) were excluded from this analysis. These data were compared with those from a representative random sample of the population of the Federal Republic of Germany from the 1987 microcensus (Chaberny et al. 1989).

The present evaluation of risk factors for melanoma is based on the data from two case control studies. The first of these studies included 1079 melanoma patients and 778 controls who were interviewed and underwent a whole-body physical examination. The controls were outpatients presenting at dermatology clinics. Patients with previous UV treatment for skin disorders or who presented because of skin cancer or melanocytic nevi were excluded from the control group (Weiß et al. 1990). In the second study using the same inclusion criteria as in the first, a whole-body documentation of pigmented skin lesions was performed in 200 melanoma patients and 200

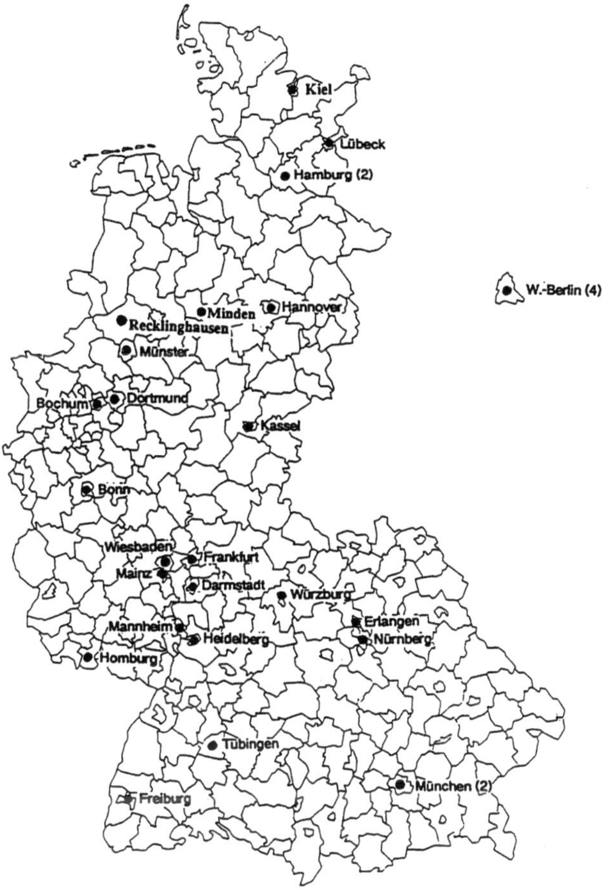

Fig. 1. Geographical distribution of the centers cooperating in the Central Malignant Melanoma Registry of the German Dermatological Society. The governmental districts are used for calculations on the basis of population statistics

controls (Garbe et al. 1989b; Krueger et al. 1992). The skin lesions were classified as common acquired melanocytic nevi, atypical melanocytic nevi, and actinic lentigines. Additionally, the subjects underwent detailed interviews on sun exposure and other potential risk factors.

Statistics. Frequency calculations and statistical comparison of frequency distributions were done with the computer program SPSS, version X. Statistical significance was tested using the χ^2-test, Wilcoxon's *U* test and the Kruskall and Wallis *H* test.

99% confidence intervals were calculated for comparing the frequency of different professions in the melanoma group and in the representative population sample. Differences were considered to be significant at the 1%

level (χ^2). Significance testing was additionally adjusted for multiple analysis according to Holm (1979).

Associations between potential risk factors and cases/controls were assessed univariately by χ^2 tests. Factors with p values below 0.1 were entered in a stepwise logistic regression analysis, which was performed using the GLIM package (Baker and Nelder 1978). Estimated odds ratios may be interpreted as relative risks in this context.

Results

The Central Malignant Melanoma Registry of the German Dermatological Society. The data from 7789 patients with malignant melanoma from 32 clinics were stored from July 1983 to February 1990. A nearly complete registration of all melanoma patients was achieved in some regions (crude

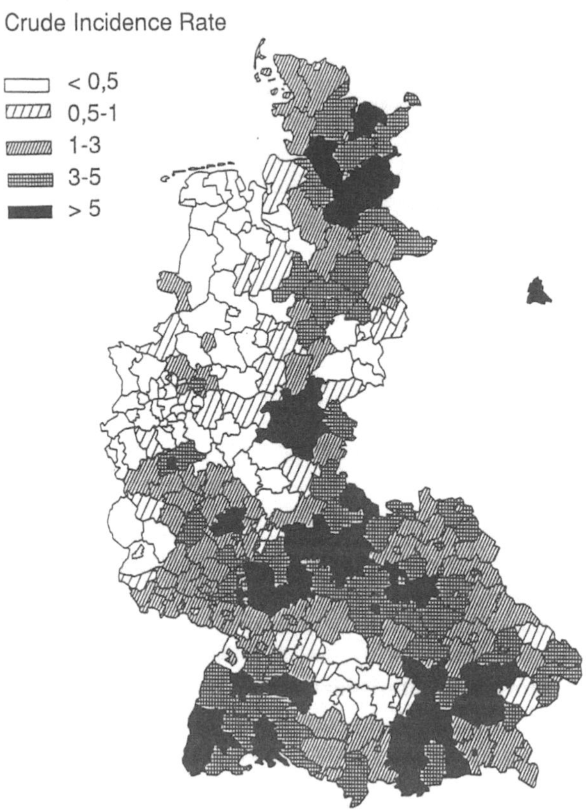

Fig. 2. Crude incidence rates of CMMR registered cases can be utilized for estimation of the completeness of melanoma registration

incidence rates >5/100 000 inhabitants and year) (Fig. 2). The proportion of women was 57.6%. Mean age at the time of diagnosis was between 52 and 53 years (males 52.7 years, females 52.0 years), and there was no significant difference in age distribution between the two sexes. 90.8% of the patients had clinical stage I tumors with only the primary tumor present and no clinical signs of metastases at the time of first diagnosis. A slightly higher proportion of men than women (10.7% vs 8.1%) already had metastases when they first presented (Table 1). The percentage of metastasizing tumors at the time of first diagnosis increases with age from 6.9% in patients under 40 to 13.4% in patients over 70 (Table 2).

Tumor thickness, which is the most important prognostic factor in stage I melanoma, also varied significantly with age. Younger patients had thinner tumors than older ones. The proportion of thin tumors (≤0.75 mm) was 43% in patients under 40 and only 26.8% in those over 70. Slightly more women than men had thin tumors (≤0.75 mm; 39.4% vs 34.1%) (Table 3).

The age distribution showed considerable variation according to the different histologic subtypes of melanoma. Median age was 50 years in patients with superficially spreading melanoma, 54 years in nodular melanoma, 64 years in acral-lentiginous melanoma, and 67 years in lentigo maligna melanoma (Fig. 3). Tumor thickness varied significantly between the different melanoma subtypes, with the highest median thickness for

Table 1. Tumor stage at the time of first diagnosis (according to TNM classification 1979)

		Males (n = 3262)	Females (n = 4449)	Total[a] (n = 7711)
I	(primary tumor)	89.3	91.9	90.8
IIa	(satellite or in transit metastases)	5.9	5.8	5.8
IIb	(regional node metastases)	3.2	1.3	2.1
III	(juxtaregional node metastases)	0.3	0.1	0.2
IV	(distant metastases)	1.4	0.9	1.1

[a] Missing data n = 78 patients.

Table 2. Tumor stage (TNM 1979) at the time of first diagnosis in relationship to age

		<40 years (n = 1706)	40–69 years (n = 4706)	≥70 years (n = 1181)
I	primary tumor)	93.1	91.0	86.6
IIa	(satellite or in transit metastases)	3.7	5.7	9.4
IIb	(regional node metastases)	2.3	2.3	2.3
IV	(distant metastases)	0.8	1.1	1.7

Missing data n = 196 patients.

Table 3. Tumor thickness (in %) at first diagnosis (according to TNM classification 1979)

	Males (n = 2945)	Females (n = 4020)	Total[a] (n = 6965)
≤0.75 mm	34.1	39.4	37.2
0.76–1.50 mm	27.7	28.0	27.9
1.51–3.0 mm	21.4	20.5	20.8
>3.0 mm	16.8	12.1	14.1

[a] Missing data n = 824 patients.

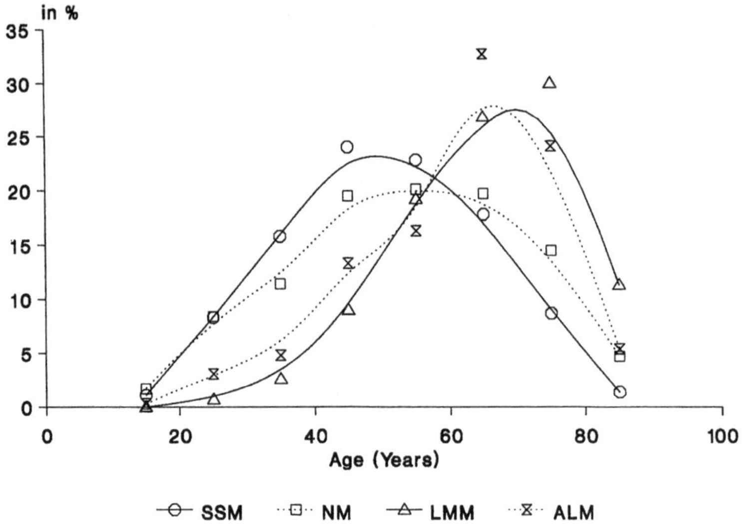

Fig. 3. Age distribution of the melanoma subtypes superficially spreading melanoma (SSM, n = 4130), nodular melanoma (NM, n = 1625), lentigo maligna melanoma (LMM, n = 630), and acral lentiginous melanoma (n = 294)

nodular melanoma and the lowest for lentigo maligna melanoma (Fig. 4). Superficially spreading melanoma and nodular melanoma were mostly located on the trunk in males (60% and 53%) and on the lower extremity in females (47% and 44%), while lentigo maligna melanoma was predominantly located on head and neck (ca. 60%) (Fig. 5).

Occupation as a Potential Risk Factor for Melanoma. 3546 patients with valid occupational data were registered from 1983 to 1988. The work performed longest was used for the analysis. Housewives, students, and pensioners were excluded from this evaluation. Occupations were registered as 3-digit codes using the classification of the Federal Employment Office with a total of 328 occupational groups. For evaluation, these groups were

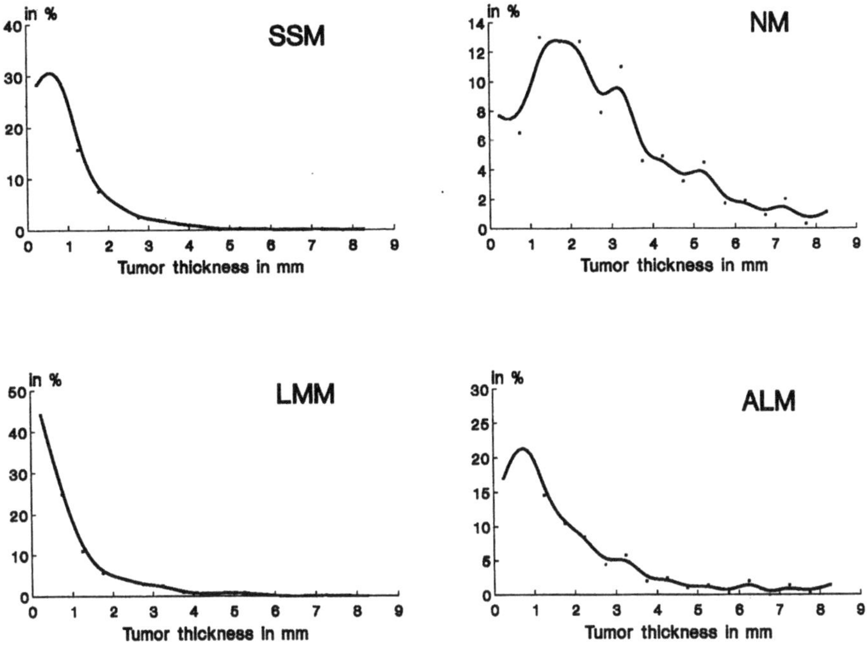

Fig. 4. Tumor thickness of the different melanoma subtypes

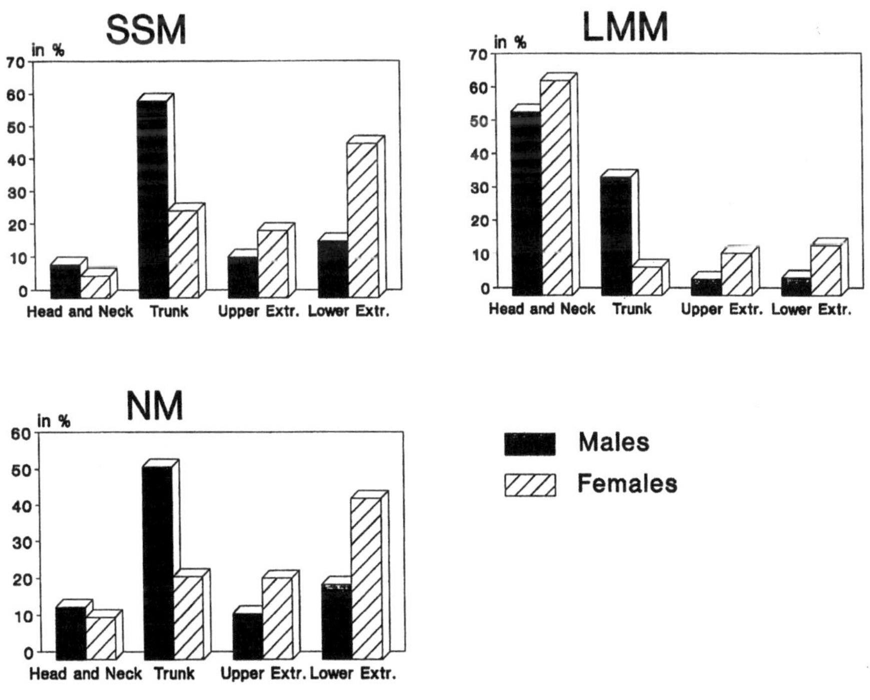

Fig. 5. Anatomical localization of the different melanoma subtypes

Table 4. Occupations of melanoma patients (MP) in comparison to a representative population-based sample (RPBS) (1% of the working population in the 1987 microcensus) of the Federal Republic of Germany

	% of MP	% of RPBS
Higher proportion of melanoma patients		
Farmers	3.5	1.7*
Scientists	0.6	0.2*
Merchants	12.6	7.8*
Administrative clerks	3.8	1.1*
Teachers	3.8	2.7*
Textile workers	3.3	0.9*
Lower proportion of melanoma patients		
Unskilled workers	0.1	3.3*
Chemical workers	0.2	0.8*
Mechanics	1.9	3.1*
Locksmiths	0.4	1.2*
Electricians	1.2	2.6*
Joiners	0.1	1.1*
Product controllers	0.2	1.3*
Policemen	1.3	2.9*

*$p < 0.01$ after adjustment for multiple testing (Holm 1979).

further condensed to 86 using 2-digit codes for registration. Representative data from the 1987 microcensus were used for comparison. This control group comprises 1% of the working population or 270940 individuals of the Federal Republic of Germany.

Significant differences between the controls and the melanoma patients were seen for 14 of the 86 professional groups. The percentage of farmers, scientists, merchants, administrative clerks, teachers, and textile workers was significantly higher among melanoma patients, while unskilled workers, chemical workers, mechanics, locksmiths, electricians, joiners, product controllers, policemen, and security guards were underrepresented in this group (Table 4).

For further evaluation, the occupational groups were subdivided into those with and those without sun exposure. These groups were then additionally classified according to socioeconomic status. Status groups were workers, employees, qualified employees, and self-employed individuals. There were significant differences between patients and controls in the frequency of these professional groups. The percentage of subjects with occupational sun exposure, employees, qualified employees, and self-employed individuals was higher in the melanoma group, while the percentage of workers was markedly lower in this group (Table 5). Interestingly, lentigo maligna melanoma and localization on the head and neck were markedly more frequent in individuals with occupational sun exposure (Table 6). Tumor thickness on first presentation also differed between these

Table 5. Occupational groups among melanoma patients (MP) in comparison to a representative population-based sample (RPBS) (1% of the working population in the 1987 microcensus) of the Federal Republic of Germany

	% of MP	% of RPBS
Occupations with sun exposure	10.9	6.9*
Workers	27.0	43.0*
Employees	37.0	33.7*
Qualified employees	16.8	11.9*
Self-employed individuals	8.3	4.2*

*$p < 0.01$ after adjustment for multiple testing (Holm 1979).

Table 6. Histologic type and tumor localization in patients with and without occupational sun exposure

	With sun exposure in % ($n = 378$)	Without sun exposure in % ($n = 3096$)
Histologic type		
Lentigo-maligna melanoma	15.3	7.0
Others	84.7	93.0*
Localization		
Head and neck	23.3	9.7
Others	76.7	90.3*

*$p < 0.0001$.

Table 7. Melanoma thickness in different occupational groups

	Median thickness (mm)
Occupations with sun exposure ($n = 344$)	1.30
Workers ($n = 872$)	1.20
Employees ($n = 1184$)	0.97
Qualified employees ($n = 547$)	1.00
Self-employed individuals ($n = 267$)	1.00

groups. Workers and individuals with occupational sun exposure had the thickest tumors. Markedly thinner tumors were seen in employees, qualified employees, and self-employed individuals (Table 7).

Significant Risk Factors in Case Control Studies. The first case control study of the CMMR included 1079 melanoma patients from 1984–1987 and 778 controls. Multivariate analysis revealed four factors that were associated

Table 8. Significant risk factors in the multicenter case control study of the German melanoma registry 1984–1987

	Adjusted relative risk (95% CI)
Total number of melanocytic nevi: >50 vs ≤10	4.8 (2.9–7.9)
Hair color: red vs black	4.7 (2.4–8.9)
Occupational sun exposure: nearly always vs none	2.7 (1.3–5.7)
Skin type: I vs IV	2.1 (1.2–3.9)

CI, confidence interval.

with a significantly increased risk of developing melanoma: total number of melanocytic nevi, hair color, occupational sun exposure, and skin type. In this study, no distinction was made between common and atypical melanocytic nevi, and the occurrence of actinic lentigines was not documented separately. The total number of melanocytic nevi in whole-body counts was clearly shown to be the most significant risk factor for the development of malignant melanoma in this study (Table 8).

In the second case control study conducted from 1988 to 1989, the occurrence of melanocytic lesions over the entire integument was documented in more detail (Garbe et al. 1989b). Pigmented lesions in this study were subclassified as common melanocytic nevi, clinically atypical melanocytic nevi, and actinic lentigines. It was shown that the total number of each of these benign melanocytic lesions independently affected the risk for melanoma in a highly significant manner. The second study also confirmed that occupational sun exposure and photosensitive skin are associated with an increased risk for the development of malignant melanoma (Table 9).

Sun Exposure as a Risk Factor for Melanoma Development. In the two case control studies presented above, occupational and recreational sun exposure were evaluated for their potential influence on the risk of developing melanoma. In the first study, from 1984 to 1987, complete data on all sun

Table 9. Significant risk factors in the case control study of the German melanoma registry 1988–1989

	Adjusted relative risk (95% CI)
Total number of melanocytic nevi: >60 vs ≤10	14.7 (5.6–38.1)
Total number of atypical melanocytic nevi: ≥1 vs 0	7.0 (3.2–15.1)
Actinic lentigines: moderate to large number vs none	6.2 (2.8–13.8)
Occupational sun exposure: nearly always vs none	11.6 (2.1–63.3)
Skin type: I vs IV	2.2 (0.8–6.2)

Table 10. Occupational sun exposure and relative risk of developing of melanoma: Case control study 1984–1987

Occupational sun exposure	Melanoma patients in % (n = 856)	Controls in % (n = 705)	Relative risk (95% CI)	Adjusted relative risk[a] (95% CI)
Amount				
None	66.6	75.5	1.0	1.0
Occasional–nearly always	33.4	24.5	1.4 (1.1–1.8)	1.1 (0.8–1.6)
Nearly always	13.0	7.7	1.4 (0.9–2.1)	2.7 (1.3–5.7)
Duration of occupational sun exposure				
<1 year	74.6	79.9	1.0	1.0
>1 year	25.4	20.1	0.9 (0.6–1.4)	0.8 (0.4–1.3)
>10 years	20.6	14.3	1.1 (0.6–2.0)	1.1 (0.6–2.2)
>20 years	13.8	6.8	2.2 (1.3–3.7)	1.4 (0.8–2.5)

[a] Adjusted for the total number of melanocytic nevi, hair color, skin type, age, and participating centers.

exposure parameters were available for 856 patients and 705 controls. Individuals who specified their occupational sun exposure as "nearly always" were shown by multivariate analysis to have a relative risk significantly increased by a factor of 2.7. Increasing duration of occupational sun exposure was associated with an increase in relative risk, but this increase was no longer significant after adjustment for other risk factors (Table 10). The second case control study, from 1988 to 1989, yielded nearly the same results on occupational sun exposure. There was again a significantly higher risk in the group characterizing their occupational sun exposure as "nearly always." Because the study population was markedly smaller in the second investigation and the percentage of patients in this group much lower, the confidence interval was much larger, with the increase in risk ranging between a factor of 2.1 and 63.3 (Table 11). In the 20.5% of the malignant melanoma patients with occupational sun exposure, the mean duration was

Table 11. Occupational sun exposure and relative risk of developing melanoma: Case control study 1988–1989

Occupational sun exposure	Melanoma patients in % (n = 200)	Controls in % (n = 200)	Relative risk (95% CI)	Adjusted relative risk[a] (95% CI)
None	79.5	87.9	1.0	1.0
Occasional–nearly always	20.5	13.1	1.4 (0.8–2.5)	1.2 (0.6–2.5)
Nearly always	5.0	1.0	5.5 (1.2–25.3)	11.6 (2.1–63.3)

[a] Adjusted for total numbers of common melanocytic nevi, atypical melanocytic nevi, and lentigines and for skin type.

3.1 years, compared to 1.7 years in the controls (13% of this group). Like in the first study, the difference in the duration of sun exposure was not significant after adjustment for other risk factors.

Subjects included in the first study from 1984 to 1987 were asked to specify the duration and intensity of their recreational sun exposure over the last years. Odds ratios revealed a slightly increased risk in subjects with intensive sun exposure and a duration of more than 12 weeks per year. The difference between melanoma patients and controls was, however, no longer significant after adjustment for the other risk factors. 7.7% of the melanoma patients and 7.1% of the controls stated that they used sun beds; this difference was not significant (Table 12). In the second case control study, from 1988 to 1989, there was likewise no significant difference in recreational sun exposure between patients and controls. Intensity evaluations did not differ significantly between the two groups, although 14% of the melanoma patients compared to only 7.5% of the controls reported intensive recreational sun exposure over the last years. Analysis of recreational activities with sun exposure revealed no significant differences in the frequency of gardening, aquatic sports, or vacations in southern Europe, the tropics, or the mountains (Table 13).

Impact of Number and Distribution of Benign Melanocytic Lesions. The impact of the total number of melanocytic nevi, the number of atypical melanocytic nevi, and the number of actinic lentigines on the risk of devel-

Table 12. Recreational sun exposure and relative risk of developing melanoma: Case control study 1984–1987

Recreational sun exposure	Melanoma patients in % ($n = 856$)	Controls in % ($n = 705$)	Relative risk (95% CI)	Adjusted relative risk[a] (95% CI)
Amount				
Minor/none	30.5	36.3	1.0	1.0
Moderate–intense	69.5	63.7	1.2 (0.9–1.5)	1.2 (0.9–1.5)
Intense	25.4	18.0	1.5 (1.1–1.9)	1.2 (0.9–1.7)
Duration (weeks/year)				
<1 week	37.7	41.0	1.0	1.0
>1 week	62.3	59.0	1.2 (0.9–1.7)	0.9 (0.5–1.6)
>4 weeks	49.9	47.8	0.7 (0.5–1.1)	0.6 (0.4–1.0)
>8 weeks	32.5	26.5	1.0 (0.7–1.5)	0.7 (0.5–1.2)
>12 weeks	20.7	12.8	1.4 (1.1–1.7)	1.1 (0.9–1.4)
Use of sun beds				
No	92.6	92.9	1.0	1.0
Yes	7.7	7.1	1.0 (0.7–1.5)	1.5 (0.9–2.4)

[a] Adjusted for the total number of melanocytic nevi, hair color, skin type, age, and participating centers.

Table 13. Recreational sun exposure and relative risk of developing melanoma: Case control study 1988–1989

	Melanoma patients in % ($n = 200$)	Controls in % ($n = 200$)
Recreational sun exposure*		
Minor/none	48.5	54.0
Moderate	37.5	38.5
Intense	14.0	7.5
Sun exposure during gardening*		
Yes	53.0	49.5
No	47.0	50.5
Sun exposure during aquatic sports*		
Yes	44.5	41.5
No	55.5	58.5
Sun exposure during vacation in Southern Europe*		
Yes	54.5	50.5
No	45.5	49.5
Sun exposure during vacation in the tropics*		
Yes	18.0	17.0
No	82.0	83.0
Sun exposure during vacation in the mountains*		
Yes	23.5	18.0
No	76.5	82.0
Number of painful sunburns lifelong*		
None	16.0	9.5
1–2	37.0	30.0
3–4	21.0	27.0
5–10	13.0	20.0
>10	13.0	13.5

*$p > 0.05$.

oping melanoma was investigated in detail in the second case control study (Garbe et al. 1989a; Krüger et al. 1992). The total number of melanocytic nevi was found to have the greatest impact (Table 14): Patients with more than 60 melanocytic nevi had a 14.7 times higher melanoma risk. The number of atypical melanocytic nevi and the number of actinic lentigines were likewise found to be highly significant independent risk factors. Subjects with one or more atypical melanocytic nevi were at a 7 times higher risk of developing malignant melanoma, and those with a moderate to high number of actinic lentigines had a 6.2 times higher risk. Thus, the number of

Table 14. Impact of the total number of melanocytic nevi, the number of atypical melanocytic nevi, and the number of actinic lentigines on adjusted relative risk for cutaneous melanoma and 95% confidence intervals (95% CI): Case control study 1988–1989

	Melanoma patients (n = 200)	Controls (n = 200)	Relative risk (95% CI)	Adjusted relative risk[a] (95% CI)
Total number of melanocytic nevi				
0–10	17.5	47.5	1.0	1.0
11–20	18.0	21.0	2.3 (1.3–4.2)	3.1 (1.6–6.1)
21–40	17.0	21.5	2.2 (1.2–3.9)	2.3 (1.1–4.7)
41–60	16.0	5.5	7.9 (3.6–17.3)	7.3 (2.9–18.3)
>60	31.5	4.5	19.0 (8.6–41.9)	14.7 (5.6–38.1)
Number of atypical melanocytic nevi				
0	55.0	95.0	1.0	1.0
⩾1	45.0	5.0	15.5	7.0 (3.2–15.1)
1–2	11.0	1.5	14.8 (4.4–50.1)	11.4 (3.1–41.6)
⩾3	34.0	3.5	17.3 (7.7–38.9)	6.1 (2.4–15.3)
Actinic lentigines				
None	42.0	64.0	1.0	1.0
Few	36.0	28.5	1.9 (1.2–3.0)	2.2 (1.2–3.9)
Moderate to large numbers	22.0	7.5	4.5 (2.3–8.5)	6.2 (2.8–13.8)

[a] Adjusted for total number of melanocytic nevi, number of atypical nevi, number of actinic lentigines, occupational sun exposure, and skin type.

melanocytic lesions was shown to be the most important risk indicator for the development of malignant melanoma.

The distribution of melanocytic nevi over the integument also showed a clear association with the risk of developing melanoma (Table 15). The influence of site-specific numbers of nevi on melanoma risk was different for the two sexes. While melanocytic nevi on the trunk were by far the most significant risk indicator in males, melanocytic nevi on the legs were the most important risk factor in females. This pattern corresponds to the distribution of melanomas in different body regions (see Fig. 5).

Discussion

The studies presented here are based on the multicenter documentation of a large number of melanoma patients. Data were recorded by malignant melanoma specialists in the participating centers and can therefore be regarded as fairly reliable and valid. The rate of missing data was low, even

Table 15. Impact of site-specific nevus counts on relative risk (RR) and 95% confidence intervals (95% CI) for cutaneous malignant melanoma in males and females of melanoma patients and controls: Case control study 1988–1989

Nevus count	Males		Females	
	RR	95% CI	RR	95% CI
Head/neck				
0–4	1.0		1.0	
>4	2.3	1.0–5.5	4.7	2.0–11.4
p	>0.05		<0.001	
Arms				
0–4	1.0		1.0	
5–10	1.3	0.6–2.9	1.5	0.8–2.8
11–20	8.0	2.7–24.1	2.3	1.1–4.8
>20	19.0	4.1–88.7	5.2	1.8–14.8
p	<0.001		<0.001	
Legs				
0–4	1.0	1.3–8.4	1.0	
5–10	3.3	5.6–33.6	1.7	0.9–3.4
11–20	9.2	5.9–126.3	9.3	4.6–18.6
>20	27.4		14.9	5.4–41.0
p	<0.001		<0.001	
Trunk				
0–4	1.0		1.0	
5–10	2.9	0.9–9.4	0.8	0.4–1.7
11–20	5.5	1.7–17.4	3.8	1.8–8.7
>20	32.6	9.7–109.5	6.1	2.2–17.3
p	<0.001		<0.001	

for such specific histologic parameters like histologic subtype and tumor thickness or prognostic parameters and risk factors.

The Central Malignant Melanoma Registry (CMMR) of the German Dermatological Society is hospital based. Complete registration is achieved in some areas but not all over the FRG. Subjects for the control groups in the case control studies were recruited by the participating centers and not selected from the general population. An advantage of this procedure is that both patients and controls underwent detailed whole-body evaluation of pigment features, while most epidemiologic studies with a representative population-based selection of controls are limited to nevus counts on the arms or legs (Holman and Armstrong 1984; Green et al. 1985a; Österlind et al. 1988a). There is no doubt that the clinic-based selection of controls in such studies may bias the results relative to the general population. However, there was good reproducibility of the results in the two case control studies presented here. The distribution of professions in the melanoma patients and the representative population sample must also be interpreted with caution, since the melanoma patient group cannot be regarded as completely representative for the entire country. It was shown that the registration of melanoma patients was fairly incomplete in some regions. This, together with a potential regional variation in the distribution of certain professions, could distort the results in a comparison with a representative population sample.

Occupation as a Potential Risk Factor for Melanoma Development. The studies presented here did not reveal an association of specific occupations or industrial areas with an increased melanoma risk. While the higher risk in textile workers might be interpreted as an indicator of such an association, the previously reported higher risk of workers in the printing industries could not be confirmed (McLaughlin et al. 1988; Lynge and Thygesen 1988). The present study clearly demonstrates an increased risk for individuals with professional sun exposure and thus confirms similar reports from Canada (Elwood et al. 1985a) and Sweden (Wiklund and Holm 1986). In our study, the proportion of farmers was nearly twice as high in the melanoma group than in the representative population sample, and there was again a higher percentage of individuals with occupational sun exposure in the melanoma group. These differences were highly significant. This observation also correlates with our findings that individuals with occupational sun exposure have significantly more lentigo maligna melanomas and a higher incidence of tumors on the neck and head.

The present data support the assumption that melanoma risk shows a closer association with the socioeconomic status than with individual professional groups. Other studies which also classified different socioeconomic groups by occupation and professional training reported similar results (Graham et al. 1985). In Sweden, a significantly elevated risk of developing melanoma was observed in white collar workers compared to blue collar workers (Vagero and Persson 1984). It is assumed that individuals with a higher socioeconomic status have different recreational habits and more often undergo intensive intermittent sun exposure. This hypothesis is supported by findings from Vagero et al. (1986) demonstrating that indoor workers have an increased risk of developing melanoma on normally clothed body regions compared to the light-exposed anatomical sites.

Significant Risk Factors in the Case Control Studies. The total number of different pigmented lesions was revealed as the most important risk factor in the two CMMR case control studies. This is in agreement with other studies including whole-body examinations of pigmented lesions (Holly et al. 1987; MacKie et al. 1989). The influence of skin type and hair color on melanoma risk was also reported by other investigators (Dubin et al. 1986; Elwood et al. 1984; Green et al. 1986; Österlind et al. 1988a). Individuals with fair skin and increased UV sensitivity, red or blond hair, and blue eyes were found to have a 2–4-fold elevated risk of developing melanoma. Since interview questions and the classification of pigmentation parameters varied between the different studies, different pigmentation features were identified as significant risk factors with different risk magnitudes. All studies, however, identified at least one of the pigmentation features revealed to be significant risk factors by multivariate analysis.

Sun Exposure as a Risk Factor for Developing Melanoma. The two CMMR case control studies revealed a clear relationship between occupational sun exposure and an increased relative risk of developing melanoma. This relationship has been subject to much discussion in the literature. Gallagher et al. (1987) described an elevated melanoma risk for individuals with mild occupational sun exposure, while no further risk increase could be detected in the group with the highest exposure. The investigators therefore raised the question as to whether intensive occupational sun exposure might even be a protective factor in respect to melanoma development (Gallagher et al. 1986). A large Australian study did not find any impact of occupational sun exposure on melanoma risk (Holman et al. 1986).

Recreational sun exposure was not associated with an increased melanoma risk in the two CMMR case control studies. While univarate analysis revealed a slight increase for individuals with intensive sun exposure or duration of more than 12 weeks per year, the differences were no longer significant after adjustment for other risk factors. MacKie and Aitchison (1982) were the first who described a relationship between the number of painful sunburns lifelong and melanoma risk based on a study including 113 case control pairs. Subsequent studies were frequently unable to reproduce this finding. A large Canadian case control study (595 cases and matched controls) found a slightly elevated melanoma risk with an increasing number of sunburns by applying univariate statistics, but this was no longer significant after adjustment for skin type (Elwood et al. 1985b; Gallagher et al. 1986). An Australian study including 183 cases and age- and sex-matched controls did report a higher risk of melanoma after repeated sunburns, but these findings were not controlled for skin type or other pigmentation features (Green et al. 1985b). Another larger Australian study (511 cases and matched controls) investigated the impact of intermittent intensive sun exposure and recorded the history of sunburns with varying degrees of severity. No significant differences between cases and cotrols in respect to sunburns were found by multivariate analysis controlled for potential confounders (Holman et al. 1986). A Swedish study including 523 melanoma patients and 505 controls observed only a small impact of sun exposure on melanoma risk, while pigmentation features such as skin type and hair color showed a strong relationship to melanoma risk (Beitner et al. 1990).

A Danish study of 474 melanoma patients and 926 population-based controls for the first time examined the correlation of sunburn with age. A significant correlation between the number of sunburns and melanoma risk was observed in children until the age of 15, while no such association was found in older individuals (Österlind et al. 1988b). Similar results were reported in an American study analyzing the impact of sunburns at age 15–20 and after 30. Only sunburns before the age of 20 were associated with a significantly increased melanoma risk (Weinstock et al. 1989). In this context, the results of a Canadian study in 913 white school children deserve special attention (Gallagher et al. 1990). The total number of melanocytic nevi was correlated to the number of previous sunburns. This finding continued to be significant after controlling for age, skin color, skin type, and degree of tanning as possible confounding factors. Possibly, sun exposure in childhood may induce melanocytic nevi. Their total number in whole-body counts is well accepted as a risk factor of developing malignant melanoma (Garbe et al. 1989b).

Impact of Number and Distribution of Benign Melanocytic Lesions. The results of the two CMMR case control studies underline the significance of the number and distribution of pigmented lesions for the risk of developing melanoma. The total number of aquired melanocytic nevi is the most important indicator for an increased melanoma risk. Independently, the presence of atypical nevi additionally increases the risk for melanoma development. Furthermore, the number of actinic lentigines significantly contributes to melanoma risk. The importance of the number of melanocytic nevi for melanoma risk was first demonstrated in studies counting nevi exclusively on the arms or legs (Reynolds et al. 1982; Beral et al. 1983; Holman et al. 1984; Green et al. 1985a). Swerdlow et al. (1986) were the first who analyzed the total number and distribution of melanocytic nevi on the whole integument in relation to melanoma risk. They found a more than 50-fold elevated risk for persons presenting with more than 50 melanocytic nevi as compared to those with less than 10 nevi. Nevus counts in different body regions were different in the degree to which they indicated melanoma risk. The highest risk values were obtained for nevus counts on the lower extremity (not separately analyzed for males and females, preponderance of females in the sample analyzed). Holly et al. (1987) found that, independently of the total number of acquired melanocytic nevi, the number of atypical nevi was additionally associated with significantly elevated melanoma risk. This finding was again confirmed by the second CMMR case control study.

The number of actinic lentigines was likewise a significant risk factor in the second CMMR case control study, whereas ephelids during childhood were not associated with an elevated melanoma risk. These two types of hyperpigmented lesions were summarized as freckles in some studies, and freckling was reported to be a significant risk factor in addition to common and atypical melanocytic nevi (MacKie et al. 1989).

Site-specific nevus counts in the CMMR case control study revealed melanocytic nevi on the trunk in males and on the lower extremities in females to be the most significant risk indicator for developing melanoma (Krüger et al. 1992). Thus, nevus counts on those body regions where melanoma predominantly develops in each sex seem to be most strongly correlated to melanoma risk. Possibly, these are the body regions which are most frequently exposed to the sun in childhood.

Conclusions

Evaluation of the data of the CMMR on occupation-associated risk factors for the development of malignant melanoma did not identify individual professional groups or industrial areas with a significantly increased risk. It was, however, shown that individuals with occupational sun exposure had a significantly increased melanoma risk. This group had significantly more lentigo maligna melanomas and they had a significantly higher proportion of melanomas on the head and neck. For the other professions, a higher socioeconomic status was found to be associated with an increasing risk. Accordingly, most blue collar workers were at a markedly lower risk for melanoma. Occupational sun exposure was identified as a significant risk factor in two of the CMMR case control studies. The risk was found to increase along with the intensity and duration of occupational sun exposure. Recreational sun exposure was shown by univariate analysis to be associated with a slightly increased melanoma risk, but the increase was no longer significant after adjustment for the other risk factors. Recreational activities with sun exposure were nearly identical in melanoma patients and controls, and there were no significant differences with respect to sports with sun exposure or the frequency of vacations in sunny regions. The lifelong number of painful sunburns was likewise not significantly different between the two groups. Less than 8% of the subjects in each group stated that they used sun beds. These results suggest that sun exposure in adulthood has no major impact on the risk of developing melanoma.

The case control studies identified the number and distribution of melanocytic lesions as the most important risk factor. The number of common melanocytic nevi was the most significant risk factor, followed by the number of atypical melanocytic nevi and the number of actinic lentigines. Nevus distribution was found to be sex-specific and in melanoma patients the highest numbers were counted in body areas most prone to melanoma development: the trunk in males and the lower legs in females. Recent studies on the induction of melanocytic nevi by sun exposure in childhood suggest that sun exposure in early life induces the development of nevi and increases the risk of melanoma development in those areas of the body which are, sex-specifically, mainly exposed to the sun in leisure time.

References

Baker RJ, Nelder JA (1978) Generalized linear interaction modelling: release 3. Numerical Algorhythm Group, Oxford

Beitner H, Norell SE, Ringborg U, Wennersten G, Mattson B (1990) Malignant melanoma: aetiological importance of individual pigmentation and sun exposure. Br J Dermatol 122:43–51

Beral V, Evans S, Shaw H, Milton G (1983) Cutaneous factors related to the risk of malignant melanoma. Br J Dermatol 109:165–172

Chaberny A, Parmentier K, Schnur P (1989) Berufsspezifische Struktur- und Entwicklungsdaten 1976–1987. Beitr Arbeitsmarkt Berufsforschung 60:1–291

Dubin N, Moseson M, Pasternack BS (1986) Epidemiology of malignant melanoma: pigmentary traits, ultraviolet radiation, and the identification of high-risk populations. Recent Results Cancer Res 102:56–75

Elwood JM, Gallagher RP, Hill GB, Spinelli JJ, Pearson JC, Threlfall W (1984) Pigmentation and skin reaction to sun as risk factors for cutaneous melanoma: Western Canada melanoma study. B M J 288:99–102

Elwood JM, Gallagher RP, Hill GB, Pearson JC (1985a) Cutaneous melanoma in relation to intermittent and constant sun exposure – the Western Canada melanoma study. Int J Cancer 35:427–433

Elwood JM, Gallagher RP, Davison J, Hill GB (1985b) Sunburn, suntan and the risk of cutaneous malignant melanoma – the Western Canada melanoma study. Br J Cancer 51:543–549

Federal Bureau of Statistics Wiesbaden (1975) Klassifizierung der Berufe. Kohlhammer, Stuttgart

Gallagher RP, Elwood JM, Hill GB (1986) Risk factors for cutaneous malignant melanoma: the Western Canada melanoma study. Recent results. Cancer Res 102:38–55

Gallagher RP, Elwood JM, Threlfall WJ, Spinelli JJ, Fincham S, Hill GB (1987) Socioeconomic status, sunlight exposure, and risk of malignant melanoma: the Western Canada melanoma study. J Natl Cancer Inst 79:647–652

Gallagher RP, McLean DI, Yang CP, Coldman AJ, Silver HK, Spinelli JJ, Beagrie M (1990) Suntan, sunburn, and pigmentation factors and the frequency of acquired melanocytic nevi in children. Similarities to melanoma: the Vancouver mole study. Arch Dermatol 126:770–776

Garbe C, Bertz J, Orfanos CE (1986) Malignes Melanom: Zunahme von Inzidenz und Mortalität in der Bundesrepublik Deutschland. Z Hautkr 61:1751–1764

Garbe C, Bertz J, Orfanos CE (1987) Das maligne Melanom im deutschsprachigen Raum in den 80er Jahren. Hautarzt 38:639–644

Garbe C, Krüger S, Stadler R, Guggenmoos-Holzmann I, Orfanos CE (1989a) Markers and relative risk in a German population for developing malignant melanoma. Int J Dermatol 28:517–523

Garbe C, Wiebelt H, Orfanos CE (1989b) Change of epidemiological characteristics of malignant melanoma during the years 1962–1972 and 1983–1986 in the Federal Republic of Germany. Dermatologica 178:131–135

Garbe C, Thieß S, Nürnberger F, Ehlers G, Albrecht G, Lindler F, Bertz J (1991) Incidence and mortality of malignant melanoma in Berlin (West) from 1980 to 1986. Acta Derm Venereol (Stockh) 71:506–511

Graham S, Marshall J, Haughey B, Stoll H, Zielezny M, Brasure J, West D (1985) An inquiry into the epidemiology of melanoma. Am J Epidemiol 122:606–619

Green A, MacLennan R, Siskind V (1985a) Common aquired naevi and the risk of malignant melanoma. Int J Cancer 35:297–300

Green A, Siskind V, Bain C, Alexander J (1985b) Sunburn and malignant melanoma. Br J Cancer 51:393–397

Green A, Bain C, McLennan R, Siskind V (1986) Risk factors for cutaneous melanoma in Queensland. Recent results. Cancer Res 102:76–97

Holly EA, Kelly JW, Shpall SN, Ciu SH (1987) Number of melanocytic nevi as a major risk factor for malignant melanoma. J Am Acad Dermatol 17:459–468

Holm S (1979) A simple sequentially rejective multiple test procedure. Scand Statist 6:65–70
Holman C, Armstrong B (1984) Pigmentary traits cthnic origin, benign nevi, and family history as risk factors for cutaneous malignant melanoma. J Natl Cancer Inst 72:257–266
Holman CDJ, Armstrong BK, Heenan PJ (1986) Relationship of cutaneous malignant melanoma to individual sunlight exposure habits. J Natl Cancer Inst 76:403–414
Holman CDJ, Armstrong BK, Heenan PJ, Blackwell JB, Cumming FJ, English DR, Holland S, Kelsall GRH, Matz LR, Rouse IL, Singh A, Ten Seldam REJ, Watt DJ, Xu Z (1986) The causes of malignant melanoma: results from the West Australian Lions melanoma research project. Recent Results Cancer Res 102:18–37
Houghton A, Flannery J, Viola M (1980) Malignant melanoma in Connecticut and Denmark. Int J Cancer 25:95–104
Krueger S, Garbe C, Buettner P, Stadler R, Guggenmoos-Holzmann I, Orfanos CE (1992) Epidemiologic evidence for the role of melanocytic nevi as risk markers and direct precursors of cutaneous malignant melanoma. Results of a case control study in melanoma patients and non-melanoma controls. J Am Acad Dermatol 26:920–926
Lynge E, Thygesen L (1988) Use of surveillance systems for occupational cancer: data from the Danish national system. Int J Epidemiol 17:493–500
MacKie RM, Aitchison T (1982) Severe sunburn and subsequent risk of primary cutaneous malignant melanoma in Scotland. Br J Cancer 46:955–960
MacKie RM, Freudenberger T, Aitchison TC (1989) Personal risk factor chart for cutaneous melanoma. Lancet 2:487–490
McLaughlin JK, Malker HS, Blot WJ, Ericsson JL, Gemne G, Fraumeni JF Jr (1988) Malignant melanoma in the printing industry. Am J Ind Med 13:301–304
Österlind A, Tucker MA, Hou-Jensen K, Stone BJ, Engholm G, Jensen OM (1988a) The Danish case-control study of cutaneous malignant melanoma: I. Importance of host factors. Int J Cancer 42:200–206
Österlind A, Tucker MA, Stone BJ, Jensen OM (1988b) The Danish case-control study of cutaneous malignant melanoma. II. Importance of UV-light exposure. Int J Cancer 42:319–324
Reynolds P, Austin D, Thomas J (1982) Familial and occupational risks associated with malignant melanoma of thc skin. Am J Epidemiol 116:570
Swerdlow HJ, English J, MacKie RM, O'Doherty CJ, Hunter JAH, Clark J, Hole DJ (1986) Benign melanocytic naevi as a risk factor for malignant melanoma. B M J 292:1555–1559
Vagero D, Persson G (1984) Risks, survival and trends of malignant melanoma among white and blue collar workers in Sweden. Soc Sci Med 19:475–478
Vagero D, Ringback G, Kiviranta H (1986) Melanoma and other tumors of the skin among office, other indoor and outdoor workers in Sweden 1961–1979. Br J Cancer 53:507–512
Weinstock MA, Colditz GA, Willet WC, Stampfer MJ, Bronstein BR, Mihm MC, Speizer FE (1989) Nonfamilalial cutaneous melanoma incidence in women associated with sun exposure before 20 years of age. Pediatrics 84:199–204
Weiß J, Garbe C, Bertz J, Biltz H, Burg G, Hennes B, Jung EG, Kreysel HW, Orfanos CE, Petzold D, Schwermann M, Stadler R, Tilgen W, Tronnier H, Völkers W (1990) Risikofaktoren für die Entwicklung maligner Melanome in der Bundesrepublik Deutschland. Hautarzt 41:309–313
Wiklund K, Holm LE (1986) Trends in cancer risks among Swedish agricultural workers. J Natl Cancer Inst 77:657–664

Fair Complexion and Risk of Malignant Melanoma of the Skin Based on Experience from the Danish Cancer Registry

A. Østerlind

Danish Cancer Registry, Institute of Cancer Epidemiology, Danish Cancer Society, Strandboulevarden 49, Box 839, DK-2100 Copenhagen, Denmark; and Department of Dermatology, Bispebjerg Hospital, Bispebjerg Bakke, DK-2400 Copenhagen NV, Denmark

Introduction

While malignant melanoma of the skin is a rare cancer in many populations, the incidence and mortality rates are increasing in most Western countries. The increase in incidence for skin melanoma is exceeding that of any other malignancy and is most pronounced among younger generations. It has been predicted that without preventive intervention this cancer will become one of the numerically most important tumours in the future (Roush et al. 1987). The current incidence and mortality rates may be easier to understand if they are expressed as a risk for the individual: Thus, currently in Denmark 1 in 100 persons will develop a skin melanoma during his or her lifetime, and each melanoma death "costs" 14–15 years of potential life lost before 65 years of age.

Melanoma is primarily a disease of Caucasians and is rare in pigmented races, i.e., Asians and blacks. In the United States the incidence in whites is approximately ten times higher than in blacks living in the same area (Muir et al. 1987). The United States and other parts of the world where different ethnic groups live together are interesting for melanoma research because people with different skin complexions are potentially exposed to the same degree of sunlight. In these areas the ethnic groups with the lightest skin have the highest risk of melanoma, i.e., a relative risk ten times higher compared to the ethnic group with the darkest complexion, as reported from Los Angeles (Muir et al. 1987). In many white populations the incidence rates increase 3%–9% per year, in contrast to the constant or only slightly increasing rates in nonwhites (Armstrong 1988).

Internationally, the incidence of malignant melanoma varies 100–200-fold (Muir et al. 1987), and as a result the morbidity and mortality vary substantially in different countries. The variation in incidence and mortality is 10-fold even within Europe. It has been known for a long time that the incidence increases with proximity to the equator, in accordance with the

Recent Results in Cancer Research, Vol. 128

sun exposure hypothesis (Lancaster 1956). This is true for North America and for Australia, but not for Europe, where the highest rates are seen in the Scandinavian countries (Muir et al. 1987). This finding may be explained by the lighter complexion of nordic people, who are therefore less protected compared to those living in southern Europe.

In 1952, McGovern first suggested that persons with fair hair and freckles who do not tan well on exposure to sunlight seem to be predisposed to malignant melanoma. An early case-control study focusing on pigmentation and sun exposure was reported from Australia in 1957 by Lancaster and Nelson (1957). They reported higher proportions of individuals with red or blond hair, fair complexion, and blue (green and grey) eyes among cases compared to the controls.

Since this early report, some 25 case-control studies have been carried out, including our own study from Denmark (Table 1), investigating the role of complexion and other host characteristics and also sun exposure. Five of the studies were conducted in Australia, eight in North America and 12 in Europe. The majority have been carried out and published during the last 10 years. The studies vary considerably, with regard to how cases and controls were recruited, how information was obtained, and how the statistical analyses were carried out. The important problem of confounding between different risk factors is not properly covered in all studies. Only five studies are truly population based.

In the following I will focus on the Danish data on complexion as a risk factor and relate our experience to data from other case-control studies. Results from the Danish melanoma study have been reported in detail elsewhere (Østerlind et al. 1988).

Material and Methods

Our study was a strictly population-based case-control study. All newly diagnosed patients from 1 October 1982 to 31 March 1985, aged 20–79, were identified from the routine notifications to the Danish Cancer Registry. The study was carried out in eastern Denmark, including Copenhagen in which 45% of the entire national Danish population of 5.1 million resides. Persons diagnosed with lentigo maligna melanoma were not included, due to the rarity of these tumours (4%) and the quite different epidemiological features from the other melanomas. Histological sections were reviewed in a standardized manner by one pathologist. A diagnosis of primary melanoma was rejected in 26 of the 577 patients initially reported as melanomas, who were then excluded. Of the 551 cases selected for the study, 35 were ineligible for study: 28 had died, six had migrated from the study area, and in one case permission to approach the patient was not obtained. The remaining 516 cases were contacted initially by mail without mentioning melanoma as the specific disease under study, then contacted within the

Table 1. Case-control studies of malignant melanoma of the skin which reported associations between individual melanoma risk and host factors

Reference	Region	Number of cases/controls	Sampling frame, cases/controls
Lancaster and Nelson 1957	Australia	173/173	H/Hc
Pack et al. 1963	New York, USA	273/78	H/Hc
Gellin et al. 1969	New York, USA	79/1037	H/Hs
Beardmore 1972	Australia	468/468	H/Hsc
Klepp and Magnus 1979	Norway	78/131	H/Hc
Adam et al. 1981	England	111/342	P/GP
Mackie and Aitchison 1982	Scotland	113/113	H/H
Beral et al. 1983	Sydney, Australia	287/574	H/H
Lew et al. 1983	Boston, USA	111/107	H/friends
Rigel et al. 1983	New York, USA	114/228	H/H
Elwood et al. 1984	Western Canada	595/595	P/P
Holman and Armstrong 1984	Western Australia	511/511	P/P
Green et al. 1985	Queensland, Australia	183/183	P/P
Graham et al. 1985	Buffalo, USA	404/521	H/Hc
Sorahan and Grimley 1985	Birmingham, UK	58/333	H/H + P
Dubin et al. 1986	New York, USA	1103/585	H/H
Elwood et al. 1986	Nottingham, UK	83/83	P/H
Cristofolini et al. 1987	Trento, Italy	103/205	H/H
Holly et al. 1987	San Francisco, USA	121/139	H/H
Østerlind et al. 1988	East Denmark	474/926	P/P
Zanetti et al. 1988	Turin, Italy	208/416	P/P
Garbe et al. 1989	Berlin, Germany	200/200	H/H
MacKie et al. 1989	Scotland	280/280	P/H
Beitner et al. 1990	Stockholm, Sweden	525/525	H/P
Elwood et al. 1990	England	195/195	P/H

H, Hospital controls (Hc, cancer patients; Hsc, skin cancer patients); P, population controls; GP, general practitioner list controls

following days by telephone or home visit to arrange for an interview; 27 patients refused to participate, ten were too ill, and five could not be contacted. The voluntary response rate was thus 474/516 (92%) and the overall participation rate 474/551 (86%).

The control group, stratified for sex and age in 5-year groups, was drawn at random in April 1984 from the National Population Register among the residents of eastern Denmark. No individual matching was undertaken. Of the 1164 controls selected for the study, 30 were ineligible for study: 16 had died and 14 had moved out of the study area. These controls were not replaced. The remaining 1134 controls eligible for study were contacted and asked to participate in exactly the same way as the cases. Refusals to participate in the study were received from 168 controls, 23 were too ill, and 17 could not be contacted. The voluntary response rate was thus 926/1134 (82%) and the overall participation rate 926/1164 (80%).

Information was collected by means of personal interviews. Four interviewers, who were unaware of the study subjects' case or control status interviewed the participants in their private residence (96%) or their workplace. No interviews were performed in hospital wards. A structured questionnaire was used to obtain information on known and suspected risk factors. Constitutional factors were evaluated by interview and by objective measurement of hair, eye, and skin colour; raised pigmented naevi were counted on the arms. Natural hair colour was graded visually against 20 samples of human hair. Bald persons or those with dyed hair were asked to select the hair sample that would provide the best colour match with their original hair colour. Interviewers assessed eye colour by inspection of the left eye, and skin colour was recorded using standardized skin colour charts (Scotto and Fears 1978). A count of pigmented raised naevi on each arm and separate counts of naevi 5 mm or more in diameter were made.

Analysis used standard methods appropriate for case-control studies including multivariate analysis, using a disease probability logistic model, to control simultaneously for several confounding variables (Breslow and Day 1980).

Results and Comments

Of the 474 melanoma patients, 280 (59%) were female; the average age at diagnosis was 52 years, with some 20% being under 40 years of age. The distribution of histological types was 75% superficial spreading melanoma, 17% nodular melanoma, and 8% unclassifiable melanoma. The cases and controls did not differ with regard to age, sex, marital status, or place of residence. Ethnicity was evaluated on the basis of country of birth of the subjects, their parents and their grandparents. No difference was found between cases and controls; 95% of cases and 96% of controls were born in Denmark. There was also no difference in the country of birth of their parents and grandparents.

The natural appearance of the skin or the complexion was categorized into three main groups: (I) The basic degree of pigmentation, which is a genetically determined constitutional characteristic reflected by the colour of the skin, hair, and eyes. (II) The pigmentary response to sunlight, the tendency to sunburn, to tan and to freckle. (III) Pigmentation characteristics, as reflected by the number of palpable pigmented naevi on the arms. Naevi may represent a genetic factor, but environmental factors alone or in combination with predisposition may also have an influence on the occurrence of such lesions.

Skin, Hair, and Eye Colour

Skin colour tended to be darkest on the dorsum of the hand, lighter on the shoulder tip, and lightest on the upper inner arm. Measurement on the upper inner arm is assumed to reflect most clearly the person's skin colour without the influence of sun exposure and the reported results are based on this measurement. In the univariate analysis persons with the lightest skin had a significant relative risk (RR) of 1.7 compared to those with dark pigmentation. This risk became non-significant after adjustment for freckling (Table 2).

Hair colour was a significant individual risk factor. A significant relative risk of 1.8 was seen for red hair compared to dark brown or black hair, whereas intermediate levels were seen in persons with light brown (RR = 1.5) and fair or blond hair (RR = 1.7) (Table 2). The effect of light brown and fair or blond hair remained significant after adjustment for freckling, but the effect of red hair disappeared. People with fair skin and fair or blond hair showed a relative risk of 2.9 compared to those with dark skin and dark hair. No relationship was found between eye colour and risk of melanoma in the Danish study (Table 2).

The increased risk of malignant melanoma in persons with light brown, fair, or blond hair colour is consistent with the results reported in most earlier studies (Adam et al. 1981; Beitner et al. 1990; Beral et al. 1983; Dubin et al. 1986; Elwood et al. 1984; Gellin et al. 1969; Graham et al. 1985; Green et al. 1985; Holman and Armstrong 1984; Lancaster and Nelson 1957; Pack et al. 1963; Rigel et al. 1983). Although the risk associated with red hair in our study is explained largely by the association with naevi and freckling, this finding is corroborated by others (Elwood et al. 1990; Holman and Armstrong 1984). Many of the studies have shown that of the three pigmentation characteristics, hair colour gives the most consistent results, perhaps because it is easier to measure than skin colour. Fair skin was associated with melanoma risk in most of the studies addressing this variable, but many only reported data from univariate analyses (Beral et al. 1983; Cristofolini et al. 1987; Elwood et al. 1984; Gellin et al. 1969; Graham et al. 1985; Lancaster and Nelson 1957; Rigel et al. 1983). In our study the association is almost completely explained by incomplete tanning ability and by freckling. The ability to tan deeply in response to sunlight may be protective and may be more important than the baseline skin colour. The lack of risk associated with eye colour in our study is similar to tendencies in recent population-based case-control studies in which eye colour only has an effect in univariate analyses and most of the associations are explained by other complexion factors (Elwood et al. 1984; Green et al. 1985; Holman and Armstrong 1984). Generally, eye colour is a weak risk factor when positive relationships are reported (Adam et al. 1981; Beitner et al. 1990; Dubin et al. 1986; Gellin et al. 1969; Graham et al. 1985; Lancaster and

Table 2. Relative risk for malignant melanoma of the skin in Denmark, 1982–1985 (from Østerlind et al. 1988)

Factor	Category	Relative risk, crude (95% confidence interval)	Relative risk, adjusted[a] (95% confidence interval)
Skin colour[b]	Dark	1.0[c]	1.0[c]
	Medium	1.4 (1.0–1.9)	1.0 (0.8–1.3)
	Light	1.7 (1.2–2.3)	1.3 (0.9–1.8)
	p value, trend test	<0.01	0.17
Hair colour	Dark brown/black	1.0[c]	1.0[c]
	Light brown	1.5 (1.2–1.9)	1.5 (1.2–1.9)
	Blond/fair	1.7 (1.0–2.9)	1.7 (1.0–2.9)
	Red	1.8 (1.1–2.7)	1.3 (0.8–2.0)
	p value, trend test	<0.001	0.04
Eye colour	Brown	1.0[c]	1.0[c]
	Grey/green	0.9 (0.6–1.2)	0.7 (0.5–1.1)
	Blue	1.1 (0.8–1.5)	0.9 (0.9–1.3)
	p value, trend test	0.33	0.96
Freckles	None	1.0[c]	1.0[c]
	Some	1.5 (1.2–1.9)	1.5 (1.2–2.0)
	Many	3.0 (2.2–4.1)	2.9 (2.1–4.1)
	p value, trend test	<0.001	<0.001
Acute reaction to sunlight	No sunburn	1.0[c]	1.0[c]
	Mild sunburn	1.3 (1.0–1.6)	1.1 (0.8–1.4)
	Painful sunburn	1.6 (1.1–2.6)	1.3 (0.8–2.1)
	Blisters	2.2 (0.9–5.0)	1.6 (0.7–3.9)
	p value, trend test	<0.001	0.16
Chronic reaction to sunlight	Deep tan	1.0[c]	1.0[c]
	Moderate tan	1.4 (1.1–1.8)	1.2 (0.9–1.6)
	Mild tan	1.8 (1.3–2.6)	1.4 (1.0–2.1)
	No tan	2.0 (1.0–3.7)	1.2 (0.6–2.5)
	p value, trend test	<0.001	0.09
Number of raised naevi on arms, total	None	1.0[c]	1.0[c]
	1	1.5 (1.1–2.1)	1.4 (1.0–2.0)
	2–4	2.3 (1.6–3.1)	2.2 (1.6–3.1)
	5+	5.4 (3.5–8.1)	5.1 (3.3–7.9)
	p value, trend test	<0.001	

[a] Estimates were mutually adjusted (number of raised naevi not included) and adjusted for sex; effect of number of raised naevi on arms adjusted for sex, freckles, and hair and skin colour.

[b] Complexion chart sample numbers 1,2,3,4,5,6,7 = dark; 8,9 = medium, 10 = light; measured on the inner surface of the left upper arm.

[c] Reference category.

Nelson 1957; Pack et al. 1963; Sorahan and Grimley 1985). Commonly, adjustments for other pigmentary characteristics are not reported.

Freckling and the Skin's Sensitivity to the Sun (Skin Type)

Freckling was used as an indicator both of the skin's sensitivity to the sun and of sun exposure. Freckling showed a strong association with melanoma, with a relative risk of 3.0 comparing those with most to those with no freckles, while a lesser degree of freckling was associated with an intermediate relative risk (Table 2). This factor remained strong and significant after adjustment for the other pigmentation factors. The skin's reaction to the sun, the tendency to sunburn and suntan, respectively, were significantly related to melanoma risk when considered on their own, with a two-fold greater risk in persons who blistered on first exposure (trend test $p < 0.001$), and freckled rather than tanned on repeated exposure (trend test $p < 0.001$). This effect, however, became insignificant when the effects of other pigmentation factors were taken into account.

The increased risk related to freckles was anticipated since freckling is most frequent in individuals with red or blond hair and light skin. The increased risk associated with freckling has previously been consistently reported and, more recently, by all investigators examining this feature (Dubin et al. 1986; Elwood et al. 1984; Elwood et al. 1986, 1990; Klepp and Magnus 1979; MacKie et al. 1989). Skin type or sensitivity to the sun is commonly shown to be associated with increased melanoma risk (Beitner et al. 1990; Dubin et al. 1986; Elwood et al. 1984, 1986; Garbe et al. 1989; Graham et al. 1985; Green et al. 1985; Holman and Armstrong 1984; Klepp and Magnus 1979; Lancaster and Nelson 1957; Lew et al. 1983; Rigel et al. 1983; Zanetti et al. 1988). In contrast, our data showed the skin's response to sunlight to be a less important determinant of melanoma, possibly because this factor is strongly related to freckling, naevi and light pigmentation.

Naevi

The most important and strongest disease determinant in the Danish study is the number of palpable pigmented naevi on the arms. The risk of melanoma was positively correlated with the number of naevi, up to a relative risk of 5.4 in persons with five or more naevi. This association remained strong and significant and was only minimally reduced after adjusting for the other pigmentation factors.

The most important and strongest disease determinant identified today is pigmented naevi. The more naevi, counted on the whole body or in a particular anatomical region such as the arms, the greater the risk of melanoma (Beral et al. 1983; Dubin et al. 1986; Elwood et al. 1986, 1990;

Garbe et al. 1989; Green et al. 1984; Holman and Armstrong 1984; MacKie et al. 1989; Sorahan and Grimley 1985). In only one study, from Italy, were naevi not related to increased melanoma risk. Although various counting techniques have been used, from simple naevus counts on the arms done by the person himself or by a lay person or a nurse to whole body examination by a trained dermatologist, it does not influence the fact that number of naevi is a strong predictor of melanoma risk.

Summary

Our Danish study shows that many pigmented naevi, a tendency to freckle and light hair colours are significant, important, and independent host factors which increase the risk of development of malignant melanoma of the skin. These results are in line with what has been consistently shown in previous and in more recent case-control studies. Light hair colour may be a measure of light complexion. The finding that individuals with a large number of naevi, a tendency to freckle and a sensitive skin constitute a risk group may be of importance. Such individuals could be warned about signs of early melanoma development and be instructed to avoid excessive sun exposure, especially damaging sunburns, with the aim of reducing melanoma mortality and melanoma incidence, respectively.

References

Adam SA, Sheaves JK, Wright NH, Mosser G, Harris RW, Vessey VP (1981) A case-control study of the possible association between oral contraceptives and malignant melanoma. Br J Cancer 44:45–50

Armstrong BK (1988) Epidemiology of malignant melanoma: intermittent or total accumulated exposure to the sun? J Dermatol Surg Oncol 14:835–849

Beardmore GL (1972) The epidemiology of malignant melanoma in Australia. In: McCarthy W (ed) Melanoma and skin cancer. Government Printer, Sidney, pp 39–64

Beitner H, Norell SE, Ringborg U, Wennersten G, Mattson B (1990) Malignant melanoma: aetiologic importance of individual pigmentation and sun exposure. Br J Dermatol 122:43–51

Beral V, Evans S, Shaw H (1983) Cutaneous factors related to the risk of malignant melanoma. Br J Dermatol 109:165–172

Breslow NE, Day NE (1980) Statistical methods in cancer research: I. The analysis of case-control studies. IARC Sci Publ 32:1–350

Cristofolini M, Franceschi S, Tasin L, Zumiani G, Piscioli F, Talamini R, La Vecchia C (1987) Risk factors for cutaneous malignant melanoma in a northern Italian population. Int J Cancer 39:150–154

Dubin NM, Moseon M, Pasternack BS (1986) Epidemiology of malignant melanoma: pigmentary traits, ultraviolet radiation, and the identification of high

risk populations. In: Gallagher RP (ed) Epidemiology of malignant melanoma. Springer, Berlin Heidelberg New York, pp 56–75
Elwood JM, Gallagher RP, Hill GB, Spinelli JJ, Pearson JCG, Threlfall W (1984) Pigmentation and skin reaction to sun as risk factors for cutaneous melanoma: Western Canada melanoma study. B M J 288:99–102
Elwood JM, Williamson C, Stapleton PJ (1986) Malignant melanoma in relation to moles, pigmentation and exposure to fluorescent and other lighting sources. Br J Cancer 53:65–74
Elwood JM, Whitehead SM, Davison J, Stewart M, Galt M (1990) Malignant melanoma in England: risks associated with naevi, freckles, social class, hair colour, and sunburn. Int J Epidemiol 19:801–810
Garbe C, Kruger S, Stadler R, Guggenmoos-Holzmann I, Orfanos CE (1989) Markers and relative risk in a German population for developing malignant melanoma. Int J Dermatol 28:517–523
Gellin GA, Kopf AW, Garfinkel L (1969) Malignant melanoma. A controlled study of possibly associated factors. Arch Dermatol 99:43–48
Graham S, Marshall J, Haughey B, Stoll H, Zielezny M, Brasure J, West D (1985) An inquiry into the epidemiology of melanoma. Am J Epidemiol 122:606–619
Green A, MacLennan R, Siskind V (1985) Common acquired naevi and the risk of malignant melanoma. Int J Cancer 35:297–300
Holly EA, Kelly JW, Shpall SN, Chiu S-H (1987) Number of melanocytic nevi as a major risk factor for malignant melanoma. J Am Acad Dermatol 17:459–468
Holman CDJ, Armstrong BK (1984) Pigmentary traits, ethnic origin, benign nevi, and family history as risk factors for cutaneous malignant melanoma. J Natl Cancer Inst 72:257–266
Klepp O, Magnus K (1979) Some environmental and bodily characteristics of melanoma patients. A case-control study. Int J Cancer 23:482–486
Lancaster HO (1956) Some geographical aspects of the mortality from melanoma in Europeans. Med J Aust 1:1082–1087
Lancaster HO, Nelson J (1957) Sunlight as a cause of melanoma. A clinical survey. Med J Aust 1:452–456
Lew RA, Sober AJ, Cook N, Marvell R, Fitzpatrick TB (1983) Sun exposure habits in patients with cutaneous melanoma: a case-control study. J Dermatol Surg Oncol 9:981–986
MacKie RM, Aitchison T (1982) Severe sunburn and subsequent risk of primary cutaneous malignant melanoma in Scotland. Br J Cancer 40:955–960
MacKie RM, Freudenberger T, Aitchison TC (1989) Personal risk-factor chart for cutaneous melanoma. Lancet 2:487–490
McGovern VJ (1952) Melanoblastoma. Med J Aust 1:139–142
Muir CS, Waterhouse JAH, Mack T, Powell J, Whelan S (eds) (1987) Cancer incidence in five continents, vol V. IARC Sci Publ 88:878–879
Østerlind A, Tucker MA, Hou-Jensen K, Stone BJ, Engholm G, Jensen OM (1988) The Danish case-control study of cutaneous malignant melanoma: I. Importance of host factors. Int J Cancer 42:200–206
Pack GT, Davis J, Oppenhein A (1963) The relation of race and complexion to the incidence of moles and melanomas. N Y Acad Sci 100:719–742
Rigel DS, Friedman RJ, Levenstein MJ, Greenwald DI (1983) Malignant melanoma and exposure to fluorescent lighting at work. Lancet 1:704
Roush GC, Holford TR, Schymura MH, White C (1987) Cancer risk and incidence trends. The Connecticut perspective. Hemisphere, Washington, pp 203–219
Scotto J, Fears TR (1978) Skin cancer epidemiology: research needs. Natl Cancer Inst Monogr 50:169–177

Sorahan T, Grimley RP (1985) The aetiological significance of sunlight and fluorescent lighting in malignant melanoma: a case-control study. Br J Cancer 52:765–769

Zanetti R, Rosso S, Faggiano F, Roffino R, Colonna S, Martina G (1988) Etude cas-temoins sur le melanome de la peau dans la province de Torino. Ital Rev Epidemiol Sante Publ 36:309–317

Dysplastic Nevi–Dysplastic Nevus Syndromes: Clinical Features and Genetic Aspects

J. Weiss[1,4], C. Garbe[2], P. Büttner[3], and E.G. Jung[1]

[1] Department of Dermatology, Mannheim Medical School, Th. Kutzer Ufer, W-6800 Mannheim, Fed. Rep. of Germany
[2] Department of Dermatology, University Medical Center Steglitz, Free University of Berlin, W-1000 Berlin, Fed. Rep. of Germany
[3] Institute of Medical Statistics, University Medical Center Steglitz, Free University of Berlin, W-1000 Berlin, Fed. Rep. of Germany
[4] Present address: Ludwig Institute for Cancer Research, San Diego Branch, 9500 Gilman Drive, La Jolla, CA 92093, USA

Introduction

The incidence of cutaneous malignant melanoma (MM) is rising tremendously worldwide in white populations. The reasons for the dramatic increase are not entirely known. A number of factors have been linked etiologically with melanoma, including host factors such as skin complexion, hair and eye color, and number of melanocytic nevi and environmental factors such as sunlight exposure and a positive family history of malignant melanoma. The last mentioned risk factor was recognized in 1978 when the groups of Clark and Lynch simultaneously reported an inherited syndrome characterized by atypical moles and melanomas. Clark et al. (1978) termed this syndrome BK mole syndrome, using the initials of his affected families, while Lynch et al. (1978) called it FAMMM (familial atypical multiple mole melanoma) syndrome. The very exciting clinical feature of these families was the finding that in affected individuals, those with atypical or dysplastic nevi, the risk for developing melanoma approached 100%. The atypical nevus therefore was regarded as the putative precursor for MM. In the following years observations on atypical moles in melanoma-prone families were generalized and applied to individuals who had no family history of the tumor. The term dysplastic nevus syndrome (DNS) was first used for this condition by Elder et al. (1980) and is now widely accepted. Since then, however, many epidemiologic studies have demonstrated a significant lower melanoma risk for these individuals compared with the classic BK mole patients. Therefore, it is now commonly accepted that dysplastic nevi are both a risk indicator and possible precursors of malignant melanomas (Elder 1988).

In 1983 a NIH conference tried to form a consensus on the clinical features and histologic criteria of dysplastic nevi (National Institutes of Health 1984). A fierce scientific controversy arose over the definition of dysplasia in the years that followed, which for research was both stimulating

Recent Results in Cancer Research, Vol. 128

and paralyzing as it limited communication between the protagonists. Recently, Kopf et al. (1990) proposed the term atypical mole syndrome in order to circumvent the dispute over the definition of dysplasia.

The clinical features and the significance of atypical nevi in different populations showed obvious racial and ethnic differences. The data presented in this paper on the location, distribution, correlation to melanoma and histologic melanoma subtypes, and associated risk are based on the results of a study of the German melanoma registry.

Since about 5% of all melanomas arise in a familial setting (Sigg et al. 1989), intensive efforts have been made to identify the genetic alterations causing the tumors. Although a melanoma gene has not yet been localized, exciting results have been obtained with heritable melanomas in fish and with other familial tumors in humans. A summary of the current state of knowledge is presented here, and an attempt is made to apply the clinical features and the analogies with other hereditary tumors to a hypothetical model for melanoma genesis, which might explain the clinical heterogeneity of familial melanoma.

Since many of the contradicting results on the predictive value of melanoma risk factors can be attributed to ethnical inhomogeneity of the examined patients, especially in countries with large immigrant populations, the German Melanoma Registry readdressed the validity of melanoma risk factors for an ethnically homogeneous population. The data on dysplastic nevi presented derive from this case-control study. More than 500 melanoma patients were recruited from the departments of dermatology of the university hospitals of Berlin-Steglitz, Bonn, Hamburg, Heidelberg, Homburg, Lübeck, Mannheim, Zürich (Switzerland), and Graz (Austria), of whom 492 could be evaluated (218 males, 274 females). They were compared with an age- and sex-matched control group of 472 persons (207 males, 265 females), consisting of dermatological in- and outpatients after exclusion of individuals treated for skin cancer or nevi. An atypical nevus was diagnosed if a melanocytic lesion fulfilled at least three out of five clinical criteria defined by the NIH consensus conference.

Clinical Features and Histologic Signs of Dysplastic Nevi

The NIH meeting was held in 1983 (National Institutes of Health 1984) in order to form a consensus on the clinical and histologic features of dysplastic nevi (Table 1). They are preferentially located on the trunk and typically have a heterogeneous appearance in the same individual. According to a study by Kelly et al. (1986), the most common clinical feature of these pigmentary lesions was an ill-defined border, which occurred in 90% of the cases; other common features were irregularly distributed pigmentation (84%), a maximal diameter greater than 5 mm (72%), and accentuated skin markings (63%). An irregular border was found in 41% of the nevi. A surrounding erythema, not a criterion defined by the NIH conference, was

Table 1. Clinical features and histologic signs of dysplastic nevi as defined by the NIH Consensus Conference, 1983 (National Institutes of Health 1984)

Clinical features	Histologic features
Size >5 mm in diameter	Cytologic atypia with hyperchromatic nuclei
Macular (and papular) component	Patchy or bandlike lymphocytic infiltrate of dermis
Variegated color	
Irregular border	Basilar melanocytic hyperplasia
Ill-defined border	Lamellar and concentric dermal fibroplasia
Tendency to occur on the trunk	Bridging between rete ridges

observed in 68% of all atypical nevi. The described features of dysplastic nevi are not unique for this benign lesion, as MM may display identical signs.

The histologic features of dysplastic nevi (Table 1) defined by the NIH consensus conference have become a source of controversy. There are no major differences regarding the architectural criteria, but the cytologic signs are fiercely disputed by some dermatopathologists (Roth et al. 1991). In contrast to the vehemence of the controversy, this issue influences the diagnosis only of a minor portion of melanocytic nevi.

It is unknown as yet whether the clinical signs and histologic features characterize the atypical nevi as a particular type of melanocytic nevi or a temporary condition of common nevi. Clark and Ackerman (1989), terming dysplastic nevi Clark's nevi, regard them as the most frequent particular type of acquired benign nevus beside the nevi of Miescher, Unna, and Spitz. Piepkorn (1990), however, proposes that they may be activated common nevi, which may terminate in melanoma.

Since there is neither a clinical sign nor a histologic feature nor an immunohistologic marker which permits an unambiguous diagnosis of atypical/dysplastic nevi, interobserver discrepancies in assigning there lesions to the particular type of common nevi are inevitable. Even very experienced examiners with identical concepts for diagnosis agreed on clinical classification only in 85% of the cases (Cooke et al. 1989). The same is true for the histologic examination. Depending on the severity of the displayed clinical features of atypical nevi, the histologic classification confirmed 75% of the clinical diagnoses in a study by Kelly et al. (1986). Recently, Klein and Barr (1990) reported that the histologic examination of common nevi which neither showed clinical signs of dysplasia nor derived from patients with other detectable dysplastic nevi showed at least some degree of dysplasia in 30%.

Prevalence of Dysplastic Nevi

These interobserver discrepancies in clinical and histologic classification partly explain the differences of the reported prevalence of dysplastic nevi between populations. First, there are racial differences, with low figures in Asians and Africans. In Caucasians a wide range for the prevalence of atypical nevi exists, the figures depending on the ethnic origin of the patients and on the criteria used for the diagnosis. Crutcher and Sagebiel (1984) detected at least one clinically atypical nevus, which also proved to be histologically dysplastic, in 5% of Californians. Using clinical criteria only, the prevalence is higher. For Northern Europe there are reports from Sweden (Augustsson et al. 1991) showing 18% and from Scotland (MacKie et al. 1989) showing 20% to be affected. In the German study, 17% of the control persons had at least one clinically dysplastic nevus. Piepkorn et al. (1989) in Utah assumed the prevalence of atypical nevi to be 50% by considering all nevi which displayed either clinical or histologic dysplasia. The estimation by Clark and Ackerman (1989) of 80%, based on histologic criteria alone, is even higher. This figure, if confirmed, would define the dysplastic nevus as the most common benign nevus in humans. The clinical relevance of dysplastic nevi is their association with MM. However, it has not yet been established which of the clinical or histologic features in particular contribute to melanoma risk.

Obviously there is a strong correlation between the numbers of dysplastic nevi and common melanocytic nevi. In patients with more than 100 nevi, the probability is higher than 60% that at least one lesion will display clinical criteria of dysplasia (Augustsson et al. 1991). According to studies of MacKie et al. (1985), the number of common nevi is age dependent, with the highest prevalence in middle age and lower figures in youth and higher ages. Cooke et al. (1989) reported a similar age dependence for dysplastic nevi in a New Zealand population, with higher numbers in the fourth decade compared to the sixth decade. It is a characteristic of dysplastic nevi that they mainly arise after puberty, later than common nevi, and also develop in individuals older than 40 years of age, which is quite uncommon for melanocytic nevi. Photographic studies by the Philadelphia group indicate that dysplastic nevi are quite stable for a long period of time (Roth et al. 1991).

Location of Dysplastic Nevi

Dysplastic nevi preferentially arise on the trunk, a characteristic referred to by the NIH consensus conference. We diagnosed in 82 of 472 (17%) control persons a total of 313 atypical nevi (Table 2). Seventy-six percent of the lesions were located on the trunk, which is significant even taking into consideration it's surface area. In the 182 melanoma patients, who had 999 atypical nevi (37%), this preference in location is still detectable, although the proportion of dysplastic nevi is higher on the limbs, especially the legs. These findings confirm the results of others, although an explanation for this phenomenon does not exist.

Table 2. Total numbers of atypical nevi and their relative proportions, diagnosed clinically in 182 (96 males, 86 females) out of 492 melanoma patients and in 82 (44 males, 38 females) out of 472 control persons

	Dysplastic nevi in 182 MM patients (n = 999)		Dysplastic nevi in 82 controls (n = 313)	
	(n)	(%)	(n)	(%)
Head/neck	5	1	11	3
Upper limbs				
proximal	89	9	23	7
distal	37	4	7	2
Upper trunk				
back	363	36	136	44
breast	121	12	47	15
Lower trunk	189	19	56	18
Lower limbs				
proximal	115	11	12	4
distal	77	8	21	7

The data of the German study show a sex difference in the prevalence of atypical nevi (Table 3). Males have dysplastic nevi significantly more often, and significantly higher numbers of them. In 33% of all examined males (21% in male controls, 44% in male melanoma patients) and in 22% of all females (14% in female controls, 31% in female melanoma patients) we diagnosed at least one atypical nevus. On average, an affected male had 6.4 atypical nevi, compared to 3.4 atypical nevi in females. This surplus of dysplastic nevi is located on the trunk, preferentially on the upper back. These results confirm findings in Australia (English et al. 1986) that in male melanoma patients the percentage of individuals with atypical nevi is higher, and observations of Sagebiel et al. (1985) that dysplastic nevi are more often surgically removed in males. Since there is no sex difference in affected individuals of families with the classic BK mole syndrome (Bergman et al. 1986), a genetic basis seems unlikely. Environmental factors such as higher numbers of sunburns in males, which was confirmed for the German patients, or possibly protective hormonal factors in females might be explanations. While a link between the numbers of common and atypical nevi and UV radiation has been assumed, these associations are apparently complex. Kopf et al. (1985) reported the numbers of nevi in DNS patients to be higher in sun-exposed body areas. In a recent study, Weinstock et al. (1991) showed a nonlinear association of dysplastic nevus risk with the sun sensitivity of the examined individuals, but failed to demonstrate con-

Table 3. Distribution of dysplastic nevi in controls and melanoma patients

	Dysplastic nevi in 124 MM females (*n* = 419)		Dysplastic nevi in 140 males (*n* = 893)	
	(*n*)	(%)	(*n*)	(%)
Head/neck	7	2	9	1
Upper limbs				
proximal	48	12	64	7
distal	24	6	20	2
Upper trunk				
back	129	31	370	42
breast	31	7	140	15
Lower trunk	88	21	167	19
Lower limbs				
proximal	49	12	78	9
distal	53	13	45	5

In all controls and melanoma patients, 124 females (22%) and 140 males (33%) showed clinically at least one atypical nevus. If affected by DN, females had in average 3.4 DN and males 6.4 DN. The table shows the absolute and relative figures of the diagnosed DN in both sexes.

nections with sun exposure measures. Since it is a characteristic of familial DNS that atypical nevi are also located in sun-protected areas, UV light might induce them both as a single agent in sporadic cases and as a cofactor in heritable cases.

Associations of Dysplastic Nevi with Malignant Melanoma

In melanoma patients, the reported frequencies of simultaneously detected atypical nevi depend on the racial and ethnic origin of the examined individuals, the mode of assessment, and the required features for diagnosis. Not surprisingly, these frequencies ranged from 14% of 50% (Elder 1988; Sigg et al. 1989). The evaluation of melanoma subtypes showed a significant association with superficial spreading melanoma (SSM), a melanoma subtype predominantly found in BK mole families. These findings were confirmed in the recently completed German study. In 37% of all melanoma patients a least one dysplastic nevus could be detected. In SSM a frequency of 50% was found, while weaker associations were found with nodular melanoma (NM) (30%), acrolentiginous melanoma (ALM) (28%), and especially with lentigo maligna melanoma (LMM) (19%). While the relationship to SSM is not explained, there might be a common genetic basis or identical causative risk factors.

Since the first descriptions of the BK mole and FAMMM syndrome, dysplastic nevi have been regarded as tumor precursors. Remnants of putative precursor nevi were found in over 90% of histologic sections of hereditary melanomas. In sporadic melanomas this figure is actually lower, with reported frequencies ranging from <5% to 40% (Elder 1988), depending again on the ethnic (racial) origin of the patients and the intensity and the methods of survey. In the German study, a nevus was contiguous with the tumor in 21% of the cases.

Even as a precursor for only a small proportion of melanomas, the presence of dysplastic nevi is an indicator for an elevated tumor risk. A decade ago dysplastic nevi were regarded as the most influential feature for MM risk; however, as more recent studies show this was an overestimate. Frequently cited figures of up to 100% tumor risk in dysplastic nevus patients (Greene et al. 1985) proved to refer only to the rather seldom families with the classical BK mole syndrome. Despite the relationship between common acquired nevi and dysplastic nevi, in patients with sporadic (nonfamilial) melanomas the number of common nevi has been shown to be a more predictive risk factor than the number of dysplastic nevi (Holly et al. 1987). It has not been confirmed that a single dysplastic nevus implies an additional melanoma risk, but higher numbers of them are unequivocally associated with an increased tumor risk (Holly et al. 1987). In the German study, the presence of more than five dysplastic nevi proved to be an independent factor with a relative risk of 4.2 (Table 4). Since there is a preferential association of dysplastic nevi with SSM, a separate risk calculation for this histologic subtype is necessary. The results proved to be similar to the values for the whole MM group with an odds ratio of 3.6 for more than five dysplastic nevi. The influence of dysplastic nevi on the risk for other melanoma subtypes has yet to be established, for the calculation

Table 4. Frequency of clinically dysplastic nevi in malignant melanoma patients and controls and the relative melanoma risk (odd's ratio) incuced (adjusted for the influence of the number of common melanocytic nevi

No. of dysplastic nevi	MM patients (n = 492)	Controls (n = 473)	Odd's ratio
0	63%	83%	1.0
1	13%	9%	1.4
2–5	14%	7%	1.6*
>5	10%	1%	4.2*

$^{*}p < 0.05$.

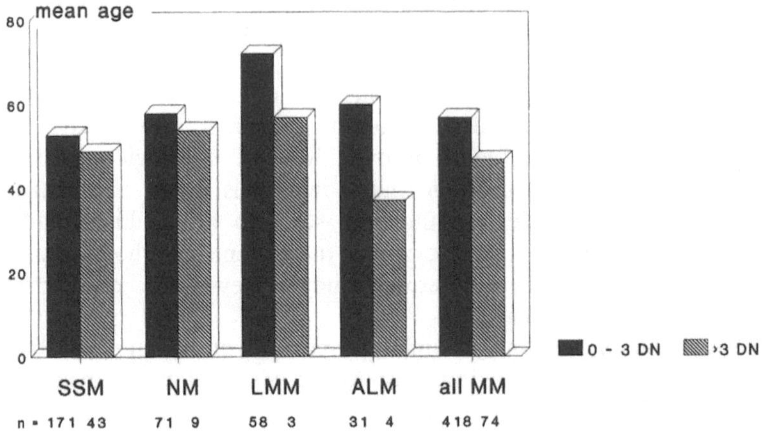

Fig. 1. Average age of melanoma manifertation in patients with 0–3 dysplastic nevi compared to melanoma patients with at least 4. Calculations were performed for the whole tumor patient group and for histologic melanoma subtypes separately

requires case-control studies with very high numbers of melanoma patients. Even the German study with 500 melanoma patients proved to be too small to make a clear decision in these groups. Recently, a study by Roush et al. (1988) suggested that the influence of dysplastic nevi might be a qualitative rather than a quantitative one, with a constant risk elevation independent of the numbers of nevi.

It is well established in many kinds of heritable cancer that tumors manifest earlier in life than in sporadic cancers. This observation has also been made in familial melanoma. Confirming a report of Sigg et al. (1989), the German study showed that this lower age of melanoma onset is also a characteristic of persons with multiple dysplastic nevi, independent of a family history of melanoma. The mean age of tumor manifestation in all patients with at least four dysplastic nevi proved to be 10 years lower than in individuals with a maximum of three nevi. This phenomenon is not restricted to a particular histologic subtype, as it can be shown in all melanoma subsets, including LMM (Fig. 1). The earlier onset of the tumors might result from chromosome instability in individuals with multiple atypical nevi, a characteristic which will be discussed in a later section.

Dysplastic Nevus Syndromes

The heritable association of two features is the broadest definition of a syndrome. The association of familial melanoma with inherited atypical nevi was therefore called BK mole or dysplastic nevus *syndrome*. Kraemer et al. (1983) extended the definition of DNS, by requiring only the presence of atypical nevi and not the manifestation of melanomas for diagnosis. He distinguished four particular types of DNS: type A with sporadic dysplastic nevi; type B with familial dysplastic nevi but without a family history of melanoma; type C with familial melanomas and sporadic dysplastic nevi; and type D, the classical BK mole syndrome, with heritable dysplastic nevi and familial melanomas. The risk for developing melanoma increases from type A to type D. In the last group this risk was reported to approach 100%. For clinical purposes Elder (1988) holds the discrimination of two types of DNS, dysplastic nevi with or without familial melanoma, to be sufficient.

There is, however, so far no consensus as to the number of dysplastic nevi required for the diagnosis of a DNS. Elder uses the presence of at least one, dysplastic nevus, Clark diagnoses the syndrome by the detection of at least two, while the NIH consensus conference required multiple atypical nevi (Ackermann 1988). In individuals with a DNS (except type A) the development of dysplastic nevi is inherited, caused by a germline mutation. This genetic alteration affects all cells and is associated with chromosome instability. The penetrance of the syndrome is variable, therefore it is possible that in particular patients one dysplastic nevus is sufficient proof for the inheritance of the genetic alterations. It should be noted, however, that single dysplastic nevi can also be caused by somatic mutations or might be induced by nongenetic alterations and be phenocopies, i.e., the pseudomelanomas. The report of a patient with a segmental (quadrant) distribution of dysplastic nevi and multiple primary melanomas by Sterry and Christophers (1988) supports this concept. In this particular case, the mutation has occurred in early embryogenesis, resulting in mosaicism. As will be discussed below, the genetic basis of dysplastic nevi and DNS is unknown, yet the pedigrees of families with DNS, irrespective of the manifestation of melanomas, indicate an autosomal dominant mode of inheritance for both. Recently, Traupe et al. (1989) challenged this hypothesis by their evaluation of mutation rates, which were only compatible with a polygenic trait. Since it is very difficult to obtain precise figures for the frequencies of dysplastic nevi and heritable melanoma, due to the lack of unambiguous features, this controversy can only be ended by the identification of the particular genes.

Cytogenetics of Melanocytic Lesions

In recent years many efforts have been undertaken to identify genetic alterations causing DNS and familial melanomas. Most work has been done in melanoma cell lines. Banding of metaphase chromosomes is a commonly used method of classical cytogenetics. This technique has been employed to determine if tumor-specific alterations are present, suggesting the localization of tumor genes. In melanoma, multiple chromosomal alterations were seen, with chromosomes 1, 6, and 7 most often affected (Sandberg 1990). Kath et al. (1989) demonstrated in cell lines of melanocytic lesions that tumor progression is associated with increasing numerical and structural alterations. Common nevi showed no obvious chromosome aberrations, whereas three out of 12 dysplastic nevi did show alterations. All melanomas had an abnormal karyotype, but a tumor-specific pattern of karyotype alterations was not found. From studies on dysplastic nevi putative localizations for the DNS gene have been proposed, but these are not consistent. Parmiter et al. (1988) reported deletions of 10q 24–26 in three cell lines from dysplastic nevi, an alteration which was also be detected in 30% of their melanoma cell lines. Cowan et al. (1988), however, demonstrated a deletion of 9p in four of 26 dysplastic nevus cell lines as well as in many melanomas. This localization was also proposed by Pedersen and Wang (1989), who showed in several melanoma metastases of one patient consistent alterations of chromosome 9. Linkage studies in DNS/MM families, however, failed to find an association of CMM risk with this chromosome (Bale and Dracopoli 1989).

DNS: A Syndrome with Chromosome Instability

After confirmation by several research groups it is now widely accepted that DNS is characterized by chromosome instability (Sandberg 1990). Unlike the classic breakage syndromes like Fanconi anemia, ataxia telangiectasia and Bloom syndrome the instability is detectable only after challenging cells from DNS patients, with or without melanoma, and cells of individuals with familial melanoma without obvious dysplastic nevi with UV light. In these persons, the chromosome fragility is not restricted to melanocytes but is also detectable in lymphocytes and fibroblasts.

The estimation of sister chromatid exchanges (SCE) is a commonly used method to assess chromosome instability. We have demonstrated (Bohnert et al. 1989; Jung et al. 1986) that the increase in SCE after exposure to UV-C light in cells from patients with multiple dysplastic nevi, with or without realized melanomas, is significant compared to control persons or patients with sporadic melanoma (Fig. 2). In DNS the increase of SCE is much more discrete than in xeroderma pigmentosum (XP-D), a well-established skin disorder prone to early onset of skin aging and tumor manifestation by UV light exposure. Unfortunately, this method does not discriminate between normals and patients, since there is a considerable interindividual variation of SCE.

Recently, Seetharam et al. (1989) proved the hypermutablity on a molecular level. They demonstrated in shuttle vector plasmids higher numbers of point mutations when transfecting them into host cells derived from DNS patients compared to host cells from control persons. While the genetic basis of the chromosome instability in these breakage syndromes is unknown,

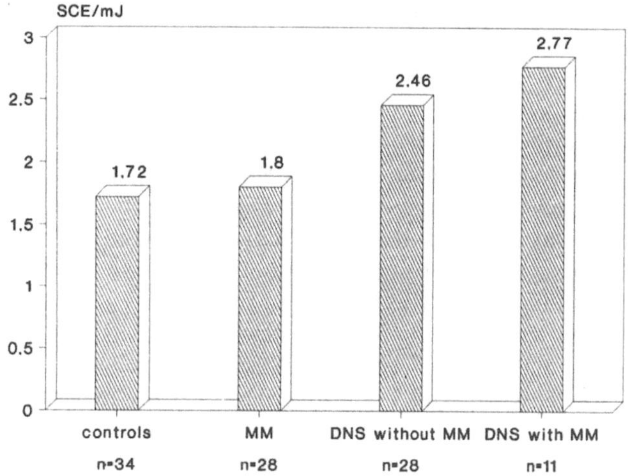

Fig. 2. Mean elevation of sister chromatid exchanges (*SCE*) per millijoule UV-C light in patients with multiple dysplastic nevi (DNS), with or without melanoma, in patients with sporadic melanoma, and in control persons

it is regarded as the reason for a possible elevated incidence of pancreas carcinomas in DNS/MM families (Bergmann et al. 1990).

The Role of Oncogenes and Tumor Suppressor Genes in Development and Progression of Melanocytic Lesions

Protooncogenes are important regulators of growth and differentiation of cells and tissues. If their expression or their gene products are altered they may take on malignant potency and become oncogenes. In recent years more than 40 specific types of oncogenes have been identified (Bishop 1987), with the *ras* family and the *myc* family being the most studied. Intensive research has shown that altered or activated *ras* genes are unlikely to influence the malignant transformation of melanocytes. In common or dysplastic nevi, *ras* alterations were found only occasionally. However, in 25% of melanoma cell lines and in 5%–6% of melanoma tissues an activation of this oncogene was demonstrated (Albino et al. 1989), mostly in late tumor stages and preferentially in tumors which arose in sun-exposed sites. In these cases point mutations were found in oncogene segments rich in pyrimidine, a well-known target of UV-light (van't Veer et al. 1989).

N-*myc*, an oncogene associated with neuroblastoma, is also involved in the regulation of the expression of MHC antigens on cell surfaces. In melanoma cells the loss of particular HLA antigens induced by an altered N-*myc* expression has been shown to be associated with tumor progression (van Duinen et al. 1988). An increased density of receptors for the epidermal growth factor (EGF receptor) on melanoma cell surfaces is considered a further marker of tumor progression. Koprowski et al. (1985) gave evidence that these cases are due to an increase in EGF receptor gene expression caused by aneuploidy of chromosome 7, the chromosome on which this gene is located.

These data, along with other reports, suggest that oncogenes may be involved in the loss of differentiation of melanoma cells. There is, however, no evidence that they may induce the malignant transformation of melanocytes. Interestingly, no heritable tumor so far has been shown to be caused by an inherited activated oncogene.

The elucidation of the mechanisms inducing retinoblastoma (RB) tumorigenesis has revolutionized current thinking about cancer genes (Hollingsworth and Lee 1991). This was the first tumor in which it could be shown that the loss or inactivation of genes was oncogenic. Since then several tumor suppressor genes have been identified as causing other heritable tumors and their sporadic counterparts. These inheritable malignancies show typical clinical features, as they have an earlier onset in life, develop multifocally, and have an autosomal dominant mode of inheritance. They are also less frequent than sporadic cases. Early in 1966 Schnyder described all these features as characteristics for heritable skin tumors, including familial melanoma (Schnyder's rule). The obvious parallels to malignancies associated with tumor suppressor genes suggest that they may play a role in melanoma development.

Since the retinoblastoma gene was the first characterized tumor suppressor gene, some work has been done to elucidate its role in malignant melanoma. Recently, Albert et al. (1990) presented a patient with bilateral retinoblastoma and DNS with multiple primary melanomas. They discussed a possible role of the *rb* gene in melanoma development, since melanomas are common secondary tumors in patients with hereditary retinoblastoma (Traboulsi et al. 1988). Investigations (Horowitz et al. 1990) in melanoma cell lines, however, failed to demonstrate any alterations of the *rb* gene or its gene product ($p110^{RB}$). These findings and the clinical observation that melanomas are not accumulated in retinoblastoma families (Olsen et al. 1990), question the participation of *rb* genes in the transformation of melanocytes. It is not out of question that an impairement of the *rb* gene might influence melanoma progression, as $p110^{RB}$, the product of the wild-type allele, seems to inactivate oncoproteins (Hollingsworth and Lee 1991). Other tumor suppressor genes such as p53, the Wilms' gene, and NF-1, the gene of von Recklinghausen's neurofibromatosis, have been characterized very recently and their role, if any, in melanoma development has yet to be determined. Clinical findings, however, suggest that these genes are not involved in initial melanoma development as there are no associations of melanoma with these tumors.

Tumor suppressor genes were identified by their loss in heritable tumors. Melanomas and melanoma cell lines were tested with a variety of DNA probes for such a loss of heterozygosity, but a specific pattern could not be detected. Dracopoli et al. (1989) investigated the vicinity of the chromosome locus 1p36 for loss of heterozygosity. This chromosome region was found to be strongly linked with melanoma risk in DNS/MM patients (Bale et al. 1989). Loss of genes was only detected in late melanoma stages, which indicates that this localization may harbor a suppressor gene regulating tumor progression, but not the initial melanoma gene (Dracopoli et al. 1989). The reinsertion of chromosomes into tumor cells is a further method for localizing tumor suppressor genes. Trent et al. (1990) showed that melanoma cell lines lost their tumorigenicity after transfection of chromosome 6, which suggests that a tumor suppressor gene is present on this chromosome. Whether or not this is the initial melanoma gene has yet to be determined.

Intense efforts are currently underway in the study of tumor suppressor genes. It can be anticipated that an understanding of their mode of action, their number, and their contribution to cancer induction will increase in the near future.

Melanoma in *Xiphophorus* Fish

Melanoma in *Xiphophorus* fish is an animal model intensively investigated by Anders and associates (1990). It is an excellent example of the cooperation of oncogenes with tumor suppressor genes in tumorigenesis. In a tumor gene complex called TU, several genes could be identified. A compartment gene and the melanophore gene regulate the development of melanocytic lesions in particular anatomic regions of the fish. A copy of a protooncogene (X-*mrk* or X-*erb B*^{a}) coding for a tyrosine kinase closely related to the EGF receptor (Wittbrodt et al. 1989) has been integrated by duplication. It stimulates unrestricted growth of these melanocytes unless suppressed by *Diff*, a tumor suppressor gene. *Diff* and the tumor gene complex TU can be separated by crossbreeding. The loss of one allele of *Diff* induces benign melanomas; malignant growth is caused by the loss of the other allele. The specific mechanisms of regulation are not yet identified.

Hypothetical Model for Melanoma Genesis

Familial melanomas display an autosomal dominant mode of inheritance. They may be associated with DNS, but in every second case no associated dysplastic nevi can be detected. In 1988 Harnett and Kefford proposed a hypothetical model to explain the genetic basis of familial melanomas which was derived from the retinoblastoma model. According to that model, dysplastic nevi arise if one allele of a melanoma suppressor gene is inactivated, the loss of the second allele inducing the malignant trans-

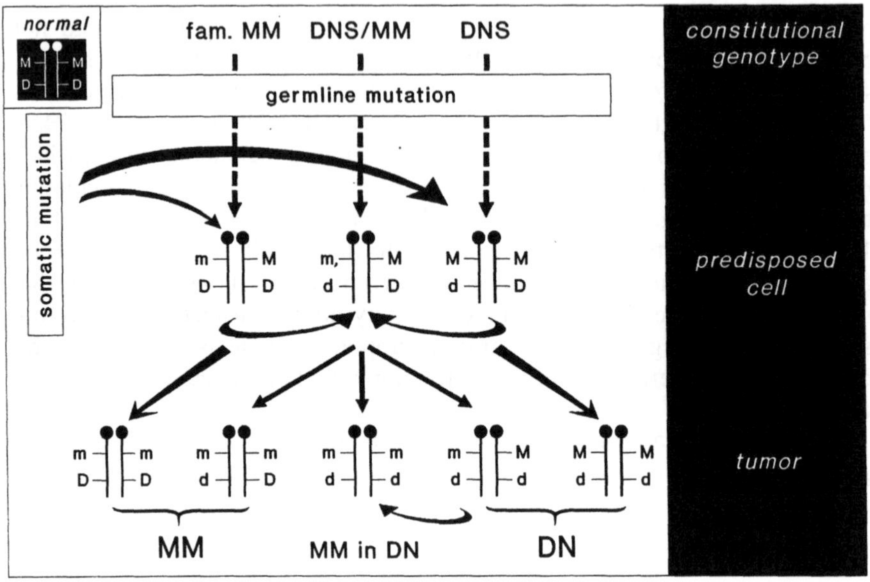

Fig. 3. A hypothetical molecular model for melanoma genesis and development of dysplastic nevi which explains the heterogeneity of the melanocytic tumors. Patients with heritable melanoma or familial melanoma/DNS have a germline mutation which inactivates one allele of the putative melanoma suppressor gene. An additional somatic mutation causes malignancy. In individuals without inherited genetic alterations, two somatic mutations are required for tumor development. The same mechanisms induce the growth of dysplastic nevi, which are inherited independently, although a combined loss of genes may occur because of the close chromosomal location (BK mole syndrome). *M*, *D*, wild-type, active suppressor genes for melanoma or dysplasia; *m*, *d*, functionally or structurally abnormal alleles of the suppressor genes

formation of the melanocytes. Parallels to melanomas in *Xiphophorus* fish are obvious. Unfortunately, this model explains neither the de novo origin of most melanomas nor the genesis of the hereditary melanomas in families without dysplastic nevi. For these tumors different genetic pathways would have to be postulated (Kefford et al. 1991).

We propose a model with a complex of at least two independent genes (Fig. 3), one of which causes dysplasia in melanocytes and the other malignant transformation. According to this model, in DNS/MM families one allele of each gene is inactivated by a germline mutation, whereas in hereditary DNS without familial MM and in hereditary melanomas without dysplastic nevi only the corresponding genes are affected. Melanocytes carrying altered genes are predisposed to develop the particular melanocytic lesions. The clinical manifestation as melanoma or as dysplastic nevi or as MM in a dysplastic nevus requires one additional somatic mutation in the remaining wild-type allele.

The development of melanomas in individuals with DNS (type A or B) without hereditary MM needs two somatic mutations in the melanoma alleles. Therefore, melanoma risk is apparently lower and the age of tumor manifestation higher than in the DNS/MM group, although these alterations may be favored by the chromosome instability of DNS. Currently no heritable tumor is known to be caused by an activated oncogene, and so the postulated DNS and MM genes in our model should be tumor suppressor genes.

This model refers only to the initial stages of transformation. Melanoma progression might be induced by both activated oncogenes and inactivated suppressor genes. It also may be relevant in the controversy on the mode of inheritance of DNS: autosomal dominant versus polygenic.

Conclusion

An atypical nevus can be easily diagnosed both clinically and histologically only if it displays all typical features. However, there are great difficulties in classifying borderline dysplastic lesions as neither histologically nor immunohistologically unambiguous signs are known which allow a distinction from common melanocytic nevi. The presence of multiple dysplastic nevi (at least six in this study) proved to increase melanoma risk in addition to the risk already indicated by the number of common nevi. These particular nevi are also associated with an alteration in tumor characteristics, as the age of melanoma onset is earlier. While the basis of this is not known, it might be related to the chromosome instability.

The characterization of these genetic alterations would provide an unequivocal sign for the recognition DNS, whose diagnosis currently is more than questionable in many cases, because of the lack of commonly acknowledged features and definitions. The elucidation of genetic alterations in these nevi would also provide information on the interesting sex differences observed in the frequencies and the location preference of dysplastic nevi. Finally, it would be of tremendous impact on educational campaigns aimed at prevention of melanoma. The rapid progress in molecular genetics and the intensive investigation in this field promise an answer in the next few years.

Acknowledgments. We have to acknowledge the efforts of the colleagues Dr. F. Bahmer (Homburg), Dr. M. Roser (Hamburg), Dr. C. Sigg (Zürich), Dr. P. Soyer (Graz), Dr. Stocker (Lübeck), Dr. W. Tilgen (Heidelberg), and Dr. J. Weckbecker (Bonn), who recruited and examined the patients in these dermatology clinics.

References

Ackermann AB (1988) What naevus is dysplastic, a syndrome and the commonest precursor of malignant melanoma? A riddle and an answer. Histopathology 13:241–256

Albert LS, Sober AJ, Rhodes AR (1990) Cutaneous melanoma and bilateral retinoblastoma. J Am Acad Dermatol 23:1001–1004

Albino AP, Nanus DM, Mentle IR et al. (1989) Analysis of ras oncogenes in malignant melanoma and precursor lesions: correlation of point mutations with differentiation phenotype. Oncogene 4:1363–1374

Anders A, Anders F, Zechel C et al. (1990) Ansätze zur Analyse der Initiation von Initialprozessen der Krebsbildung am Melanom-Modell von Xiphophorus. Arch Geschwulstforsch 60:249–263

Augustsson A, Stierner U, Suurküla M, Rosdahl I (1991) Prevalence of common and dysplastic naevi in a Swedish population. Br J Dermatol 124:152–156

Bale SJ, Dracopoli NC (1989) Chromosome 9p and hereditary cutaneous malignant melanoma. J Natl Cancer Inst 81:70

Bale SJ, Dracopoli NC, Tucker MA et al. (1989) Mapping the gene for hereditary cutaneous malignant melanoma-dysplastic nevus to chromosome 1p. N Engl J Med 320:1367–1372

Bergmann W, Palan A, Went LN (1986) Clinical and genetic studies in six Dutch kindreds with the dysplastic naevus syndrome. Ann Hum Genet 50:249–258

Bergmann W, Watson P, de Jong J et al. (1990) Systemic cancer and the FAMMM syndrome. Br J Cancer 61:932–936

Bishop JM (1987) The molecular genetics of cancer. Science 235:305–311

Bohnert E, Weiß J, Jung EG (1989) Cytogenetische Auffälligkeiten bei Melanompatienten. Akt Dermatol 15:96–98

Clark WH, Ackerman AB (1989) An exchange of views regarding the dysplastic nevus controversy. Semin Dermatol 8:229–250

Clark WH, Reimer RR, Greene M et al. (1978) Origin of familial malignant melanomas from heritable melanocytic lesions. Arch Dermatol 114:732–738

Cooke KR, Spears GFS, Elder DE, Greene MH (1989) Dysplastic naevi in a population-based survey. Cancer 63:1240–1244

Cowan JM, Halaban R, Francke U (1988) Cytogenetic analysis of melanocytes from premalignant nevi and melanomas. J Natl Cancer Inst 80:1159–1164

Crutcher WA, Sagebiel RW (1984) Prevalence of dysplastic naevi in a community practice. Lancet I:729

Dracopoli NC, Harnett P, Bale SJ et al. (1989) Loss of alleles from the distal short arm of chromosome 1 occurs late in melanoma tumor progression. Proc Natl Acad Sci USA 86:4614–4618

English DR, Menz J Heenan et al. (1986) The dysplastic naevus syndrome in patients with cutaneous malignant melanoma in Western Australia. Med J Aust 145:194–198

Elder DE (1988) Dysplastic nevus syndrome – biological significance. Semin Oncol 15:529–540

Elder DE, Goldman LI, Goldman SC et al. (1980) Dysplastic nevus syndrome: a phenotypic association of sporadic cutaneous melanoma. Cancer 46:1787–1794

Greene MH, Clark WH, Tucker MA et al. (1985) High risk of malignant melanoma in melanoma-prone families with dysplastic nevi. Ann Intern Med 102:458–465

Harnett P, Kefford RF (1988) Molecular models of tumorigenesis: application to familial and sporadic melanoma. Semin Oncol 15:549–557

Hollingsworth RE, Lee WH (1991) Tumor suppressor genes: new prospects for cancer research. J Natl Cancer Inst 83:91–96

Holly EA, Kelly JW, Shpall SN, Shu-Hui Chiu MS (1987) Number of melanocytic nevi as a major risk factor for malignant melanoma. J Am Acad Dermatol 17:459–468
Horowitz JM, Park SH, Bogenmann E et al. (1990) Frequent inactivation of the retinoblastoma anti-oncogene is restricted to a subset of human tumor cells. Proc Natl Acad Sci USA 87:2775–2779
Jung EG, Bohnert E, Boonen H (1986) Dysplastic nevus syndrome: ultraviolet hypermutability confirmed in vitro by elevated sister chromatid exchanges. Dermatologica 173:297–300
Kath R, Rodeck U, Menssen HD et al. (1989) Tumor progression in the human melanocytic system. Anticancer Res 9:865–872
Kefford RF, Salmon J, Shaw HM et al. (1991) Hereditary melanoma in Australia: variable association with dysplastic nevi and absence of genetic linkage to chromosome 1p. Cancer Genet Cytogenet 51:45–55
Kelly JW, Crutcher WA, Sagebiel RW (1986) Clinical diagnosis of dysplastic melanocytic nevi. J Am Acad Dermatol 14:1044–1052
Klein LJ, Barr RJ (1990) Histologic atypia in clinically benign nevi. J Am Acad Dermatol 22:275–282
Kopf AW, Lindsay AC, Rogers GS et al. (1985) Relationship of melanocytic nevi to sun exposure in dysplastic nevus syndrome. J Am Acad Dermatol 12:656–662
Kopf AW, Friedman RJ, Rigel DS (1990) Atypical mole syndrome. J Am Acad Dermatol 22:117–118
Koprowski H, Herlyn M, Balaban G et al. (1985) Expression of the receptor for epidermal growth factor correlates with increased dosage of chromosome 7 in malignant melanoma. Somat Cell Mol Genet 11:297–302
Kraemer KH, Tucker M, Tarone R et al. (1983) Cutaneous melanoma risk in dysplastic nevus syndrome types A and B. Lancet II:1076–1077
Lynch HT, Frichot BC, Lynch JF (1978) Familial atypical multiple mole melanoma syndrome. J Med Genet 15:352–356
MacKie RM, English J, Aitchison TC et al. (1985) The number and distribution of benign pigmented moles (melanocytic naevi) in a healthy British population. Br J Dermatol 113:167–174
MacKie RM, Freudenberger T, Aitchison TC (1989) Personal risk-factor chart for cutaneous melanoma. Lancet II:487–490
National Institutes of Health Consensus Development Conference Statement (1984) Precursors to malignant melanoma. J Am Acad Dermatol 10:683–687
Olsen JH, Winther J, Brown PN (1990) Risk of nonocular cancer in first-degree relatives of retinoblastoma patients. Hum Genet 85:283–287
Parmiter AH, Balaban G, Clark WH, Nowell PC (1988) Possible involvement of the chromosome region 10q 24–26 in early stages of melanocytic neoplasia. Cancer Genet Cytogenet 30:313–317
Pedersen MI, Wang N (1989) Chromosomal evolution in the progression and metastasis of human malignant melanoma. A multiple lesion study. Cancer Genet Cytogenet 41:185–201
Piepkorn M (1990) A hypothesis incorporating the histologic characteristics of dysplastic nevi into the normal biological development of melanocytic nevi. Arch Dermatol 126:514–518
Piepkorn M, Meyer LJ, Goldgar D et al. (1989) The dysplastic nevus: a prevalent lesion that correlates poorly with clinical phenotype. J Am Acad Dermatol 20:407–415
Roth ME, Grant-Kels JM, Ackerman AB et al. (1991) The histopathology of dysplastic nevi. Am J Dermatopathol 13:38–51
Roush GC, Nordlund JJ, Forget B et al. (1988) Independence of dysplastic nevi from total nevi in determining risk for nonfamilial melanoma. Prev Med 17:273–279

Sagebiel RW, Banda PW, Schneider JS, Crutcher WA (1985) Age distribution and histologic patterns of dysplastic nevi. J Am Acad Dermatol 13:975–982

Sandberg AA (1990) Malignant melanoma. In: Sandberg AA (ed) The chromosomes in human cancer and leukemia, 2nd edn. Elsevier, New York, pp 917–923

Schnyder UW (1966) Tumoren der Haut in genetischer Sicht. Praxis 6:1478–1482

Seetharam S, Waters HL, Seidman MM, Kraemer KH (1989) Ultraviolet mutagenesis in a plasmid vector replicated lymphoid cells from a patient with the melanoma-prone disorder dysplastic nevus syndrome. Cancer Res 49:5918–5921

Sigg C, Pelloni F, Schnyder UW (1989) Gehäufte Mehrfachmelanome bei sporadischem und familiärem dysplastischen Nävuszellnävus-Syndrom. Hautarzt 40:548–552

Sterry W, Christophers E (1988) Quadrant distribution of dysplastic nevus syndrome. Arch Dermatol 124:926–929

Traboulsi EI, Zimmermann LE, Manz HJ (1989) Cutaneous malignant melanoma in survivors of heritable retinoblastoma. Arch Ophthalmol 106:1059–1061

Traupe H, Macher E, Hamm H, Happle R (1989) Mutation rate estimates are not compatible with autosomal dominant inheritance of the dysplastic nevus syndrome. Am J Med Genet 32:155–157

Trent JM, Stanbridge EJ, McBride HL et al. (1990) Tumorigenicity in human melanoma cell lines controlled by introduction of human chromosome 6. Science 247:568–571

van Duinen SG, Ruiter DJ, Broecker EB et al. (1988) Level of HLA antigens in locoregional metastases and clinical course of the disease in patients with melanoma. Cancer Res 48:1019–1025

van't Veer LJ, Burgering BM, Versteeg R et al. (1989) N-ras mutations in human cutaneous melanoma form sun-exposed body sites. Mol Cell Biol 9:3114–3116

Weinstock MA, Stryker WS, Stampfer MJ et al. (1991) Sunlight and dysplastic nevus risk. Results of a clinic-based case-control study. Cancer 67:1701–1706

Wittbrodt J, Adam D, Malitschek B et al. (1989) Novel putative receptor tyrosine kinase encoded by the melanoma-inducing Tu locus in Xiphophorus. Nature 341:415–421

Integrins and Melanoma Progression

E.H.J. Danen, G.N.P. van Muijen, P.J.M. ten Berge, and D.J. Ruiter

Department of Pathology, University Hospital Nijmegen, P.O. Box 9101, 6500 HB Nijmegen, The Netherlands

Introduction

Tumor (or neoplastic) progression is one of the crucial events in the development of cancer. It is defined as the acquisition of permanent, irreversible, and qualitative changes of one or more characteristics in a neoplasm and its precursor lesions (Nowell 1986). Confronted with selective pressure imposed by host defense and/or therapy, tumor progression favors relentless emergence of new subpopulations with enhanced growth and metastatic capacities, creating tumor heterogeneity (Fidler 1988). Tumor heterogeneity is based on both genetic and epigenetic changes and on differences in development and maturation of the tumor cell population. A better understanding of the pathogenesis of neoplastic progression is likely to provide new clues for diagnosis and therapy aimed at the aggressive tumor cell populations.

In human cutaneous melanoma different stages of the process of tumor progression have been identified, clinically, histopathologically, and immunologically (Clark et al. 1984). The accessibility of these lesions in patients, and the availability of many well-characterized human melanoma cell lines make human melanoma an ideal candidate to study tumor progression.

In the last decade a number of monoclonal antibodies has been developed that recognize determinants on melanocytic cells that have preference for one or few stages in the process of tumor progression (Bröcker et al. 1985; Holzmann et al. 1985, 1987; Ruiter et al. 1985). Therefore, the antigens recognized have been named melanoma-associated progression antigens. Immunochemical and molecular biological analyses have revealed that most antigens characterized are either a cellular adhesion molecule or a growth factor receptor (Bröcker et al. 1985; Holzmann et al. 1985, 1987; Ruiter et al. 1985).

Theoretically, progression antigens could be involved in local tumor

Recent Results in Cancer Research, Vol. 128

growth or in the process of metastasis. Progression antigens related to local growth probably are the transferrin receptor (Van Muijen et al. 1990) and the epidermal growth factor receptor (EGF-R) (Real et al. 1986; Herlyn et al. 1987; DeWit et al. 1992). Tumor metastasis is based on a series of distinct sequential steps that are selective and have stochastic elements (Fidler 1988). These steps include tumor invasion, transportation through lymph or blood channels, adhesion to vessel walls in target organs, invasion at that site, and proliferation to a secondary growth. The progression antigens identified as cellular adhesion molecules may thus be involved in one or more steps of tumor metastasis (Johnson et al. 1989). Further studies are necessary to clarify the structure and function of these molecules and the nature of the counterstructure they react with.

The expression of one of the cellular adhesion molecules on human melanoma cells can be markedly upregulated by interferon-γ (Johnson et al. 1989). This suggests that this molecule plays a role in the local immune response to melanoma, similar to HLA class II antigens (Bröcker et al. 1985; Holzmann et al. 1987). It is very intriguing that molecules involved in cellular immune response when expressed on melanoma cells are related to the process of tumor progression as well.

Immunohistochemistry using monoclonal antibodies that recognize progression antigens has provided additional prognostic information in melanoma patients (Bröcker et al. 1985). The expression of these different progression antigens, one of them being an adhesion molecule (Klein et al. 1991), in primary melanoma lesions correlated with a high incidence of metastasis (Bröcker et al. 1985). It also may be expected that immunohistochemistry using a panel of monoclonal antibodies recognizing progression markers contributes to the diagnostic discrimination of benign and malignant melanocytic tumors.

In this contribution we shall discuss the expression of adhesion molecules on human melanoma and other tumors, with emphasis on the integrins. Expression both on cell lines and tumor lesions in patients will be dealt with.

Structure of Integrins

The last few years a group of cell surface receptors called integrins has been extensively studied and characterized, as elucidated in exellent reviews (Hynes 1987; Ruoslahti and Pierschbacher 1987; McDonald 1989). Integrins consist of a superfamily of transmembrane receptor molecules. They mediate cell–cell and cell–extracellular matrix (ECM) contacts. Structurally, each integrin is a heterodimer consisting of an α subunit noncovalently bound to a β subunit (Table 1). Both integrin subunits are glycoproteins with a large extracellular domain, a transmembrane domain, and a short cytoplasmic domain. Complete sequence information has been obtained for most α and β subunits (Hemler 1990; Erle et al. 1990). The amino acid sequences of

Table 1. The integrin superfamily

Subunits	Name	Ligands	RGD
$\alpha_1\beta_1$	VLA-1	CO-I, CO-IV, LM	
$\alpha_2\beta_1$	VLA-2	CO-I, CO-IV, LM	
$\alpha_3\beta_1$	VLA-3	CO-I, LM, FN	
$\alpha_4\beta_1$	VLA-4	FN, VCAM	
$\alpha_4\beta_p$	LPAM-2	Peyer's patch addressin	
$\alpha_5\beta_1$	VLA-5	FN	+
$\alpha_6\beta_1$	VLA-6	LM	
$\alpha_6\beta_4$		?	
$\alpha_V\beta_1$		FN	+
$\alpha_V\beta_3$	VNR	VN, FB, VWF, OP, BSP-1	+
$\alpha_V\beta_5$		VN	+
$\alpha_V\beta_6$		?	
$\alpha_{IIb}\beta_3$	gpIIbIIIa	FN, VN, VWF, FB	+
$\alpha_L\beta_2$	LFA-1	ICAM-1, ICAM-2	
$\alpha_M\beta_2$	MAC-1	C3bi, FX, FB	
$\alpha_X\beta_2$	P150, 195	?	

The known subunit combinations, their names, and their known ligands. The RGD specificity of integrins binding to this sequence is also indicated. CO, collagen; LM, laminin; FN, fibronectin; VCAM, vascular cell adhesion molecule; VN, vitronectin; FB, fibrinogen; VWF, von Willebrand factor; OP, osteopontin; BSP-1, bone sialoprotein 1; ICAM, intercellular adhesion molecule; C3bi, complement component C3bi; FX, factor X. For references see text.

seven β subunits have a 32%–48% homology and the positions of cysteine residues are highly conserved. Sequence homology between the α subunits is far less. There are two major clusters of α subunits (Hemler 1990), namely those which are posttranslationally cleaved and those which contain an insert of 180–200 amino acids that is homologous to a domain in a number of collagen binding proteins (Pytela 1988).

The association of the α and the β subunits is promoted by divalent cations (Ginsberg et al. 1988), and transport of newly synthesized receptor molecules to the cell surface takes place after combination of the subunits (Cheresh and Spiro 1987). Integrin interactions with their ligands are cation-dependent and require both subunits (Hemler 1988). The best studied amino acid sequence in the integrin ligands is the Arg-Gly-Asp (RGD) sequence. It is found within fibronectin, fibrinogen, thrombospondin, vitronectin, laminin, and collagen type I (Ruoslahti and Pierschbacher 1987). Intracellularly, the integrins are linked to the cytoskeleton. Interaction with actin filaments is thought to occur through indirect linkage, involving talin, vinculin, α-actinin (Burridge et al. 1988), and others (Geiger and Ginsberg 1991). Recent findings have demonstrated that focal contacts, in which integrins are connected with actin filaments, are not the only possible structures for integrin signalling. The integrin $\alpha_6\beta_4$ has been shown to be part of an epithelial adhesive structure, distinct from focal adhesions, the hemidesmosome complex (reviewed by Quaranta and Jones 1991). In this complex the extremely long cytoplasmic part of the β_4 chain might reach deep into the intermediate filament region.

Interaction of the β_1 subunit with talin appears to be metabolically regulated (Burn et al. 1988) and a potential integrin regulation site is formed by a tyrosine phosphorylation site in the cytoplasmic sequences of the β_1 and β_3 subunits (Tamkun et al. 1986). Phorbol ester and triggering through a protein kinase C-mediated pathway have been shown to influence the function of β_2 integrins (Van Kooyk et al. 1989), probably through changes in association of integrin with the cytoskeleton (Kupfer and Singer 1989). Apart from phosphorylation events recent studies have demonstrated a posible role for glycosylation processes in integrin function regulation. The extent of glycosylation on the β_1 integrin "very late antigen" (VLA) 6 regulates binding of laminin and vice versa (Chammas et al. 1991), and the extent of glycosylation on the "intercellular adhesion molecule" (ICAM) I affects binding to the β_2 integrin MAC-1 (Diamond et al. 1991).

Functions of Integrins

Diversity within the superfamily of integrins is generated by a large number of α subunits which form heterodimers with at least seven different β subunits (Table 1) (Erle et al. 1990). Until recently it was generally accepted that the type of β subunit defines the nature of the family and that each β subunit interacts with a specific subset of α subunits. This provided a useful basis for classification: VLA molecules are α subunits associated with the β_1 subunit (Hemler 1988; Hemler et al. 1987), leukocyte integrins are $\alpha\beta_2$ complexes (Kishimoto et al. 1989) and cytoadhesins consist of α subunits associated with the β_3 subunit (Ginsberg et al. 1988). While the β_1 and β_3 families have been thought to be involved almost exclusively in cell contacts with ECM components (Akiyama et al. 1990) the β_2 family is thought to play a role primarily in cell–cell contacts (Kishimoto et al. 1989).

The findings of new β subunits, which include β_4 (Hemler et al. 1989), β_5 (Cheresh et al. 1989), β_6 Sheppard et al. (1990), β_7 (Erle et al. 1990), and β_p (Holzmann et al. 1989), and the finding that one α subunit can associate with more than one β subunit (Krissansen et al. 1990; Vogel et al. 1990) suggest that the current classification scheme for integrins needs revision. In addition, it has been demonstrated that the β subunit plays an important role in determining the ligand specificity of the complex (Cheresh et al. 1989; Vogel et al. 1990). The finding that the binding specificities of a certain integrin may vary, depending on the cell type involved, also strongly enhances the complexity of the integrin superfamily. In particular, binding of endothelial cells to laminin and fibronectin is mediated by $\alpha_2\beta_1$, whereas the same molecule on platelets does not bind to these proteins (Kirchhofer et al. 1990).

Until recently VLA antigens were mainly supposed to be receptors for basement membranes. Blocking of cell adhesion to ECM components with antibodies and affinity chromatography experiments have demonstrated that β_1 integrins may serve as a receptor for a single ECM protein (VLA-4, VLA-5, and VLA-6) or as a receptor for two or more ECM proteins (VLA-1, VLA-2, and VLA-3) (Hemler 1990).

The VLA-5 fibronectin receptor binds to a region in fibronectin containing the RGD sequence (Ruoslahti and Pierschbacher 1987). In contrast, cell adhesion to the CS-I alternatively spliced domain of fibronectin is mediated by VLA-4 (Wayner et al. 1989; Guan and Hynes 1990). However, apart from being a fibronectin receptor VLA-4 is also the lymphocyte receptor for vascular cell adhesion molecule (VCAM) I (Elices et al. 1990). Recently, Komoriya et al. (1991) have narrowed down the binding site for melanoma cell adhesion to CS-I to a tripeptide Leu-Asp-Val (LDV) which is also present in VCAM-I (Osborn et al. 1989).

It has been demonstrated that more VLA proteins can play a role in cell–cell contacts. In a number of human cell lines (fibroblast, carcinoma, sarcoma) VLA-3 has been demonstrated to be localized at cell–cell contact sites (Kaufmann et al. 1989). In cultured keratinocytes α_2 and α_3 subunits have been found to accumulate in areas of cell–cell contacts (Larjava et al. 1990). In addition, serum- or calcium-induced aggregation of keratinocytes results in relocation of VLA-2 and VLA-3 from sites of focal adhesion to cell–cell contact sites and anti-VLA-3 antibodies have been shown to inhibit homotypic cell aggregation (Carter et al. 1990). By mediating cell–cell as well as cell–substratum interactions of keratinocytes these molecules might play a major role in the morphogenesis of the epidermis.

Apart from their role in mediating contact of cells with the ECM or with each other β_1 integrins are also involved in the assembly of the ECM. Antibodies directed towards the cytoplasmic domain of the integrin β_1 subunit have been demonstrated to inhibit fibronectin fibril formation in vivo during development (Darribère et al. 1990), and fibronectin matrix assembly is inhibited in vitro by RGD synthetic peptides (McDonald et al. 1987), and by anti-α_5 or anti-β_1 antibodies (Akiyama et al. 1989).

The Role of Integrins in Tumor Progression

During the process of metastasis tumor cells must adhere to and penetrate basement membranes and interstitial tissues. Specific interactions between tumor cell surface receptors and ECM components might therefore play an important role in metastasis, and complex changes in cell–cell and cell–substratum interactions are to be expected.

To metastasize melanoma cells have to interact with and penetrate basement membranes three times (Fig. 1). These are: (1) The epidermal basement membrane in order to invade the dermis at the site of the primary

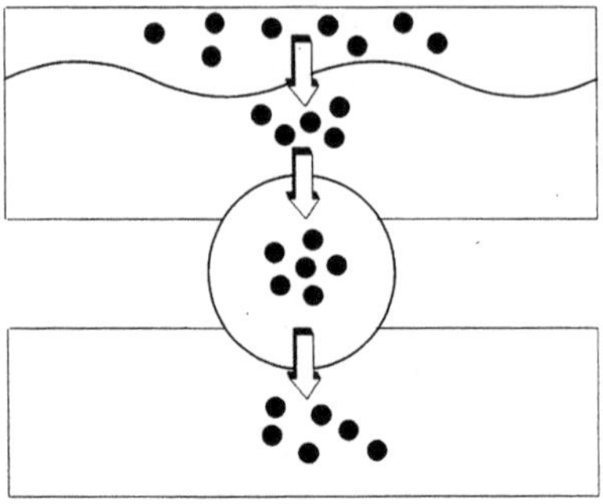

Fig. 1. Schematic representation of invasion and hematogenic metastasis of melanoma cells (*black dots*). In order to invade the dermis, enter a blood vessel, and leave the blood vessel after transportation to a distant organ, tumor cells have to penetrate a basal lamina three times (*arrows*)

tumor; (2) the endothelial basement membrane during intravasation; and (3) the endothelial basement membrane during extravasation. Invading tumor cells should therefore express the right panel and adequate levels of basement membrane receptors such as integrins. It seems likely that the expression patterns of these receptors might be different for invasive and metastatic cells compared to normal cells and/or noninvasive tumor cells. One example is the discovery that a gene encoding for a member of the immunoglobulin superfamily with high homology to the adhesion molecule NCAM was altered or absent in 70% of colorectal cancers (Fearon et al. 1990). Another example is the recent finding that E-cadherin, a member of the cadherin cell adhesion receptors (Takeichi 1991), can act as an invasion suppressor molecule (Vleminckx et al. 1991). Data from several studies strongly suggest that similar changes in integrin expression or function are involved in tumor progression. Most data have been obtained for melanoma but other types of cancer have also been investigated.

Nonmelanoma

Only a few immunohistological studies have been performed to compare the expression of the integrin receptors in normal human tissues and in benign and malignant neoplasms. The expression of VLA-2 and to a lesser extent of other integrins has been found to be decreased in adenocarcinomas of the breast compared with expression on epithelium of the ducts and ductules of normal breast tissue (Zutter et al. 1990). Furthermore, a 67-kDa non-integrin receptor with high affinity for laminin has been shown to be intimately associated with tumor invasion and metastasis of human breast carcinoma cells (Terranova et al. 1983).

Metastatic murine sarcoma cell lines have been demonstrated to adhere preferentially to type IV collagen using laminin as an attachment protein and preincubation of the metastatic cells with antibodies directed to laminin prior to injection into mice reduced the number of pulmonary metastases (Terranova et al. 1982) indicating a role for laminin in the metastatic process. In addition, a study by Aresu et al. (1991) in which osteosarcoma cell lines derived from BALB/c mice were used demonstrated in an in vitro chemoinvasion assay that a chemotactic response to laminin is a property of high and not low metastatic cell lines.

A study on the integrin expression on Lewis lung carcinoma cells has demonstrated that the expression of the $\alpha_6\beta_4$ integrin is associated with the metastatic phenotype (Perrotti et al. 1990). Recently, this finding has been confirmed and extended for cultured human squamous sarcoma cells (Van Waes et al. 1991).

Chemical transformation of a human osteogenic sarcoma cell line that is nontumorigenic in nude mice leads to increased VLA-1, VLA-2, and VLA-6 expression and increased invasion through a reconstituted basement membrane (Dedhar and Saulnier 1990). Oncogenic transformation of rodent cells leads to a reduced level of expression of the $\alpha_5\beta_1$ fibronectin receptor whereas expression of VLA-3 is unchanged (Plantefaber and Hynes 1989). These last results have been extended by Giancotti and Ruoslahti (1990). They have demonstrated that elevated levels of VLA-5 expression can suppress the transformed phenotype of hamster ovary cells. Recently, the importance of another integrin, VLA-2, in the process of metastasis has been demonstrated (Chan et al. 1991). Transfection of human rhabdomyosarcoma cells with VLA-2 led to the formation of substantially more metastatic tumor colonies in nude mice both after intravenous and after subcutaneous inoculation.

Melanoma

During the metastatic process melanoma cells invade the dermis, enter a blood vessel, are transported in the bloodstream, extravasate, and grow out to form a new tumor. During this process different phenotypes might be needed for each specific step. Therefore strong intratumor heterogeneity is expected. Anichini et al. (1990a,b) have demonstrated that this is indeed the case. A marked heterogeneity for susceptibility to lysis by autologous cytotoxic T cells and heterologous peripheral blood cells, for ICAM-1 expression, for invasive ability, and for VLA profile was found among 19 clones isolated from a human metastatic melanoma. After selection for resistance to lysis the surviving melanoma cells showed reduced expression of ICAM-1 and VLA.

In an immunohistological study Albelda et al. (1990) compared the expression of integrins in benign and malignant human melanocytic lesions. No differences were found in expression of β_1 integrins between cells from radial growth phase, vertical growth phase, metastatic cells, and nevus cells.

Elevated expression of the β_3 subunit, however, appeared to be associated with tumor progression to vertical growth. The presence of IIb–IIIa (α_{IIb}-β_3)-like glycoproteins, which had been thought to be exclusively present on platelets, has been demonstrated on human metastatic melanomas but not on benign melanocytes (McGregor et al. 1989). That the integrin involved is α_{IIb}-β_3 and not another β_3 integrin has recently been reported by Chen et al. (1991).

Johnson et al. (1989) have demonstrated ICAM-1, a ligand for the β_2 integrin LFA-1, to be a useful marker for melanoma progression and Natali et al. (1990) have confirmed this finding in a survival study of stage I melanoma patients.

Analysis of human primary and metastatic melanoma cell cultures has demonstrated an increased expression of VLA-1, VLA-2, and VLA-6 on cultures derived from metastatic lesions (Mortarini et al. 1991). An immunohistochemical study has shown that VLA-2 may be a progression marker in human melanocytic lesions (Bröcker et al. 1985; Klein et al. 1991). This finding has not been confirmed by Albelda et al. (1990), possibly because of differences between the antibodies used or because of differences in the sensitivity of the procedures. We have recently found additional evidence for VLA-2 to be a progression marker in human melanoma (Van Muijen et al. 1991). In a nude mouse model it appeared that highly metastatic human melanoma cell lines show high VLA-2 expression, whereas poorly metastatic human melanoma cell lines show low VLA-2 expression (E.H.J. Danen et al., manuscript submitted). In an immunohistochemical study we have investigated integrin expression on melanocytic lesions from different stages of tumor progression (E.H.J. Danen et al., manuscript submitted). We find correlated expression of the α_5- and β_3-subunits and emergence of these integrins in advanced primary and metastatic melanoma lesions. We also find increased VLA-2 expression in advanced primary and metastatic melanomas compared to early primary melanomas. However, common nevi often show VLA-2 expression as well.

Conclusion

In conclusion, a number of studies strongly suggest an important role for integrins in the metastatic process. Both the α_2 and β_3 integrin subunits appear to be correlated with melanoma tumor progression. Possibly there is not one metastatic phenotype, but rather a subtle equilibrium exists in which a large panel of integrins plays a role. Further investigations will probably demonstrate the involvement of more integrins and other adhesion molecules in the metastatic process.

Acknowledgments. We gratefully acknowledge Dr. A. Sonnenberg for C17 monoclonal antibodies, Dr. C.E. Klein for A1.43 and MT78 monoclonal

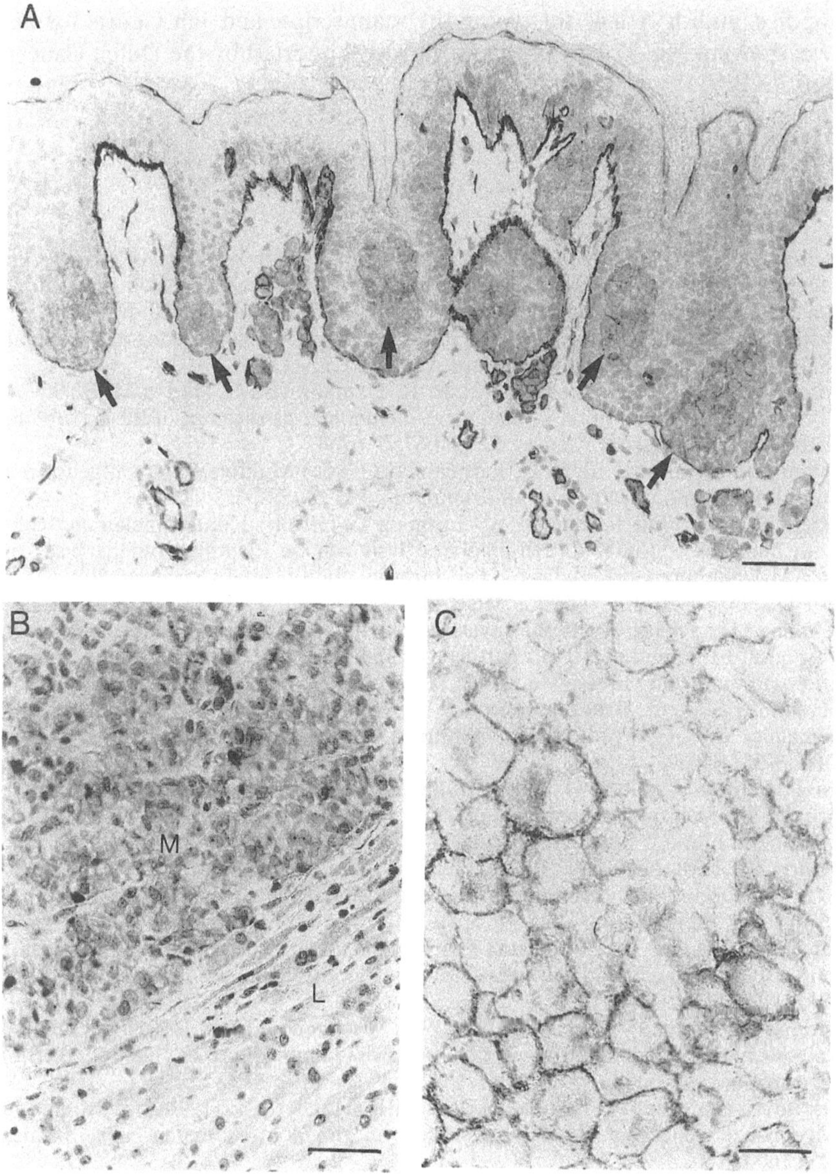

Fig. 2A–C. Immunohistochemical staining of human cutaneous lesions reveals integrin expression on melanocytic cells. Frozen sections were stained with anti-integrin subunit monoclonal antibodies using an immunoperoxidase-AEC technique. Nuclei were counterstained with hematoxylin. **A** Nevus stained with MT78 anti-α_6 monoclonal antibodies (Klein et al. 1990). *Arrows* indicate nevus cells. *Bar* is 17 μm. **B** Melanoma liver metastasis stained with C17 anti-β_3 monoclonal antibodies (Tetteroo et al. 1983). *M*, melanoma; *L*, liver parenchyma. Melanoma cells show a moderate membraneous reaction with the antibodies. *Bar* is 13 μm. **C** Primary melanoma stained with A1.43 anti-α_2 monoclonal antibodies (Klein et al. 1991). *Bar* is 11 μm

antibodies, Judith Ariëns for typing the manuscript, and Jan Geurts for his help in drawing Fig. 1. Part of this work was supported by the Dutch Cancer Society (KWF).

References

Akiyama S, Yamada SS, Chen W, Yamada KM (1989) Analysis of fibronectin receptor function with monoclonal antibodies: roles in cell adhesion, migration, matrix assembly, and cytoskeletal organization. J Cell Biol 109:863–875

Akiyama SK, Nagata K, Yamada KM (1990) Cell surface receptors for extracellular matrix components. Biochim Biophys Acta 1031:91–110

Albelda SM, Mette SA, Elder DE, Stewart R, Damjanovich L, Herlyn M, Buck CA (1990) Integrin distribution in malignant melanoma: association of the β_3 subunit with tumor progression. Cancer Res 50:6757–6764

Anichini A, Mortarini R, Berti E, Parmiani G (1990a) Multiple VLA antigens on a subset of melanoma clones. Hum Immunol 28:119–122

Anichini A, Mortarini R, Supino R, Parmiani G (1990b) Human melanoma cells with high susceptibility to cell-mediated lysis can be identified on the basis of ICAM-1 phenotype, VLA profile and invasive ability. Int J Cancer 46:508–515

Aresu O, Nicolò G, Allavena G, Melchiori A, Schmidt J, Kopp JB, d'Amore E, Chader GJ, Albini A (1991) Invasive activity, spreading on and chemotactic response to laminin are properties of high but not low metastatic mouse osteosarcoma cells. Invest Metastasis 11:2–13

Bröcker EB, Suter L, Brüggen J, Ruiter DJ, Macher E, Sorg C (1985) Phenotypic dynamics of tumor progression in human malignant melanoma. Int J Cancer 36:29–35

Burn P, Kupfer A, Singer J (1988) Dynamic membrane-cytoskeletal interactions: specific association of integrin and talin arises after phorbol ester treatment of peripheral blood lymphocytes. Proc Natl Acad Sci USA 85:497–501

Burridge K, Fath K, Kelly T, Nuckolls G, Turner C (1988) Focal adhesions: transmembrane junctions between the extracellular matrix and the cytoskeleton. Ann Rev Cell Biol 4:487–525

Carter WG, Wayner EA, Bouchard TS, Kaur P (1990) The role of integrins α2β1 and α3β1 in cell-cell and cell-substrate adhesion of human epidermal cells. J Cell Biol 110:1387–1404

Chammas R, Veiga SS, Line S, Potocnjak P, Brentani RR (1991) Asn-linked oligosacharide-dependent interaction between laminin and gp 120/140. J Biol Chem 266:3349–3355

Chan BMC, Matsuura N, Takada Y, Zetter BR, Hemler ME (1991) In vitro and in vivo consequences of VLA-2 expression on rhabdomyosarcoma cells. Science 251:1600–1602

Chen YQ, Nelson KK, Fitzgerald LA, Honn KV (1991) Detection of αIIbβ3 integrin in melanoma cells and its correlation with tumor cell metastasis. Proc Am Assoc Cancer Res 32:3–3

Cheresh DA, Spiro RC (1987) Biosynthetic and functional properties of an Arg-Gly-Asp-directed receptor involved in human cell attachment to vitronectin, fibrinogen, and von Willebrand factor. J Biol Chem 262:17703–17711

Cheresh DA, Smith JW, Cooper HM, Quaranta V (1989) A novel vitronectin receptor integrin (αvβx) is responsible for distinct adhesive properties of carcinoma cells. Cell 57:59–69

Clark WH Jr, Elder DE, Guerry D, Epstein ME, Greene MH, Van Horn MH (1984) A study of tumor progression. The precursor lesions of superficial spreading and nodular melanoma. Hum Pathol 15:1147–1156
Darribère T, Guida K, Larjava H, Johnsos KE, Yamada KM, Thiery J, Boucaut J (1990) In vivo analysis of integrin β1 subunit function in fibronectin matrix assembly. J Cell Biol 110:1813–1823
Dedhar S, Saulnier R (1990) Alterations in integrin receptor expression on chemically transformed human cells: specific enhancement of laminin and collagen receptor complexes. J Cell Biol 110:481–489
DeWit PEJ, Moretti S, Koenders PE, Weterman MAJ, Van Muijen GNP, Gianotti B, Ruiter DJ (1992) Increasing epidermal growth factor receptor expression in human melanocytic tumor progression. J Invest Dermatol 99:168–173
Diamond MS, Staunton DE, Martin SD, Springer TA (1991) Binding of the integrin Mac-1 (CD11b/CD18) to the third immunoglobulin-like domain of ICAM-1 (CD54) and its regulation by glycosylation. Cell 65:961–971
Elices MJ, Osborn L, Takada Y, Crouse C, Lubkowskyi S, Hemler ME, Lobb RR (1990) VCAM-1 on activated endothelium interacts with the leucocyte integrin VLA-4 at a site distinct from the VLA-4/fibronectin binding site. Cell 60:577–584
Erle DJ, Ruegg C, Sheppard D, Pytela R (1990) Complete amino acid sequence of an integrin β subunit (β7) identified in leucocytes. J Biol Chem 266:11009–11016
Fearon ER, Cho KR, Nigro JM, Kern SE, Simons JW, Ruppert JM, Hamilton SR, Preisinger AC, Thomas G, Kinzler KW, Vogelstein B (1990) Identification of a Chromosone 18q gene that is altered in colorectal cancers. Science 247:49–56
Fidler IJ (1988) The biology of melanoma metastasis. J Dermatol Surg Oncol 14:875–881
Geiger B, Ginsberg D (1991) The cytoplasmic domain of adherens type junctions. Cell Motil Cytoskeleton 20:1–6
Giancotti FG, Ruoslahti E (1990) Elevated levels of the α5β1 fibronectin receptor supress the transformed phenotype of chinese hamster ovary cells. Cell 60:849–859
Ginsberg MH, Loftus JC, Plow EF (1988) Cytoadhesins, integrins, and platelets. Thromb Haemost 59:1–6
Guan J, Hynes RO (1990) Lymphoid cells recognize an alternatively spliced segment of fibronectin via the integrin receptor α4β1. Cell 60:53–61
Hemler ME (1988) Adhesive protein receptors on hematopoietic cells. Immunol Today 41:109–113
Hemler ME (1990) VLA proteins in the integrin family: structures, functions, and their role on leucocytes. Ann Rev Immunol 8:365–400
Hemler ME, Huang C, Schwarz L (1987) The VLA protein family: characterization of five distinct cell surface heterodimers each with a common 130,000 molecular weight β subunit. J Biol Chem 262:3300–3309
Hemler ME, Crouse C, Sonnenberg A (1989) Association of the VLA α6 subunit with a novel protein: a possible alternative to the common VLA β1 subunit on certain cell lines. J Biol Chem 264:6529–6535
Herlyn M, Clark WH Jr, Rodeck U, Mancianti ML, Jambrosic J, Koprowski H (1987) Biology of tumor progression in human melanocytes. Lab Invest 66:461–474
Holzmann B, Johnson JP, Kaudewitz P, Riethmuller G (1985) In situ analysis of antigens on malignant and benign cells of the melanocytic lineage. J Exp Med 161:366–377
Holzmann B, Bröcker E-B, Lehmann J, Ruiter DJ, Sorg C, Riethmuller G, Johnson JP (1987) Tumor progression in human malignant melanoma: four sequential progression stages defined by their antigenic phenotypes. Int J Cancer 39:466–471

Holzmann B, McIntyre BW, Weissman IL (1989) Identification of a murine Peyers Patch-specific lymphocyte homing receptor as an integrin molecule with an α chain homologous to human VLA-4α. Cell 56:37–46

Hynes RO (1987) Integrins: a family of cell surface receptors. Cell 48:549–554

Johnson JP, Stade BG, Holzmann B, Schwable W, Riethmuller G (1989) De novo expression of intercellular-adhesion molecule 1 in melanoma correlates with increased risk of metastasis. Proc Natl Acad Sci USA 86:641–644

Kaufmann R, Frosch D, Westphal C, Weber L, Klein CE (1989) Integrin VLA-3: ultrastructural localization at cell-cell contact sites of human cell cultures. J Cell Biol 109:1807–1815

Kirchhofer D, Languino LR, Ruoslahti E, Pierschbacher MD (1990) α2β1 Integrins from different cell types show different binding specificities. J Biol Chem 265:615–618

Kishimoto TK, Larson RS, Corbi AL, Dustin ML, Staunton DE, Springer TA (1989) The leucocyte integrins. Adv Immunol 46:149–182

Klein CE, Steinmeyer T, Mattes J, Kaufmann R, Weber L (1990) Integrins of normal human epidermis: differential expression, synthesis and molecular structure. Br J Dermatol 123:171–178

Klein CE, Steinmeyer T, Kaufmann D, Weber L, Brocker EB (1991) Identification of a melanoma progression antigen as integrin VLA-2. J Invest Dermatol 96:281–284

Komoriya A, Green LJ, Mervic M, Yamada SS, Yamada KM, Humphries MJ (1991) The minimal essential sequence for a major cell type-specific adhesion site (CS1) within the alternatively spliced type III connecting segment domain of fibronectin is leucine-aspartic acid-valine. J Biol Chem 266:15075–15079

Krissansen GW, Elliot MJ, Lucas CM, Stomski FC, Berndt MC, Cheresh DA, Lopez AF, Burns GF (1990) Identification of a novel integrin β subunit expressed on cultured monocytes (macrophages). J Biol Chem 265:823–830

Kupfer A, Singer J (1989) Cell biology of cell couples. Ann Rev Immunol 7:309–337

Larjava H, Peltonen J, Akiyama SK, Yamada SS, Gralnick HR, Uitto J, Yamada KM (1990) Novel function for β1 integrins in keratinocyte cell-cell interactions. J Cell Biol 110:803–815

McDonald JA (1989) Receptors for extracellular matrix components. Am J Physiol 257:L331–L337

McDonald JA, Quade BJ, Broekelmann TJ, LaChance R, Forsman K, Hasegawa E, Akiyama S (1987) Fibronectin's cell-ahesive domain and an amino-terminal matrix assembly domain participate in its assembly into fibroblast pericellular matrix. J Biol Chem 262:2957–2967

McGregor BC, McGregor JL, Weiss LM, Wood GS, Hu C, Boukerche H, Warnke R (1989) Presence of cytoadhesins (IIb-IIIa-like glycoproteins) on human metastatic melanomas but not on benign melanocytes. Am J Clin Pathol 92:495–499

Mortarini R, Anichini A, Parmiani G (1991) Heterogeneity for integrin expression and cytokine-mediated VLA modulation can influence the adhesion of human melanoma cells to extracellular matrix proteins. Int J Cancer 47:551–559

Natali P, Nicotra M, Cavaliere R, Bigotti A, Romano G, Temponi M, Ferrone S (1990) Differential expression of intercellular adhesion molecule 1 in primary and metastatic melanoma lesions. Cancer Res 50:1271–1278

Nowell PC (1986) Mechanisms of tumor progression. Cancer Res 46:2203–2207

Osborn L, Hession C, Tizard R, Vassallo C, Luhowskyj S, Chi-Rosso G, Lobb RR (1989) Direct cloning of vascular cell adhesion molecule-1, a cytokine induced endothelial protein that binds to lymphocytes. Cell 59:1203–1211

Perrotti D, Cimino L, Tibursi RFG, Gentileschi MP, Sacchi A (1990) Metastatic phenotype: growth factor dependence and integrin expression. Anticancer Res 10:1587–1598

Plantefaber LC, Hynes R (1989) Changes in integrin receptors on oncogenically transformed cells. Cell 56:281–290
Pytela R (1988) Amino acid sequence of the murine Mac-1 α chain reveals homology with the integrin family and an additional domain related to von Willebrand factor. EMBO J 7:1371–1378
Quaranta V, Jones JCR (1991) The internal affairs of an integrin. Trends Cell Biol 1:2–4
Real FX, Rettig WJ, Garin Chesa P, Melamed MR, Old LJ, Mendelsohn J (1986) Expression of epidermal growth factor receptor in human cultured cells and tissues. Cancer Res 46:4726–4731
Ruiter DJ, Dingjan GM, Steylen PM, Van Beveren-Hooijer M, De Graaff-Reitsma CB, Bergman W, Van Muyen GNP, Warnaar SO (1985) Monoclonal antibodies selected to discriminate between malignant melanomas and nevocellular nevi. J Invest Dermatol 85:4–8
Ruoslahti E, Pierschbacher MD (1987) New perspectives in cell adhesion. Science 283:491–497
Sheppard D, Rozzo C, Starr L, Quaranta V, Erie DJ, Pytela R (1990) Complete amino acid sequence of a novel integrin β subunit (β6) identified in epithelial cells using the polymerase chain reaction. J Biol Chem 265:11502–11507
Springer TA (1990) Adhesion receptors of the immune system. Nature 346:425–434
Takeichi M (1991) Cadherin cell adhesion receptors as a morphogenetic regulator. Science 251:1451–1455
Tamkun JW, DeSimone DW, Fonda D, Patel RS, Buck C, Horwitz AF, Hynes RO (1986) Structure of integrin, a glycoprotein involved in the transmembrane linkage between fibronectin and actin. Cell 46:271–282
Terranova VP, Liotta LA, Russo RG, Martin GR (1982) Role of laminin in the attachment and metastasis of murine tumor cells. Cancer Res 42:2265–2269
Terranova VP, Rao CN, Kalebic T, Margulies IMK, Liotta LA (1983) Laminin receptor on human breast carcinoma cells. Proc Natl Acad Sci USA 80:444–451
Tetteroo PAT, Lansdorp PM, Leeksma OC, Von dem Borne AEG (1983) Monoclonal antibodies against human platelet glycoprotein IIIa. Br J Haematol 55:509
Van Kooyk Y, van de Wiel-van Kemenade P, Weder P, Kuijpers TW, Figdor CG (1989) Enhancement of LFA-1-mediated cell adhesion by triggering through CD2 or CD2 on T lymphocytes. Nature 342:811–813
Van Muijen GNP, Ruiter DJ, Hoefakker S, Johnson JP (1990) Monoclonal antibody PAL-M1 recognizes the transferrin receptor and is a progression marker in melanocytic lesions. J Invest Dermatol 95:65–69
Van Muijen GNP, Cornelissen LMHA, Jansen CFJ, Figdor CG, Johnson JP, Bröcker E, Ruiter DJ (1991) Antigen expression of metastasizing and non-metastasizing human melanoma cells xenografted into nude mice. Clin Exp Metastasis 9:259–272
Van Waes C, Kozarsky KF, Warren AB, Kidd L, Paugh D, Liebert M, Carey TE (1991) The A9 antigen associated with aggressive human squamous carcinoma is structurally and functionally similar to newly defined integrin α6β4. Cancer Res 51:2395–2402
Vleminckx K, Vakaet L, Mareel M, Fiers W, Van Roy F (1991) Genetic manipulation of E-cadherin expression by epithelial tumor cells reveals an invasion supressor role. Cell 66:107–119
Vogel BE, Tarone G, Giancotti FG, Gailit J, Ruoslahti E (1990) A novel fibronectin receptor with an unexpected subunit composition (αvβ1). J Biol Chem 265:5934–5937
Wayner EA, Garcia-Pardo A, Humphries MJ, McDonald JA, Carter WG (1989) Identification and characterization of the T-lymphocyte adhesion receptor for an

alternative cell attachment domain (CS-1) in plasma fibronectin. J Cell Biol 109:1321–1330
Zutter MM, Mazouijan G, Santoro SA (1990) Decreased expression of integrin adhesive receptors in adenocarcinoma of the breast. Am J Pathol 137:863–870

*Growth Regulation in Normal and Malignant Melanocytes**

R. Halaban

Yale University School of Medicine, Department of Dermatology, 500 LCI, P.O. Box 3333, New Haven, CT 06510-8050, USA

Introduction

The biochemical events responsible for the progression of normal melanocytes into preneoplastic cells, such as in dysplastic nevi, and further on into early malignant state such as in thin-radial melanoma, into nodular melanoma and culminating in metastatic disease are not yet known. One of the most common characteristics of melanoma cells grown in vitro from nodular primary or metastatic melanoma lesions is an acquired autonomy from growth factors required by their normal counterparts and possibly by melanocytes from primary melanomas of the radial growth phase. In view of the fact that normal human melanocytes depend on several growth factors, it is possible that progression to melanoma is due to inappropriate production of one or more of these factors, to mutations that cause constitutive activation of the receptors for these growth factors, or to constitutive activation of other components of the signal transduction pathway. Therefore knowledge of growth factors/receptors and their substrates operative in normal human melanocytes may provide clues for the biochemical basis of transformation to melanomas. The following review focuses on growth factor and receptor activity in normal and malignant melanocytes.

Melanocyte Proliferation

In order to proliferate in vitro, normal human melanocytes need at least two mutually synergistic factors in addition to the common growth factors

* A version of this article appeared in *Critical Reviews in Oncogenesis* (Halaban and Moellmann 1991).

Recent Results in Cancer Research, Vol. 128

required by all mammalian cells. The mitogenic peptides identified thus far that support human melanocytes in vitro are several members from the fibroblast growth factor (FGF) family, i.e., basic FGF (bFGF) (Halaban et al. 1987), acidic FGF (aFGF) (Halaban 1988, 1989), K-FGF/Hst-1 (Halaban et al. 1988), FGF-5, and FGF-6 (Halaban 1989; Halaban et al. 1991), and the unrelated hepatocyte growth factor (HGF) (Matsumoto et al. 1991; Rubin et al. 1991; Halaban et al. 1992) and mast cell growth factor (MGF, also known as Kit-ligand, stem cell growth factor and steel factor; Anderson et al. 1990a; Copeland et al. 1990; Flanagan et al. 1990; E. Huang et al. 1990; Martin et al. 1990; Williams et al. 1990; Zsebo et al. 1990a,b). All are known to stimulate receptors with tyrosine kinase activity (Coughlin et al. 1988; Friesel et al. 1989; Lee et al. 1989; Ruta et al. 1989; Dionne et al. 1990; Johnson et al. 1990; Safran et al. 1990; Bottaro et al. 1991; Naldini et al. 1991). These factors act as mitogens only in synergy with stimulators of protein kinase A (PKA) such as dibutyryl cyclic adenosine monophosphate (dbcAMP), or protein kinase C (PKC) such as TPA (12-*O*-tetradecanoylphorbol-13-acetate) (Halaban 1988, 1989, 1991; Halaban et al. 1987; Halaban et al. 1988b, 1991; Matsumoto et al. 1991; Rubin et al. 1991). bFGF and HGF also act in synergy with each other (Matsumoto et al. 1991; Halaban et al. 1992).

bFGF appears to play a central role in melanocyte biology. In situ, the peptide is provided by basal keratinocytes (Schulze-Osthoff et al. 1990; Scott et al. 1991). Unlike other cells that respond to bFGF, normal melanocytes do not produce this peptide on their own. bFGF is expressed neither at the messenger (m)RNA nor at protein level (Halaban et al. 1988a; Halaban 1989; Albino et al. 1991; Rodeck et al. 1991). In fact, melanocytes do not produce any mitogen that stimulates their own growth (our unpublished results), which is the reason for their failure to proliferate in media suitable for other cell types, including metastatic melanoma cells. In contrast, proliferating fibroblasts and keratinocytes produce bFGF and, in coculture with melanocytes, maintain melanocyte viability (De Luca et al. 1988; Halaban et al. 1988b; Scott and Haak 1991). Like purified bFGF, mitogenicity of whole-cell extracts of fibroblasts and keratinocytes depends on dbcAMP, indicating that in vivo, melanocyte proliferation is restricted by the absence of a complementary mitogen. UVB irradiation of keratinocytes doubles the level of their mitogenic activity due to increase in bFGF (Halaban et al. 1988; Halaban et al. 1993). In addition, UVB irradiation of pure melanocyte cultures causes an increase in [^{3}H]thymidine incorporation but only when the culture medium is supplemented with TPA or bFGF, indicating that UVB light provides the cAMP requirements (Halaban et al. 1988b; our unpublished results). These findings suggest that, in vivo, melanocytes are regulated by keratinocyte-derived mitogens, the abundance of which is augmented by at least one agent that also induces pigmentation, namely UVB irradiation.

Melanocyte Differentiation

Exogenous growth factors promote not only melanocyte proliferation but also differentiation. bFGF, for example, stimulates the expression of the melanocytic phenotype in embryonic quail dorsal root ganglia (Stocker et al. 1991), and MGF increases the level of melanin production in human fetal melanocytes (unpublished results). In fact, any substance that stimulates the proliferation of normal or malignant melanocytes on addition to the culture medium also stimulates the production of melanocyte-specific mRNAs, the enzyme tyrosinase, and the final product, melanin (Halaban et al. 1983; Kwon et al. 1987, 1988). Therefore, signal transduction from exogenous growth factors triggers a cascade of events leading to proliferation and expression of melanocytic differentiated functions.

Signal transduction from endogenous growth factors that accumulate in the cells due to absence of a signal peptide may abrogate the expression of differentiated functions. The introduction of bFGF complementary (c)DNA into the murine melanocyte line L-B10.BR via a recombinant retrovirus conferred, as expected, autonomous growth in culture (Dotto et al. 1989). Not necessarily expected was the loss of all differentiated functions, including pigmentation, expression of tyrosinase (the key enzyme in melanin synthesis), synthesis of melanosomes (the subcellular organelles in which melanin is normally deposited), and formation of dendrites. The bFGF-transformed melanocyte no longer resembles its original counterpart but rather appears like a fibroblast or endothelial cell (Dotto et al. 1989). Though independent of exogenous growth factor in vitro, the transformants were not malignant in that they failed to grow as tumors in syngeneic or nude mice. Instead, in vivo, they regained their differentiated functions, including the ability to produce melanin, and behaved in all respects like normal melanocytes. These observations suggest that differentiation of melanocytes is dependent on continuous stimulation at the cell surface and, possibly, endocytosis. The endogenous bFGF produced in transfected melanocytes appears to activate a pathway that maintains only proliferation but not differentiation. Whether this pathway is the same as the one that is part of the transduction cascade after external stimulation is not known. As mentioned before, bFGF does not have a signal peptide and is probably not transported by the same subcellular route as the membrane-bound glycoprotein receptors that circulate to and from the cell surface.

Surface Receptors and Signal Transduction

Both high- and low-affinity classes of receptor for basic and acidic FGF have been identified and their cDNAs cloned. The high-affinity receptors are tyrosine protein kinases of 125 and 145 kDa (Neufeld and Gospodarowicz

1985; Huang and Huang 1986; Imamura et al. 1988; Coughlin et al. 1988; Friesel et al. 1989; Lee et al. 1989; Ruta et al. 1989; Johnson et al. 1990; Bottaro et al. 1990; Safran et al. 1990; Hattori et al. 1990; Dionne et al. 1990; Kiefer et al. 1990; Eiseman et al. 1991; Partanen et al. 1991; Avivi et al. 1991; Keegan et al. 1991). There are at least four different genes encoding variants of FGF-R. They are designated *FGF-R1*, *FGF-R2* (formerly *flg* and *bek*), *FGF-R3*, and *FGF-R4*. The amino acid sequences deduced from the respective cDNAs show that all four receptors belong to the immunoglobulin superfamily of proteins. The significance of the FGF receptor variants is not clear, but perhaps the different isoforms play a role in different tissues, or during different developmental stages, as shown already for FGF-R1 and FGF-R4 (Partanen et al. 1991; Barnard et al. 1991). In addition, an mRNA species encoding only the extracellular domain of the FGF receptor has been cloned (Johnson et al. 1990; Eiseman et al. 1991), suggesting the existence of a soluble FGF binding protein whose function is also not yet known.

The low-affinity receptor was shown to be a membrane-bound heparan sulfate proteoglycan (HSPG) (Kiefer et al. 1990), and the suggestion was made that binding of bFGF to cell surface HSPG was obligatory for binding to high-affinity receptors, because a Chinese hamster ovary (CHO) cell mutant expressing the high- but not the low-affinity receptors did not bind bFGF unless heparan sulfate was included in the binding medium (Yayon et al. 1991). Indeed, direct involvement of surface heparin sulfate was demonstrated in fibroblasts' growth and myoblasts' differentiation by treating the cells with agents that remove heparan sulfate or block sulfation, such as heparitinase and sodium chlorate, respectively (Rapraeger et al. 1991). However, the significance of high- versus low-affinity FGF receptors is clearly not fully understood, since an HSPG with high affinity to aFGF has recently been identified in a rat parathyroid cell line (Sakagushi et al. 1991).

The integral membrane high-affinity glycoprotein FGF receptors are tyrosine kinases, which undergo autophosphorylation and induce a cascade of activation phosphorylations of target proteins (see Yarden and Ullrich 1988 for review on receptor tyrosine kinases). Binding of bFGF and aFGF to NIH 3T3 cells induces autophosphorylation of 125- and 145-kDa receptor proteins and phosphorylation of additional proteins of 145, 90, 46, and 42 kDa (Huang and Huang 1986; Imamura et al. 1988; Coughlin et al. 1988; Friesel et al. 1989). The additional 145-kDa phosphoprotein was identified as phospholipase Cγ (Coughlin et al. 1988; Burgess et al. 1990; Cuadrado and Molloy 1990). This enzyme hydrolyzes the membrane phospholipid phosphatidylinositol-4,5-bisphosphate (PIP_2) to form two second messengers: 1,2-diacylglycerol (DG), which activates protein kinase C, and inositol triphosphate, which causes release of calcium from internal stores (Berridge and Irvine 1984). Stimulation of protein kinase C by bFGF was demonstrated in bovine aortic endothelial cells (Presta et al. 1989).

The 40–42-kDa phosphoproteins were identified as extracellular signal-regulated kinases (ERKs), also known as microtubule-associated protein kinases (MAP kinases), a group of related enzymes that are common intermediates in cell surface receptor signal transduction (Ahn and Krebs 1990; Anderson et al. 1990b; Boulton and Cobb 1991; Boulton et al. 1991a,b; Kawakami et al. 1991; L'Allemain et al. 1991). ERKs are serine/threonine kinases that integrate signals from more then one phosphorylation pathway because they require phosphorylation on tyrosyl and threonyl residues for activation. They phosphorylate and activate S6 kinase, leading to phosphorylation of ribosomal protein S6 and concomitant acceleration of protein synthesis (Sturgill et al. 1988; Gregory et al. 1989; Ahn and Krebs 1990). Recently, two other substrates for MAP kinases were identified, Raf-1, also a serine/threonine kinase whose activation is mediated by growth factors (Anderson et al. 1991; Lee et al. 1992) and c-Jun (Pulverer et al. 1991). Therefore, activation of the FGF receptor tyrosine kinase leads to stimulation of possibly two serine/threonin kinases and a transcription factor, a pattern observed also with other receptor tyrosine kinases (reviewed in Cantley et al. 1991).

In melanocytes, the same intermediates are probably operative because bFGF elicits the appearance of 125- and 40–42-kDa phosphoproteins and causes an increase in MAP kinase activity (Funasaka et al. 1992). In addition, melanoma cells expressing bFGF (see below) also have higher basal levels of MAP kinase activity, suggesting that this enzyme is important for melanocyte proliferation (Funasaka et al. 1992).

The role of exogenous FGFs may not be restricted to activation of the FGF receptors at the cell surface. Both basic and acidic FGF have been localized in the nucleus (Baldin et al. 1990; Imamura et al. 1990; Tessler and Neufeld 1990). Two aFGF gene products with mutations at the nuclear targeting domain that abolish nuclear localization were unable to initiate cell proliferation and DNA synthesis in NIH 3T3 fibroblasts, even though they were able to bind to the FGF receptor, stimulate the phosphorylation of membrane bound and cytosolic proteins, and induce *c-fos* expression, an early response of endothelial cells to aFGF (Imamura et al. 1990). On the other hand, a six-amino-acid deletion in the amino acid sequence similar to that proposed to target aFGF to the nucleus did not affect the mitogenic activity of bFGF toward several cell types, including NIH 3T3 fibroblasts, but reduced by two orders of magnitude the ability of the peptide to stimulate the production of plasminogen activator in endothelial cells (Isacchi et al. 1991). In this experiment, the cellular localization of the bFGF was not determined, but others have shown that the various forms of bFGF, all fully mitogenic, display different cellular localization, the smallest form occurring predominantly in the cytosol, while the higher molecular weight forms of 22, 22.5 and 24 kDa are associated with the nucleus and ribosomes; the nuclear localization of the higher molecular weight forms resides within the NH_2-terminal extension (Quarto et al.

1991). Thus, the detailed molecular pathways by which FGFs stimulate their target cells is not entirely elucidated. Knowledge of these pathways may, however, be important for learning the reason why bFGF, aberrantly produced intracellularly by bFGF-transfected melanocytes or metastatic melanoma cells (see below), causes extinction of differentiated functions, whereas when supplied extracelluarly, it induces and maintains the melanocytic phenotype.

FGFs and Malignant Transformation

Basic FGF is probably the principal factor that stimulates growth of melanocytes in melanocytic lesions. mRNA for bFGF can be detected in dysplastic and dermal nevi, as well as in primary and metastatic melanomas, by in situ hybridization with a bFGF riboprobe (Scott et al. 1991). Mitogenic activity toward normal human melanocytes was verified in freshly excised dermal nevi (our unpublished results) and in cultures of advanced primary and metastatic melanoma cells (Moscatelli et al. 1986; Lobb et al. 1986; Halaban et al. 1987, 1988a; Ogata et al. 1987). Melanoma cells that proliferate in culture autonomously depend on intrinsic bFGF, because internalized neutralizing anti-bFGF antibodies (Halaban et al. 1988a) and antisense, but not sense, oligodeoxynucleotides targeted against human bFGF mRNA (Becker et al. 1989) inhibit their growth. Antisense oligodeoxynucleotides to nerve growth factor mRNA and insulin-like growth factor I mRNA are not inhibitory, suggesting that the respective peptides, which are produced by melanoma cells, are not sufficient to give autocrine growth advantage to melanomas in vitro (Becker et al. 1989).

Intrinsic bFGF appears to stimulate melanoma cells through an internal loop, because bFGF neutralizing antibodies inhibit melanoma growth only when injected into the cells but not by simple addition to the culture medium (Halaban et al. 1988a). As mentioned above, expression of intrinsic bFGF alone was insufficient to confer the malignant phenotype on melanocytes in vivo (Dotto et al. 1989). Likewise, the melanocytes in dysplastic nevi that express bFGF mRNA (Scott et al. 1991) are not malignant. People with the dysplastic nevus syndrome, who may have hundreds of dysplastic nevi known to be precursors for melanoma, develop at best only a small number of primaries (Greene et al. 1985). The spontaneous expression of bFGF in melanomas is probably due to gene activation rather than amplification or rearrangement (Theillet et al. 1989; Halaban et al. 1991). The gene for bFGF has been mapped to human chromosome region 4q26-q27 (Mergia et al. 1986; Lafage-Pochitaliff et al. 1990) but chromosome 4 is not among those known to be affected in melanomas (Balaban et al. 1984; Cowan et al. 1988; Trent et al. 1990a; Cowan and Francke 1991).

bFGF receptor kinase activity is critical for the proliferation of melanomas, because synthetic bFGF peptides that span the receptor's ligand-binding domain and act as bFGF antagonists inhibit melanoma cell growth (Halaban et al. 1988a). Sequences from nonrelevant domains do not have this effect (Halaban et al. 1988a). Likewise, internalized anti-phosphotyrosine antibodies and anti-sense FGF-R mRNA inhibit melanoma cell growth (Halaban et al. 1988a; Becker et al. 1993), again suggesting growth inhibition via abrogation of receptor activity. In agreement with the importance of bFGF receptor activity in melanoma growth is our recent finding that the bFGF receptor is constitutively phosphorylated in metastatic human melanomas (Halaban et al. 1991). The receptor appeared to be encoded by *flg*, resulting in a 125-kDa protein compatible with the two-loop form of receptor (Halaban et al. 1991). *FGF-R1* and *-R2* genes (*flg* and *bek*) are not amplified or rearranged in nine metastatic melanomas so tested (Halaban et al. 1991; Becker et al. 1993) and the receptor protein is not expressed at abnormally high levels (Becker et al. 1993). Taken together, the data indicate that melanoma growth is due to intrinsic, intracellular activation but not overexpression of the bFGF receptor.

Southern blot analysis of other genes from the FGF family has shown that two of the 15 melanomas tested contained amplification of the linked FGF-related oncogenes *int-2* and *K-FGF/hst* (Adelaide et al. 1988; Halaban et al. 1991). However, in one such melanoma, YU SIT1, with 12-fold amplification of the *int-2* and *K-FGF* genes, both known to encode secreted factors (Moore et al. 1986; Delli Bovi and Basilico 1987; Taira et al. 1987), there was no mitogenic activity in the culture medium toward normal human melanocytes (Halaban 1991; Halaban et al. 1991) and the corresponding mRNAs were not detectable on Northern blot. The cell-associated mitogenic activity toward melanocytes in this melanoma was neutralized by antibodies specific for bFGF (Halaban 1991; Halaban et al. 1991). These results suggest that the amplification of the *int-2* and *K-FGF/hst* genes was of no consequence to the viability of the melanoma cells. More recently, the polymerase chain reaction (PCR) was used to detect low levels of transcripts for several growth factors in 19 melanoma and 14 normal pigment cell lines (Albino et al. 1991). This study confirmed the reports, discussed above, on the pattern of expression of mRNAs for bFGF and K-FGF. Furthermore, it showed that mRNAs for aFGF and FGF-5 were present in 15% and 25%, respectively, of the melanomas cell lines tested but not in normal melanocytes, whereas mRNA for KGF, a peptide not mitogenic for normal melanocytes, was expressed in almost all of the normal and malignant melanocyte lines (Albino et al. 1991).

Other Growth Factors for Melanocytes, and Their Relationship to the FGF Family of Peptides

Because a single growth factor is not sufficient to sustain melanocyte proliferation, and because activation of FGF receptors by internal bFGF is not sufficient to confer tumorigenicity, it is likely that, in vivo, additional receptor kinases play a synergistic role. MGF and HGF, the two melanocyte mitogens not related to the FGFs, stimulate the tyrosine-kinase receptors known as c-KIT and MET, respectively. c-KIT, like the FGF receptors, is a member of the immunoglobulin superfamily of genes (Yarden et al. 1987; Qiu et al. 1988; Chabot et al. 1988; Geissler et al. 1988), and MET is a member of the insulin growth factor receptor family (Bottaro et al. 1991; Naldini et al. 1991).

MGF and its receptor are known to be important for optimal melanoblast viability. Mice with mutations at the dominant white spotting (*W*) and steel (*Sl*) loci, encoding c-*kit* and *mgf*, respectively (Yarden et al. 1987; Qiu et al. 1988; Chabot et al. 1988; Geissler et al. 1988; Copeland et al. 1990; Flanagan and Leder 1990; E. Huang et al. 1990; Zsebo et al. 1990a), have a deficiency either in the receptor-tyrosine kinase or its ligand (Nocka et al. 1989, 1990; Reith et al. 1990; Tan et al. 1990; Brannan et al. 1991; Flanagan et al. 1991). In addition to the white spots, *W* and *Sl* mutations in mice cause anemia and sterility by reducing the proliferation and differentiation of hematopoietic and germ cells (Nocka et al. 1989, 1990; Reith et al. 1990; Tan et al. 1990; Brannan et al. 1991; Flanagan et al. 1991). Human melanocytes are also dependent on c-KIT kinase for normal distribution because several missense mutations, deletions, and duplications causing dysfunction of KIT have been identified in some human piebaldism (Giebel and Spritz 1991; Fleischman et al. 1991; Spritz et al. 1992a,b; Fleischam 1992; Bernstein et al. in preparation).

v-*kit*, the oncogenic form of c-*kit*, induces sarcomas in cats (Yarden et al. 1987; Qiu et al. 1988) and a chimeric molecule, composed of the extracellular portion of the EGF receptor and the transmembrane and cytoplasmic domain of c-Kit, confers an EGF-dependent transformed phenotype on NIH 3T3 cells (Bottaro et al. 1991). *MET* has been identified as an oncogene by transfection of NIH-3T3 cells with DNA from a carcinogen-treated human osteosarcoma cell line (Cooper et al. 1984; Bottaro et al. 1991; reviewed in gherandi and Stoker 1991). It was, therefore, of particular interest to determine the role of *KIT* and *MET* gene products in melanomas.

We found that c-KIT, activated by MGF, is one of the most abundant tyrosine-phosphorylated proteins in normal human melanocytes. MGF triggers the tyrosine phosphorylation of several proteins, the most prominent one being c-KIT itself. Among the KIT-kinase substrates and intermediates identified so far in normal human melanocytes is MAP2 kinase (Funasaka et al. 1992). Several metastatic melanoma cell lines, however, were not stimulated by MGF, and in these, c-*KIT* mRNA was expressed only at normal levels in three out of 12 melanomas (Funasaka et al. 1992). Although MGF, the ligand of c-KIT, was aberrantly expressed by several of the melanoma cell lines tested (it was not expressed in normal melanocytes), the growth factor probably did not contribute to autonomous growth, because these cells lacked the receptor (Funasaka et al. 1992). The growth of melanoma lines expressing normal levels of c-*KIT* mRNA and proteins in which MGF stimulated c-KIT phosphorylation was not stimulated but rather inhibited by the ligand (Funasaka et al. 1992; Zakut et al. 1993). Therefore, c-KIT receptor kinase activity does not positively regulate melanoma proliferation and its absence may actually contribute to their dedifferentiated phenotype, because MGF promoted melanization, as mentioned above.

MET, phosphorylated in response to HGF, activates in melanocytes several substrates and intermediates through a cascade of tyrosine phosphorylations (Halaban et al. 1992). In melanomas, MET is not constitutively activated but, as in normal melanocytes, is stimulated by exogenous ligand, suggesting that melanoma cells do not themselves express the growth factor (Halaban et al. 1992). MET activation through extrinsic HGF probably promotes melanoma growth in synergy with intrinsic bFGF because the two peptides stimulate conversing pathways in melanocytes. Because HGF is known to be not only a growth but also a cell-scatter factor, and to increase the motility of melanocytes and other cell types, including keratinocytes (Lev et al. 1990), the peptide may contribute to the dissemination of melanoma cells from primary to ectopic, metastatic sites. Preferential metastasis to the liver was shown to be the result of a melanoma growth factor produced by hepatocytes (Sargent et al. 1988). This growth factor may be HGF.

Concluding Remarks

Extensive studies in vitro on growth factors and growth factor receptors in normal and malignant melanocytes have shown so far that expression of bFGF and activation of the bFGF-R is probably necessary, but not sufficient, to confer tumorigenicity. The other receptors active in the melanocyte system, c-KIT and MET, are not constitutively active in melanomas and therefore their activity does not positively contribute to the malignant phenotype. The question still remains what are the cooperating factors that act in synergy with bFGF. It is possible that future work may unravel a new growth factor/receptor system that plays a critical role in human melanocyte biology. A receptor from the EGF receptor family, *erbB*-like, was shown to be a constitutively active tumor gene in fish (Anders et al. 1984; Zechel et al. 1988; Wittbrodt et al. 1989), and its homolog has recently been identified in mammalian cells (Schartle et al., unpublished). It is not yet clear, however, whether it is constitutively active in melanoma cells. In transgenic mice, expression of mutant *ret*, also encoding a constitutively active receptor tyrosine kinase related to c-*KIT*, caused the appearance of melanoma in adult animals (Iwamoto et al. 1991); however, expression of c-*RET* mRNA is not widespread in human cells and was shown to be at high levels only in three of 28 different human tumors not including melanomas.

Alternatively, a cooperating factor could be loss of a tumor suppressor gene implied to exist in mammalian melanocytes because tumorigenicity is suppressed in somatic cell hybrids made between normal and malignant cells, and in melanoma cells after transfer of normal chromosome 6 (Fougère et al. 1972; Straus et al. 1976; Halaban et al. 1980; Trent et al. 1990b; Wakeling et al. 1992). The fish melanoma model mentioned above clearly provides genetic evidence for the existence of a tumor suppressor gene because the development of melanomas was dependent on the loss of a tissue-specific gene which has not yet been characterized (Anders et al. 1984; Zechel et al. 1988; Wittbrodt et al. 1989). More recently, a gene, *nm23*, that suppresses melanoma metastatic spread, but not tumor growth, was identified in murine and human cells (Leone et al. 1991). The gene encodes a protein of 17 kDa that shares approximately 75% identity with the product of the *awd* gene in *Drosophila*, which had been shown to control morphogenesis and to have a nucleotide diphosphate kinase activity, associated with microtubule polymerization. Another type of tumor suppressor gene, not yet identified in melanomas, could be a protein tyrosine phosphatase (Hunter 1990; Fischer et al. 1991), since absence of such an enzyme could enhance the tyrosine kinase activity of the FGF receptor.

A full account of events participating in the progression from preneoplastic lesions to metastatic melanomas should also take environmental influences into account. Tumor cells in vivo can be restrained by environmental factors, as shown in the case of melanoma formation by melanocytes expressing the *neu* oncogene encoding a transmembrane receptor with a constitutively active tyrosine protein kinase, aborted by the cografting of keratinocytes but not fibroblasts (Dotto et al. 1989). In another study, a B16 murine melanoma inhibitor was found to be secreted by excised embryonic mouse skin (10- to 14-day-old embryos) but not by the skin of newborn mice (Gerschenson et al. 1986). More recently, Cornil and his collaborators (1991) showed that dermal fibroblasts repressed the growth of melanocytes from early stages of primary melanoma, but stimulated the growth of melanocytes from advanced metastatic melanomas. The nature of the melanoma inhibitors was identified as Interleukin 6 (Lu et al. 1992). Future research will undoubtly contribute further to our understanding of factors controlling malignant transformation of melanocytes.

References

Adelaide J, Mattei M-G, Marics I, Raybaud F, Planche J, De Lapeyriere O, Birnbaum D (1988) Chromosomal localization of the *hst* oncogene and its co-amplification with the *int*.2 oncogene in human melanoma. Oncogene 2:413–416

Ahn NG, Krebs EG (1990) Evidence for an epidermal growth factor-stimulated protein kinase cascade in Swiss 3T3 cells. J Biol Chem 265:11495–11501

Albino AP, Davis BM, Nanus DM (1991) Induction of growth factor RNA expression in human malignant melanoma: markers of transformation. Cancer Res 51:4815–4820

Anders F, Schartl M, Barnekow A, Anders A (1984) *Xiphophorus* as an *in vivo* model for studies on normal and defective control of oncogenes. Adv Cancer Res 42:191–275

Anderson DM, Lyman SD, Baird A, Wignall J, Eisenman J, Rauch C, March CJ, Boswell HS, Gimpel SD, Cosman D, Williams DD (1990a) Molecular cloning of mast cell growth factor, a hematopoietin that is active in both membrane bound and soluble forms. Cell 63:235–243

Anderson NG, Maller JL, Tonks NK, Sturgill TW (1990b) Requirement for integration of signals from two distinct phosphorylation pathways for activation of MAP kinase. Nature 343:651–653

Anderson NG, Li P, Marsden LA, Williams N, Roberts TM, Sturgill TW (1991) Raf-1 is a potential substrate for mitogen-activated protein kinase in vivo. Biochem J 277:573–576

Avivi A, Zimmer Y, Yayon A, Yarden Y, Givol D (1991) Flg-2, a new member of the family of fibroblast growth factor receptors. Oncogene 6:1089–1092

Balaban G, Herlyn M, Guerry IV D, Bartolo R, Koprowski H, Clark WH, Nowell PC (1984) Cytogenetics of human malignant melanoma and premalignant lesions. Cancer Genet Cytogenet 11:429–439

Baldin V, Roman A-M, Bosc-Bierne I, Almaric F, Bouche G (1990) Translocation of bFGF to the nucleus is G_1 phase cell cycle specific in bovine aortic endothelial cells. EMBO J 9:1511–1517

Becker D, Meier CB, Herlyn M (1989) Proliferation of human malignant melanomas is inhibited by antisense oligodeoxynucleotides targeted against basic fibroblast growth factor. EMBO J 8:3685–3691

Becker D, Lee PL, Rodeck U, Herlyn M (1992) Inhibition of the fibroblast growth factor receptor 1 (FGFR-1) gene in human melanocytes and malignant melanomas leads to inhibition of proliferation and signs indicative of differentiation. Oncogene 7:2303–2313

Berridge MJ, Irvine RF (1984) Inositol triphosphate, a novel second messenger in cellular signal transduction. Nature 312:315–320

Barnard O, Li M, Reid HH (1991) Expression of two different forms of fibroblast growth factor receptor 1 in different mouse tissues and cell lines. Proc Natl Acad Sci USA 88:7625–7629

Bottaro DP, Rubin JS, Ron D, Finch PW, Florio C, Aaronson SA (1990) Characterization of the receptor for keratinocyte growth factor. J Biol Chem 265:12767–12770

Bottaro DP, Rubin JS, Faletto DL, Chan A, M-L, Kmiecik TE, Vande Woude GP, Aaronson SA (1991) Identification of the HGF receptor as the *c-met* protooncogene product. Science 251:802–804

Boulton TG, Cobb MH (1991) Identification of multiple extracellular signal-regulated kinases (ERKs) with antipeptide antibodies. Cell Regul 2:357–371

Boulton TG, Gregory JS, Cobb MH (1991a) Purification and properties of extracellular signal-regulated kinase 1, an insulin-stimulated microtubule-associated protein 2 kinase. Biochemistry 30:278–286

Boulton TG, Nye SH, Robbins DJ, Ip NY, Radziejewska E, Morgenbesser SD, DePinho RA, Panayotatos N, Cobb MH, GD, Yancopoulos GD (1991b) ERKs: a family of protein-serine/threonine kinases that are activated and tyrosine phosphorylated in response to insulin and NGF. Cell 65:663–675

Brannan CI, Lyman SD, Williams DE, Eisenman J, Anderson D, Cosman D, Bedell MA, Jenkins NA, Copeland NG (1991) Steel-Dickie mutation encodes a c-Kit ligand lacking transmembrane and cytoplasmic domains. Proc Natl Acad Sci USA 88:4671–4674

Burgess WH, Dionne CA, Kaplow J, Mudd R, Friesel R, Zilberstein A, Schlessinger J, Jaye M (1990) Characterization and cDNA cloning of phospholipase C-g, a

major substrate for heparin-binding growth factor 1 (acidic fibroblast growth factor)-activated tyrosine kinase. Mol Cell Biol 10:4770–4777
Cantley LC, Auger KR, Carpenter C, Duckworth B, Graziani A, Kapeller R, Soltoff S (1991) Oncogenes and signal transduction. Cell 64:281–302
Chabot B, Stephenson DA, Chapman VM, Besmer P, Bernstei A (1988) The proto-oncogene c-kit encoding a transmembrane tyrosine kinase receptor maps to the mouse *W* locus. Nature 335:88–89
Cooper CS, Park M, Blair DG, Tainsky MA, Huebner K, Croce CM, Vande Woude GF (1984) Molecular cloning of a new transforming gene from a chemically transformed human cell line. Nature 311:29–33
Copeland N, Gilbert DJ, Cho BC, Donovan PJ, Jenkins NA, Cosman D, Anderson D, Lyman SD, Williams DE (1990) Mast cell growth factor maps near the steel locus on mouse chromosome 10 and is deleted in a number of steel alleles. Cell 63:175–183
Cornil I, Theodorescu D, Man S, Herlyn M, Jambrosic J (1991) Fibroblast cell interactions with human melanoma cells affect tumor growth as a function of tumor progression. Proc Natl Acad Sci USA 88:6028–6032
Coughlin SR, Barr PJ, Cousens LS, Fretto LJ, Williams LT (1988) Acidic and basic fibroblast growth factors stimulate tyrosine kinase activity *in vivo*. J Biol Chem 263:988–993
Cowan JM, Francke U (1991) Cytogenetic analysis in melanoma and nevi. In: Nathanson L (ed) Melanoma research: genetics, growth factors, metastases, and antigens. Kluwer, Boston, pp 3–16
Cowan JM, Halaban R, Francke U (1988) Cytogenetic analysis of melanocytes from premalignant nevi and melanomas. J Natl Cancer Inst 80:1159–1164
Cuadrado A, Molloy CJ (1990) Overexpression of phospholipase C-γ in NIH 3T3 fibroblasts results in increased phosphatidylinositol hydrolysis in response to platelet-derived growth factor and basic fibroblast growth factor. Mol Cell Biol 10:6069–6072
De Luca M, D'Anna F, Bondanza S, Franzi AT, Cancedda R (1988) Human epithelial cells induce human melanocyte growth in vitro but only skin keratinocytes regulate its proper differentiation in the absence of dermis. J Cell Biol 107:1919–1926
Delli Bovi P, Basilico C (1987) Isolation of a rearranged human transforming gene following transfection of Kaposi sarcoma DNA. Proc Natl Acad Sci USA 84:5660–5664
Dionne CA, Crumley G, Bellot F, Kaplow JM, Searfoss G, Ruta M, Burgess WH, Jaye M, Schlessinger J (1990) Cloning and expression of two distinct high affinity receptors cross-reacting with acidic and basic fibroblast growth factors. EMBO J 9:2685–2692
Dotto P, Moellmann G, Ghosh S, Edwards M, Halaban R (1989) Transformation of murine melanocytes with basic fibroblast growth factor cDNA and oncogenes and selective suppression of the transformed phenotype in a reconstituted cutaneous environment. J Cell Biol 109:3115–3128
Eiseman A, Ahn JA, Graciani G, Tronick SR, Ron D (1991) Alternative splicing generates at least 5 different isoforms of the human bFGF-receptor. Oncogene 6:1195–1202
Fischer EH, Charbonneau H, Tonks NK (1991) Protein kinase phosphatases: a diverse family of intracellular and transmembrane enzymes. Science 253:401–406
Flanagan JG, Leder P (1990) The *kit* ligand: a cell surface molecule altered in steel mutant fibroblasts. Cell 63:185–194
Flanagan JG, Chan DG, Leder P (1991) Transmembrane form of the *kit* ligand growth factor is determined by alternative splicing and is missing in the Sl^d mutant. Cell 64:1025–1035

Fleischman RA (1992) Human piebald trait resulting from a dominant negative mutant allele of the c-*kit* membrane receptor gene. J Clin Invest 89:1713–1717
Fleischman RA, Saltman DL, Stastny V, Zneimer S (1991) Deletion of the c-*kit* protooncogene in the human developmental defect piebald trait. Proc Natl Acad Sci USA 88:10885–10889
Fougère C, Ruiz F, Ephrussi B (1972) Gene dosage dependence of pigment synthesis in melanoma x fibroblast hybrids. Proc Natl Acad Sci USA 69:330–334
Friesel R, Burgess WH, Maciag T (1989) Heparin-binding growth factor 1 stimulates tyrosine phosphorylation in NIH 3T3 cells. Mol Cell Biol 9:1857–1865
Funasaka Y, Boulton T, Cobb M, Yosef Y, Fan B, Lyman SD, Williams DE, Anderson DM, Zakut R, Mishima Y, Halaban (1992) c-Kit-kinase induces a cascade of protein tyrosine phosphorylation in normal human protein melanocytes in response to mast cell growth factor and stimulates mitogen-activated kinase, but is down regulated in melanomas. Mol Biol Cell 3:197–209
Geissler EN, Ryan MA, Housman DE (1988) The dominant-white spotting (*W*) locus of the mouse encodes the c-*kit* proto-oncogene. Cell 55:185–192
Gerschenson M, Graves K, Carson SD, Wells RS, Pierce B (1986) Regulation of melanoma by the embryonic skin. Proc Natl Acad Sci USA 83:7307–7310
Gherardi E, Stoker M (1991) Hepatocyte growth factor-scatter factor: mitogen, motogen, and *met*. Cancer Cells 3:227–232
Giebel LB, Spritz RA (1991) Mutation of the c-kit (mast/stem cell growth factor receptor) proto-oncogene in human piebaldism. Proc Natl Acad Sci USA 88:8696–8699
Greene MH, Clark WH Jr, Tucker MA, Kraemer KH, Elder DE, Fraser MC (1985) High risk of malignant melanoma in melanoma-prone families with dysplastic nevi. Ann Intern Med 102:458–465
Gregory J, Boulton T, Sang BC, Cobb J (1989) An insulin-stimulated ribosomal protein S6 kinase from rabbit liver. J Biol Chem 264:18377–18401
Halaban R (1988) Responses of cultured melanocytes to defined growth factors. Pigm Cell Res 1:18–26
Halaban R (1989) Growth regulation in normal and malignant melanocytes. In: Ferrone S (ed) Human melanoma. Springer, Berlin Heidelberg New York, pp 3–14
Halaban R (1991) The regulatory role of fibroblast growth factor in melanomas. In: Nathanson L (ed) Melanoma 5. Kluwer, Norwell, pp 19–40 (Cancer treatment and research series)
Halaban R, Moellmann G (1991) Proliferation and malignant transformation of melanocytes. Crit Rev Oncogen 2:247–258
Halaban R, Moellmann G, Godawska E, Eisenstadt J (1980) Pigmentation and tumorigenicity of reconstituted, cybrid and hybrid mouse cells. Exp Cell Res 130:427–435
Halaban R, Pomerantz SH, Marshall S, Lambert DT, Lerner AB (1983) Regulation of tyrosinase in human melanocytes grown in culture. J Cell Biol 97:480–488
Halaban R, Ghosh S, Baird A (1987) bFGF is the putative natural growth factor for human melanocytes. In Vitro Cell Dev Biol 23:47–52
Halaban R, Kwon BS, Ghosh S, Delli Bovi P, Baird A (1988a) bFGF as an autocrine growth factor for human melanomas. Oncogene Res 3:177–186
Halaban R, Langdon R, Birchall N, Cuono C, Baird A, Scott G, Moellmann G, McGuire J (1988b) Basic fibroblast growth factor of keratinocytes is a natural mitogen for normal human melanocytes. J Cell Biol 107:1611–1619
Halaban R, Funasaka Y, Lee P, Rubin J, Ron D, Birnbaum D (1991) Fibroblast growth factors in normal and malignant melanocytes. Ann NY Acad Sci 638:232–243

Halaban R, Rubin J, Funasaka Y, Cobb M, Boulton T, Faletto D, Rosen E, Chan A, Yoko K, White W, Cook C, Moellmann G (1992) Met and hepatocyte growth factor/scatter factor signal transduction in normal melanocytes and melanoma cells. Oncogene 7:2195–2206

Halaban R, Tyrrell L, Longley J, Yarden Y, Rubin J (1993) Pigmentation and Proliferation of Human Melanocytes and the Effect of MSH and UVB Light. Ann NY Acad Sci (in press)

Hattori Y, Odagiri O, Nakatani H, Miyagawa K, Naito K, Sakamoto H, Katoh O, Yoshida T, Sugimura T, Terada M (1990) K-*sam*, an amplified gene in stomach cancer, is a member of the heparin-binding growth factor receptor genes. Proc Natl Acad Sci USA 87:5983–5987

Huang E, Nocka K, Beier DR, Chu T-Y, Buck J, Lahm H-W, Wellner D, Leder P, Besmer P (1990) The hematopoietic growth factor KL is encoded at the *Sl* locus and is the ligand of the c-*kit* receptor, the gene product of the *W* locus. Cell 63:225–233

Huang SS, Huang JS (1986) Association of bovine brain-derived growth factor receptor with protein tyrosine kinase activity. J Biol Chem 261:9568–9571

Hunter T (1989) Protein-tyrosine phosphatases: the other side of the coin. Cell 58:1013–1016

Imamura T, Tokita Y, Mitsui Y (1988) Purification of basic FGF receptors from rat brain. Biochem Biophys Res Commun 155:583–590

Imamura T, Engleka K, Zhan X, Tokita Y, Forough R, Roder D, Jackson A, Mailer JAM, Hla T, Maciag T (1990) Recovery of mitogenic activity of a growth factor mutant with a nuclear translocation sequence. Science 249:1567–1570

Isacchi A, Statuto M, Chiesa R, Bergonzoni L, Rusnati PS, Ragnotti G, Presta M (1991) A six-amino acid deletion in basic fibroblast growth factor dissociates its mitogenic activity from its plasminogen activator-inducing capacity. Proc Natl Acad Sci USA 88:2628–2633

Iwamoto T, Takahashi M, Ito M, Hamatani K, Ohbayashi M, Wajjwalku W, Isobe K, Nakashima I (1991) Aberrant melanogenesis and melanocytic tumour development in transgenic mice that carry a metallothionein/*ret* fusion gene. EMBO J 10:3167–3175

Johnson DE, Lee PL, Lu J, Williams LT (1990) Diverse forms of a receptor for acidic and basic fibroblast growth factors. Mol Cell Biol 10:4728–4736

Kawakami M, Nishida E, Tobe K, Hoshi M, Kadowaki T, Kasuga M, Sakai H (1991) Activation of MAP kinase and enhanced phosphorylation of the 350-kDa protein by mitogenic stimuli in quiescent Balb/3 3T3 cells. Exp Cell Res 193:120–126

Keegan K, Johnson DE, Williams LT, Hayman MJ (1991) Isolation of additional member of the fibroblasts growth factor receptor family, FGFR-3. Proc Natl Acad Sci USA 88:1095–1099

Kiefer MC, Stephans JC, Crawford K, Okino K, Barr PH (1990) Ligand-affinity cloning and structure of a cell surface heparan sulfate proteoglycan that binds basic fibroblast growth factor. Proc Natl Acad Sci USA 87:6985–6989

Kwon BS, Halaban R, Kim GS, Usack L, Pomerantz S, Haq AK (1987) A melanocyte-specific cDNA clone whose expression is inducible by melanotropin and isobutylmethyl xanthine. Mol Biol Med 4:339–355

Kwon BS, Wakulchik M, Haq AK, Halaban R, Kestler D (1988) Sequence analysis of murine tyrosinase cDNA and the effect of melanotropin on its gene expression. Biochem Biophys Res Commun 153:1301–1309

Lafage-Pochitaloff M, Galland F, Simonetti J, Prats H, Mattei M-G, Birnbaum D (1990) The human basic fibroblast growth factor gene is located on the long arm of chromosome 4 bands q26–q27. Oncogene Res 5:241–244

L'Allemain G, Pouyssegur J, Weber MJ (1991) p42/Mitogen-activated protein kinase as a converging target for different growth factor signaling pathways: use of pertussis toxin as a discrimination factor. Cell Regul 2:675–684

Lee PL, Johnson DE, Cousens LS, Fried VA, Williams LT (1989) Purification and complementary DNA cloning of a receptor for basic fibroblast growth factor. Science 245:57–60

Lee R-M, Cobb MH, Blackshear PJ (1992) Evidence that extracellular signal-regulated kinases (ERKs) are the insulin-activated Raf-1 kinase kinases. J Biol Chem 267:1088–1092

Leone V, Flatow U, King CR, Sandee MA, Margulies IMK, Liotta LA, Steeg PS (1991) Reduced tumor incidence, metastatic potential, and cytokine responsiveness of *nm*23-transfected melanoma cells. Cell 65:25–35

Lev S, Yarden Y, Givol D (1990) Receptor functions and ligand-dependent transforming potential of a chimeric *kit* proto-oncogene. Mol Cell Biol 10:6064–6068

Lobb R, Sasse J, Sullivan R, Shing Y, D'Amore P, Jacobs J, Klagsbrun M (1986) Purification and characterization of heparin-binding endothelial cell growth factors. J Biol Chem 261:1924–1926

Lu C, Vickers MF, Kerbel RS (1992) Interleukin 6: a fibroblast-derived growth inhibitor of human melanoma cells from early but not advanced stages of tumor progression. Proc Natl Acad Sci USA 89:9215–9219

Martin FH, Sugs SV, Langley KE, Lu HS, Ting J, Okino KH, Morris CF, McNiece IK, Jacobsen FW, Mendiaz EA, Birkett NC, Smith KA, Johnson MJ, Parker VP, Flores JC, Patel AC, Fisher E, Erjavec HO, Herrera CH, Wypych J, Sachdev RK, Pope JA, Leslie I, Wen D, Lin C-H, Cupples RL, Zsebo K (1990) Primary structure and functional expression of rat and human stem cell factor DNAs. Cell 63:203–210

Matsumoto K, Tajima H, Nakamura T (1991) Hepatocyte growth factor is a potent stimulator of human melanocyte DNA synthesis and growth. Biochem Biophys Res Commun 17:45–51

Mergia A, Eddy R, Abraham JA, Fiddes JC, Shows TB (1986) The genes for basic and acidic fibroblast growth factors are on different human chromosomes. Biochem Biophys Res Commun 138:644–651

Moore R, Casey G, Brookes S, Dixon M, Peters G, Dickson C (1986) Sequence, typography and protein coding potential of mouse *int*-2: a putative oncogene activated by mouse mammary tumour virus. EMBO J 5:919–924

Moscatelli D, Presta M, Joseph-Silverstein J, Rifkin DB (1986) Both normal and tumor cells produce basic fibroblast growth factor. J Cell Physiol 129:273–276

Naldini L, Vigna E, Narsimhan RP, Gaudino G, Zarnegar R, Michaolopoulos GK, Comoglio PM (1991) Hepatocyte growth factor (HGF) stimulates the tyrosine kinase activity of the receptor encoded by the proto-oncogene c-Met. Oncogene 6:501–504

Neufeld G, Gospodarowicz D (1985) The identification and partial characterization of the fibroblast growth factor receptor of baby hamster kidney cells. J Biol Chem 260:13860–13868

Nocka K, Majumder S, Chabot B, Ray P, Cervone M, Bernstein A, Besmer P (1989) Expression of c-*kit* gene products in known cellular targets of *W* mutations in normal and *W* mutant mice – evidence for an impaired c-*kit* kinase in mutant mice. Genes Dev 3:816–826

Nocka K, Tan JC, Chiu E, Chu TY, Ray P, Traktman P, Besmer P (1990) Molecular bases of dominant negative and loss of function mutations at the murine c-*kit*/white spotting locus: W^{37}, W^{v}, W^{41} and *W*. EMBO J 9:1805–1813

Ogata S, Furuhashi Y, Eisinger M (1987) Growth stimulation of human melanocytes: identification and characterization of melanoma-derived growth factor (M-McGF). Biochem Biophys Res Commun 146:1204–1211

Partanen J, Mäkelä TP, Eerola E, Korhonen J, Hirvonen H, Claesson-Welsh L, Alitalo K (1991) FGFR-4, a novel acidic fibroblast growth factor receptor with a distinct expression pattern. EMBO J 10:1347–1354

Presta M, Maier JAM, Ragnotti G (1989) The mitogenic signaling pathway but not the plasminogen activator-inducing pathway of basic fibroblast growth factor is mediated through protein kinase C in fetal bovine aortic endothelial cells. J Cell Biol 109:1877–1884

Pulverer BJ, Kyriakis JM, Avruch J, Nikolakaki E, Woodgett JR (1991) Phosphorylation of c-*jun* mediated by MAP kinases. Nature 353:670–674

Qiu F, Ray P, Brown K, Barker PE, Jhanwar S, Ruddle FH, Besmer P (1988) Primary structure of c-*kit*: relationship with the CSF-1/PDGF receptor kinase family-oncogenic activation of v-*kit* involves deletion of extracellular domain and c-terminus. EMBO J 7:1003–1011

Quarto N, Finger FP, Rifkin DB (1991) The NH_2-terminal extension of high molecular weight bFGF is a nuclear targeting signal. J Cell Physiol 147:311–318

Rapraeger AC, Krufka A, Olwin BB (1991) Requirement of heparan for bFGF-mediated fibroblast growth and myoblast differentiation. Science 252:1705–1708

Reith AD, Rottapel R, Giddens E, Brady C, Forrester L, Bernstein A (1990) *W* mutant mice with mild or severe developmental defects contain distinct point mutations in the kinase domain of the c-*kit* transmembrane receptor. Genes Dev 4:390–400

Rodeck U, Melber K, Kath R, Menssen HD, Varello M, Atkinson B, Herlyn M (1991) Constitutive expression of multiple growth factor genes by melanoma cells but not normal melanocytes. J Invest Dermatol 97:20–26

Rubin JS, Chan AM-L, Bottaro DP, Burgess WH, Taylor WG, Cech AC, Hirschfield WD, Wong J, Miki T, Finch PW, Aaronson SA (1991) A broad spectrum human lung fibroblast-derived mitogen is a variant of hepatocyte growth factor. Proc Natl Acad Sci USA 88:415–419

Ruta M, Burgess W, Givol D, Epstein J, Neiger N, Kaplow J, Crumley G, Dionne C, Jaye M, Schlessinger J (1989) Receptor for acidic fibroblast growth factor is related to the tyrosine kinase encoded by the *fms*-like gene (FLG). Proc Natl Acad Sci USA 86:8722–8726

Safran A, Avivi A, Orr-Urtereger A, Neufeld G, Lonai P, Givol D, Yarden Y (1990) The murine *flg* gene encodes a receptor for fibroblast growth factor. Oncogene 5:635–643

Sakagushi K, Yanagishita M, Takeuchi Y, Auerbach GD (1991) Identification of heparan sulfate proteoglycan as a high affinity receptor for acidic fibroblast growth factor (aFGF) in a parathyroid cell line. J Biol Chem 266:7270–7278

Sargent NS, Oestreicher M, Haidvogl H, Madnick HM, Burger MM (1988) Growth regulation of cancer metastases by their host organ. Proc Natl Acad Sci USA 85:7251–7255

Schulze-Osthoff K, Risau W, Vollmer E, Clemens S (1990) *In situ* detection of basic fibroblast growth factor by highly specific antibodies. Am J Pathol 173:85–92

Scott GA, Haak A (1991) Keratinocytes regulate melanocyte number in human fetal and neonatal skin Equivalent. J Invest Dermatol 97:776–781

Scott G, Stoler M, Sarkar S, Halaban R (1991) Localization of basic fibroblast growth factor mRNA in melanocytic lesions by *in situ* hybridization. J Invest Dermatol 96:318–322

Spritz RA, Giebel LB, Holmes SA (1992a) Dominant negative and loss of function mutations of the c-*kit* (mast/stem cell growth factor receptor) proto-oncogene in human piebaldism. Am J Hum Genet 50:261–269

Spritz RA, Droetto S, Fukushima Y (1992b) Deletion of the *kit* and *Pdgfra* genes in a patient with piebaldism. Am J Hum Genet (in press)
Stocker KM, Sherman L, Rees S, Ciment G (1991) Basic FGF and TGF-β1 influence commitment to melanogenesis in neural crest-derived cells of avian embryos. Development 111:635–641
Straus DS, Jonasson J, Harris H (1976) Growth *in vitro* of tumor cell x fibroblast hybrids in which malignancy is suppressed. J Cell Sci 25:73–86
Sturgill TW, Ray B, Erikson E, Maller JL (1988) Insulin-stimulated MAP-2 kinase phosphorylates and activates ribosomal protein S6 kinase II. Nature 334:715–718
Taira M, Yoshida T, Miyagawa K, Sakamoto H, Terada M, Sugimura T (1987) cDNA sequence of human transforming gene *hst* and identification of the coding sequence required for transforming activity. Proc Natl Acad Sci USA 84:2980–2984
Takahashi M, Buma Y, Taniguchi M (1990) Identification of the *ret* proto-oncogene products in neuroblastoma and leukemia cells. Oncogene 5:126–130
Tan JC, Nocka K, Ray P, Traktman P, Besmer P (1990) The dominant W^{42} *spotting* phenotype results from a missense mutation in the c-*kit* receptor kinase. Science 247:209–212
Tessler S, Neufeld G (1990) Basic fibroblast growth factor accumulates in the nuclei of various bFGF producing cell types. J Cell Physiol 145:310–317
Theillet C, Le Roy X, De Lapeyrière O, Grosgeorges J, Adnane J, Raynaud SD, Simony-Lafontaine J, Goldfarb M, Escot C, Birnbaum D, Gaudray P (1989) Amplification of *FGF*-related genes in human tumors: possible involvement of *HST* in breast carcinomas. Oncogene 4:915–922
Trent JM, Meyskens FL, Salmon SE, Ryschon K, Leong SPL, Davis JR, McGee DL (1990a) Relation of cytogenetic abnormalities and clinical outcome in metastatic melanoma. N Engl J Med 322:1508–1511
Trent JM, Stanbridge EJ, McBride HL, Meese EU, Casey G, Araujo DE, Witkowski CM, Nagle RB (1990b) Tumorigenicity in human melanoma cell lines controlled by introduction of human chromosome 6. Science 247:568–571
Wakeling WF, Greetham LM, Bennett DC (1992) Suppression of properties associated with malignancy in murine melanoma-melanocyte hybrid cells. Br J Cancer 65:529–537
Williams DE, Eisenman J, Baird A, Rauch C, Van Ness K, March CJ, Park LS, Martin U, Mochizuki DY, Boswell HS, Burgess GM, Cosman D, Lyman SD (1990) Identification of a ligand for the c-*kit* proto-oncogene. Cell 63:167–174
Wittbrodt J, Adam D, Malitschek B, Mäueler W, Raulf F, Telling A, Robertson SM, Schartl M (1989) Novel putative receptor tyrosine kinase encoded by the melanoma-inducing *Tu* locus in *Xiphophorus*. Nature 341:415–421
Yarden Y, Ullrich A (1988) Growth factor receptor tyrosine kinases. Ann Rev Biochem 57:443–478
Yarden Y, Kuang W-J, Yang-Feng T, Coussens L, Munemitsu S, Dull TJ, Chen E, Schlessinger J, Francke U, Ullrich A (1987) Human proto-oncogene c-*kit*: a new cell surface receptor tyrosine kinase for an unidentified ligand. EMBO J 6:3341–3351
Yayon A, Klagsbrun M, Esko J, Leder P, Ornitz DM (1991) Cell surface, heparin-like molecules are required for binding of basic fibroblast growth factor to its high affinity receptor. Cell 64:841–848
Zakut R, Perlis R, Eliahu S, Yarden Y, Givol D, Lyman SD, Halaban R (1993) KIT-ligand (sast cell growth factor) inhibits the growth of *KIT*-expressing melanoma cells. Oncogene (in press)
Zechel C, Schleenbecker U, Anders A, Anders F (1988) v-*erb*B related sequences in *Xiphophorus* that map to melanoma determining Mendelian loci and overexpress in a melanoma cell line. Oncogene 3:605–617

Zsebo K, Williams DA, Geissler EN, Broudy VC, Martin FH, Atkins HL, Hsu R-Y, Birkett NC, Okino KH, Murdock DC, Jacobsen FW, Langley KE, Smith KA, Takeishi T, Cattanach BM, Galli SJ, Suggs S (1990a) Stem cell factor is encoded at the *Sl* locus of the mouse and is the ligand for the c-*kit* tyrosine kinase receptor. Cell 63:213–224

Zsebo KM, Wypych J, McNiece IK, Lu HS, Smith KA, Karkare SB, Sadchev RK, Yuschenkoff VN, Birkett NC, Williams LR, Satyagal VN, Tung W, Bosselman RA, Mendiaz EA, Langley KE (1990b) Identification, purification, and biological characterization of hematopoietic stem cell factor from buffalo rat liver-conditioned medium. Cell 63:195–201

III. Keratinocyte Carcinogenesis

Keratinocyte Carcinogenesis: Introduction

I. Moll

Department of Dermatology, Mannheim Medical School, Postbox 100023, W-6800 Mannheim, Fed. Rep. of Germany

Skin keratinocytes may give rise to a broad variety of benign and malignant epithelial tumors. Among these, basal cell carcinoma and squamous cell carcinoma are the most frequent. Up to 60% of squamous cell carcinomas are preceded by precancerous lesions, mostly by actinic keratoses and rarely by Bowen's disease. All these lesions have risen in frequency during the past decades, mainly due to enhanced sunlight exposure and certain chemical carcinogens. Basal cell carcinomas may be induced by UV light and inorganic arsenic. The correlation between UV radiation and squamous cell carcinoma, however, is more direct, and there is also a correlation with heat exposure. Chemical carcinogens inducing squamous cell carcinoma are soot, tar products, shale oil, and inorganic arsenic.

A large body of knowledge has accumulated on the various molecular mechanisms of keratinocyte carcinogenesis. Normal keratinocytes show various stages of differentiation, both in the vertical as well as in the horizontal level. Important systems of molecular differentiation markers are the cytokeratins and certain junction proteins. Within the epidermis, seven cytokeratin polypeptides are present, nos. 1, 2, 5, 10–11, 14 and 15. Of these cytokeratins, 5 and 14 are expressed in the basal keratinocytes which, in addition, are characterized by hemidesmosomal proteins, pemphigus vulgaris antigen, and the EGF receptor. In contrast, the suprabasal keratinocytes express keratinization-associated cytokeratins, mostly nos. 1, 10, 11, and, in addition, desmosomal proteins, pemphigus vulgaris antigen, and certain proteins involved in the terminal epidermal differentiation, such as filaggrin, loricrin, and involucrin. During malignant transformation these differentiation markers may be maintained, but also certain changes may occur. In general, in keratinocyte-derived tumors, mostly the differentiation markers of basal keratinocytes predominate. However, part of the tumor cells may focally undergo a limited degree of maturation. Thus, in squamous cell carcinoma, cytokeratins 1, 10–11 and involucrin can be focally detected. In addition, these tumors abundantly express cytokeratins 6 and 16, which

Recent Results in Cancer Research, Vol. 128

are typical for high proliferation. In some cases, particularly those with poor morphological differentiation, tumor cell subpopulations may even embark on aberrant routes of differentiation and, in addition, express certain simple-epithelial cytokeratins (nos. 7, 8, 18, 19) or the mesenchymal intermediate filament protein vimentin. The latter process seems to be associated with a highly malignant behavior. The divergence of differentiation within tumor cells gives rise to tumor cell heterogeneity, the biological significance of which for tumor invasion and tumor metastasis are current important subjects of investigation.

*Diversity of Epithelial Skin Tumors: Thoughts and Comments on Some Basic Principles**

U. Wollina

Klinik und Poliklinik für Hautkrankheiten, Friedrich-Schiller-Universität Jena, Erfurter Straße 35, O-6900 Jena, Fed. Rep. of Germany.

Tumor Cell Heterogeneity: Fact or Fiction?

The diagnosis of any skin tumor depends upon a spectrum of clinical and histopathological criteria which must be fitted by the individual case. This means that both the classification scheme and the use of analogy only work if the tumors were different from each other. On the other hand, we know that at least some if not all epithelial skin tumors have a certain amount of intraindividual heterogeneity.

Tumor cell heterogeneity (TCH) as discussed here is a pattern of diversification of the cellular phenotype. The phenotype – the manifestation of genes in an individual – is a mere vehicle of transmission. This is important to note, since skin tumors may arise from a single precursor cell, i.e., they are the product of clonal growth (e.g., porokeratosis, squamous cell carcinoma).

TCH can develop through various different mechanisms, some of which will be discussed in this paper. Although they represent basic biological processes, please bear in mind that the choice of topics was of course subjective and not comprehensive. Subheadings are used to focus on certain aspects of TCH, but one must not forget that a single cause, a unique mechanism is never sufficient to describe TCH in any given tumor. Reassembling of thoughts is therefore essential because, as Aristotle said, "the whole is more than the sum of the parts".

Functional Heterogeneity of Normal Epithelial Cells

Pinkus first formulated the idea of epidermal symbiosis (Pinkus 1958). This use of a biological term emphasizes the fact that the mature human

*Dedicated to Prof. Dr. med Dr. h.c. G.K. Steigleder on the occasion of his birthday.

a
b

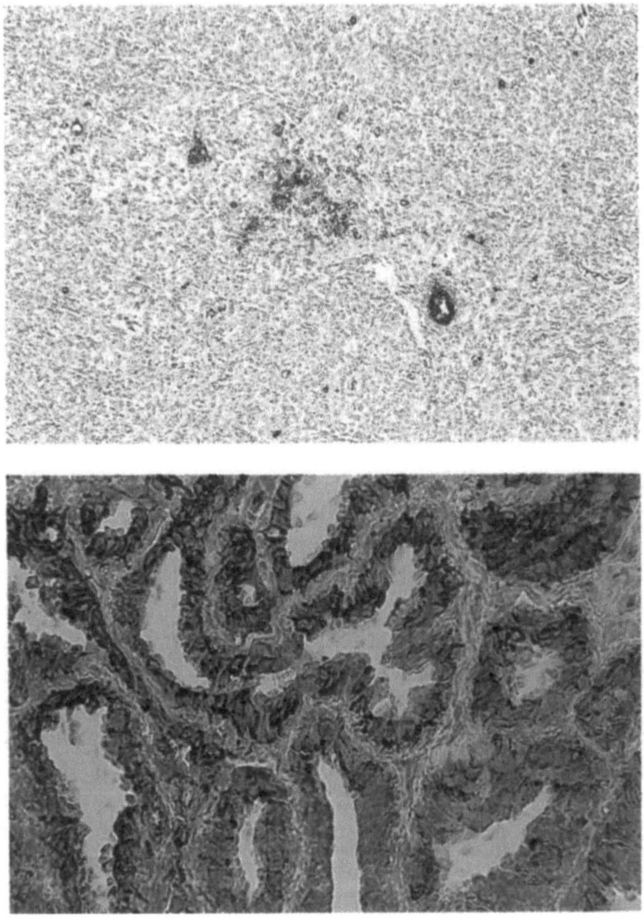

Fig. 1a,b. Polarity in adnexal skin tumors. **a** Calmodulin reactivity in luminal and preluminal formations of dermal cylindroma (polyclonal antibody ACAM). **b** Expression of simple-type ("glandular") keratins in most epithelia of syringocystadenoma papilliferum (monoclonal antibody Cam 5.2 against simple-type keratins). Unlabeled perxidase technique with amino-ethylcarbazole on cryostat (**a**) and formalin-fixed (**b**) tissue sections. Original magnification **a** ×100, **b** ×250

epidermis is built up by cells derived from more than one germ layer: keratinocytes, Langerhans cells, melanocytes, Merkel cells, and adnexal epithelial cells. In adnexal tumors, well-differentiated forms have usually emerged from the preexisting structures, so different cellular phenotypes are retained within one lesion. On the other hand, more immature tumor types are thought to arise form pluripotential stem cells, but even in the adnexal carcinomas a certain diversification of the cellular phenotypes might be seen (Hashimoto et al. 1987; Nakhleh et al. 1990; Heenan et al. 1990; Fig. 1).

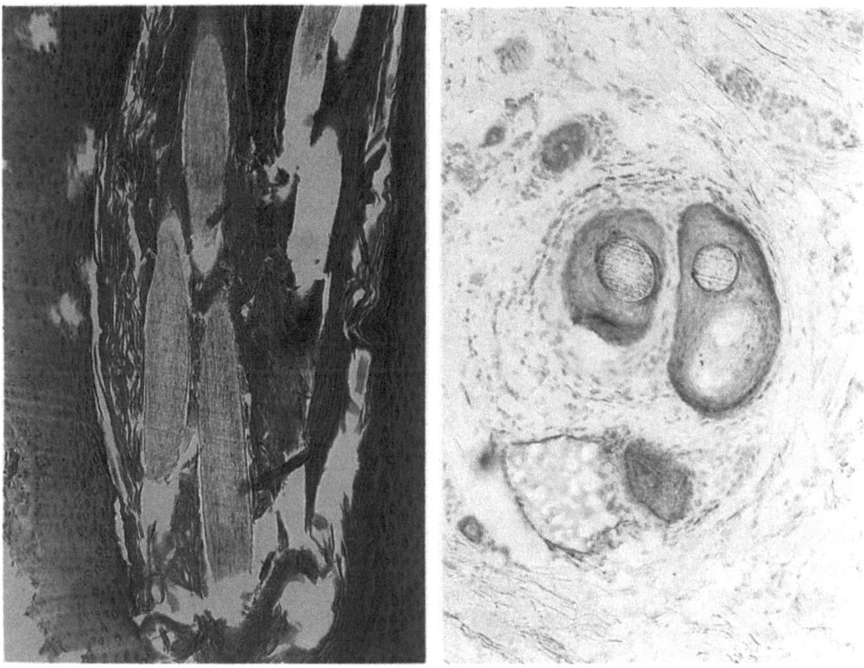

a b

Fig. 2a,b. Bundle hair nevus with several hairs within one follicle ostium. **a** Hematoxylin-eosin stained section, **b** demonstration of keratin 10 expression (unlabeled peroxidase technique with aminoethylcarbazole and monoclonal antibody RKSE 60). (From Wollina et al. 1991c) Original magnification ×100

Neviform tumors like the nevus sebaceus of Jadassohn, the hair follicle nevus, or the apocrine nevus mimic this symbiosis to greater or lesser degrees (Hashimoto et al. 1987). A very complex structure which is clearly composed of different cellular elements of ectodermal and mesodermal origin can be formed, as in bundle hair nevus (Fig. 2). The phenotypic

Table 1. Phenotypic characteristics of supraseboglandular outer hair root sheath in bundle hair nevus (from Wollina et al. 1991c)

Basal cells	Suprabasal cells
RKSE 60 (keratin 10)[a]	K8.12 (keratins 13, 16)[a]
ACAM	ACAM[a]
	Filaggrin
	RKSE 60 (only weak)[a]

[a] Abberations in the cellular phenotype of bundle hair and normal hair epithelium.

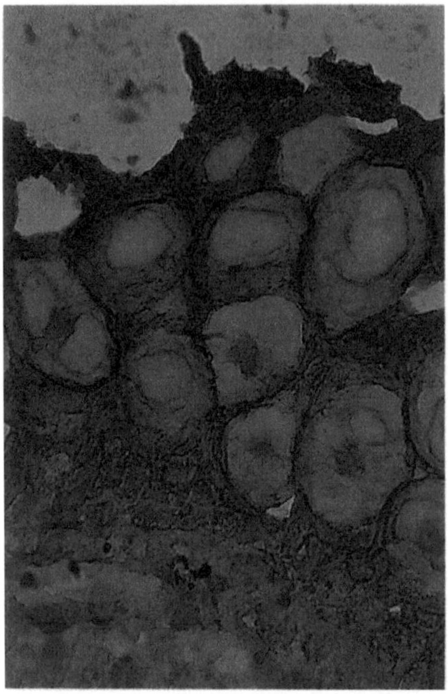
a

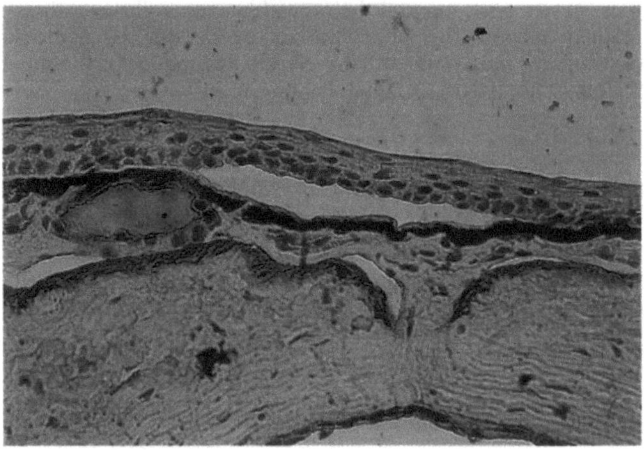
b

Fig. 3a,b. Phylogenetic variation in the distribution of calmodulin-reactive skin cells. The animals adapted to an aqueous environment have more superficial reactivity (**a** *Ambystoma mexicanum*) and species with a more terrestrial lifestyle show calmodulin immunorectivity in deeper compartments of skin (**b** *Rana ridibunda)*. Unlabeled peroxidase staining with aminoethylcarbazole and polyclonal antibody ACAM on cryostat sections. Original magnification ×250

pattern of epithelial cells forming the outer hair root sheath, however, differs from that of normal follicles (Wollina et al. 1991c; Table 1).

A central function of eccrine sweat glands is their involvement in osmoregulation. We have been studying the immunohistochemistry of calmodulin over recent years. Several lines of investigation have provided evidence that calmodulin-reactive cells are the elements responsible for osmoregulation in the skin (Fig. 3). Using an indirect immunofluorescence technique on unfixed or acetone-fixed frozen sections of normal human skin, topographic "mapping" was performed. Positive reactions were given by the basal cells of both normal interfollicular epidermis and the outer hair root sheath. In eccrine skin glands, inner ductal and myoepithelial cells were stained with appropriate antibodies, whereas secretory cells remained nonreactive (Wollina et al. 1989b, 1990, 1991d,e).

As calmodulin reactivity could be useful in characterization of adnexal tumors, clear cell acanthoma, poroma, chondroid hidradenoma, and dermal cylindroma were choosen to investigate the distribution of immunoreactive cells. It was found that in poromas and clear cell acanthomas, certain cells (in the former only squamoid cells) were stained by anti-calmodulin, suggesting a ductal differentiation in some of these tumors (Schaarschmidt and Wollina 1990). Intraepidermal poromas, however, remained completely negative, making their acrosyringial differentiation questionable. The majority of tumor cells in clear cell acathomas and poromas are immature, resembling basal cells. Such a view is further supported by studies of keratin expression (Iki 1990). Within chondroid hidradenoma, there was a predominance of calmodulin-reactive cells in the center of the adenoid structures and of keratin on the margins (Wollina and Schaarschmidt 1990a). The findings are in keeping with further immunohistochemical and ultrastructural studies showing myoepithelial, epithelial (ductal?), and hyaline cells (Hashimoto et al. 1987; Iki 1990). In cylindroma, luminal and preluminal epithelia were stained for calmodulin, supporting the idea of residual eccrine duct formation resembling the embryonic structures. In conclusion, the TCH found in these adnexal tumors seems to be a consequence of the variable differentiation of progenitor cells during tumor progression. The diversification of the phenotype could be remarkably independent of the mono- or polyclonal nature of neoplasms (Hashimoto et al. 1987). At first glance, the aformentioned examples speak in favor of basal cells being pluripotential. On closer examination, this holds true only for immature carcinomas, while the well-differentiated neoplasms seem to arise from their corresponding structures (Mehregan 1985).

One source of support for this thesis comes from pharmacological studies. It has been suggested that a large proportion of human tumors result from exposure to hazardous procarcinogens. One of the most important enzyme systems for metabolically activating carcinogens is the group of mixed function oxidases. P-450 isoenzymes have been detected in the skin of various mammals including man (for overview see Mukhtar and Khan 1989). Cytochrome P-450 expression in vitro and in vivo is a function of differentiation and extracellular calcium concentration. In a murine skin model, raising the calcium concentration from 0.04 m*M* to 1.2 m*M* resulted in a prompt and marked increase of 7-ethoxyresorufin-7-deethylase and 7-ethoxycoumarin-*O*-deethylase. The lowest and highest activities of the monooxygenases were detected in basal and most highly differentiated spinous keratinocytes (Reiners et al. 1990). Additionally, Guo et al. (1990a) reported rat skin keratinocytes expressing microsomal aryl hydrocarbon hydroxylase and cytochrome P-450 in vitro and in vivo after exposure to benz(a)anthracene. Again, the more highly differentiated cells expressed higher levels of enzyme activities than basal cells.

The nonuniform distribution of metabolizing enzyme activities among skin epithelia can be related to tumorigenesis. As Merk et al. (1987a) detected remarkable aryl hydrocarbon hydroxylase, 7-ethoxyresorufin deethylase, and cytochrome P-450-IA1 activities in basal epidermal keratinocytes and hair follicles, this casts light upon the induction of hair follicle tumors like basal cell carcinoma (see Mukhtar et al. 1989; Merk 1990; Merk et al. 1987b). Based upon their findings, it is conceivable that basal cell carcinoma arises from the outer hair root sheath, at least sometimes, primarily due to the pattern of enzyme expression in the follicle epithelium and not due to the presence of undifferentiated embryonic cells (primary epithelial germ cells) (see Lever and Schaumburg-Lever 1990; Mehregan 1985).

Assuming that the development of cell polarity is the foundation of the main stem cell lineages in embryology, loss of polarity should be a wide spread phenomenon in heterogeneous stem cell tumors. Polarity is initiated by asymmetric cell–cell contacts and assymmetric ion currents, which are followed by movement of sodium-coupled transport systems to the apical plasma membrane and modulated by uvomorulin (Wiley et al. 1990). Certain integrins in human epidermis also have a polar distribution, e.g., the $\alpha_6\beta_4$ integrin receptor, which is found at microvillous projections on the basement attachment site of basal keratinocytes (Klein et al. 1990). In basal cell carcinoma, the expression of $\alpha_2\beta_1$ and $\alpha_3\beta$ heterodimers is markedly elevated compared with normal basal cells but similar to that seen in the hair bulb and outer hair root sheath. It was suggested that the high level of integrin expression may account for the growth characteristics of this tumor and support its originating from hair follicle epithelium (Stamp and Pignatelli 1991).

In summary, TCH is facilitated by physiological heterogeneity of skin cells. However, the phenotypic mimicry of normal (functional) cellular heterogeneity by TCH is more or less incomplete.

Programmed Cell Death and Epithelial Skin Tumors

Death is one of the basic cellular processes. Cell death may arise from injury, as a degenerative phenomenon, but it can also occur as a controlled event. Only the latter form will be discussed here. I refer to it as apoptosis. It seems to be active self-destruction rather than passive degeneration (Wyllie et al. 1980). Apoptosis is implicated in steady-state kinetics of healthy adult tissues such as the epidermis, in embryology, and in metamorphosis, but it is involved in epithelial tumorigenesis as well (Wyllie 1988).

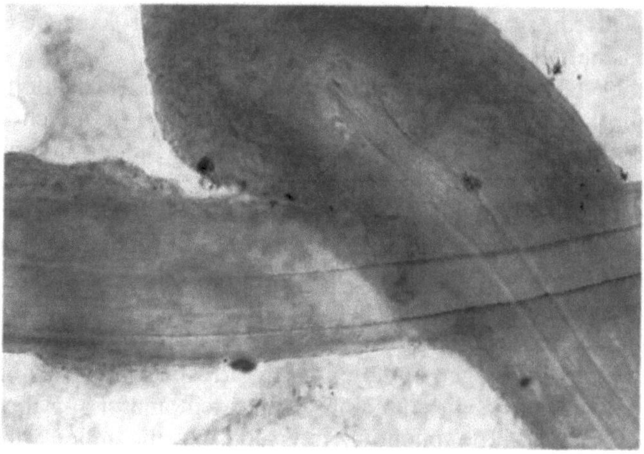

a

Fig. 4a,b. Immunostaining of Merkel cells in the outer hair root sheath of normal human skin with monoclonal antibodies against simple-type keratins: **a** CK2, **b** 5D3. **a** Unfixed epidermis preparation, view on the undersurface (APAAP). **b** Merkel cells along the hair bulb, frozen acetone-fixed section (Peroxidase technique with aminoethylcarbazole). Original magnification ×250

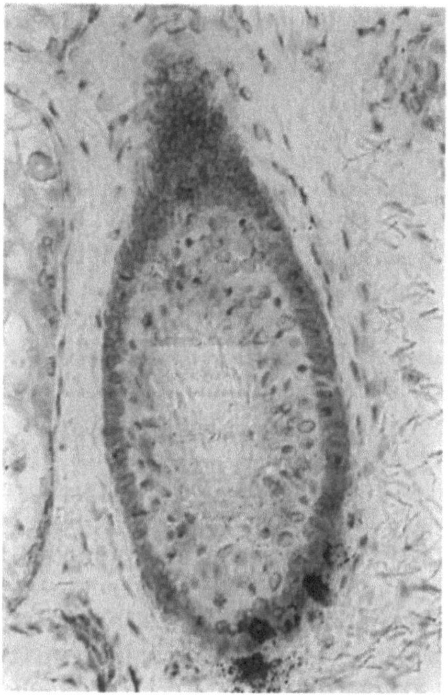

b

Apoptosis can be modulated by appropriate hormonal stimulation. It seems reasonable to assume that hair growth represents an endocrine-dependent example of programmed cell death (see Cotsarelis et al. 1990; Wollina et al. 1991d). In the outer hair root sheath of anagen follicles, the frequency of Merkel cells varies between the anagen subphases and parallels the proliferative activity as measured by staining with Ki67 (Wollina et al. 1991d; Fig. 4). It is thought that Merkel cells might be involved in the growth control. Since these cells have paracrine functions, it is possible that they will contribute to apoptosis, too. However, current evidence is only circumstantial.

Other factors must considered as well, like activation of heat shock proteins, random mutation, T-cell killing, or virus infection (Wyllie 1988; Wyllie et al. 1980). The tumor necrosis factor, like other cytokines or local growth factors, was assumed to play a role in apoptosis (Wyllie 1986). Effective focal depletion of trophic factors could be a manifestation of tumor cell heterogeneity, either through local reductions in their release, or through receptor defects.

Kinetic data indicate that a high rate of cell loss is characteristic of nearly all human tumors. Besides necrosis, apoptosis is an important factor contributing to prolonged tumor growth, irrespective of an increased growth fraction, as occurs in squamous cell carcinomas (El-Labban and Osorio-Herrera 1986). The phenomenon seems to be more widespread among skin tumors than currently assumed. Apoptosis, if it occurs in tumors, might argue for the existence of growth control in some tumor cells. Unfortunately, apoptosis alone is not sufficient to limit neoplastic growth significantly.

Developmental Conversion of Germ Layer Products

In the embryological development of eccrine sweat glands, both the mesenchyme and the neurohumoral system have inductory effects at the epidermal undersurface (Hashimoto et al. 1966). Considering the proliferative and differentiation qualities of eccrine germs, they are likely to be of mesectodermal origin (for overview see Wollina 1991b). Indeed, there are many interesting findings suggesting that ectodermal cells are converted into mesectodermal eccrine glands (Table 2). The pattern formation and thereby the physiological compartmentation of different functions in mesectoderm is lost even in benign neoplasms, indicating the need for complex regulation of mesectodermal differentiation (see Oriol 1987; Wollina et al. 1990). The random pattern of ductal and myoepithelial differentiation in chrondroid hidradenoma is an example of the loss of inductory factors controlling and propagating the mesectodermal phenotype (Fig. 5). In cylindroma, we observed an increasing loss of lumen formation, the process stopping at the stage of preluminal cells (see Hashimoto et al. 1966). These structures were positive for lysozyme and α_1-antichymotrypsin. On the other hand, they coexpressed vimentin and simple types of keratin, like mature myoepithelial cells (Wollina et al. 1992; Wollina 1991a; Fig. 6).

The induction of hair germs (epithelial germs) and hair germ-like structures is related to mesenchymal forces and tractions: Epithelial responses include morphogenetic (epidermal downgrowth) and biochemical alterations (Stolar et al. 1989; Wollina et al. 1991a). Again, the formation of hair germ-like structures in varieties of basal cell carcinoma involves mesenchymal

Table 2. Differences between eccrine glands and the pilosebaceous unit (from Wollina 1991b)

	Eccrine glands	Pilosebaceous unit
1. Anlagen		
Time of formation	2nd trimenon	1st trimenon
Mode of growth	Perpendicular	Straight
Direction of growth	Dermal and epidermal	Dermal
Differentiation	Epithelial and endocrine	Epithelial
Mesenchymal condensation	Absent	Essential
2. Mature appendage		
Gene control (ABH/Le)	H, Le (duct) Se (coiled portion)	H
Cytokeratins	Simple-type Epithelia-like	Stratified Epithelia-like
Expression of neuroendocrine antigens	Present	Absent
Regeneration	From the dermal duct	From the stratum basale

condensation. Trichilemmal keratinization depends upon the presence of inner root sheath cells (Henle and Huxley cells), which develop trichohyaline granules. Trichilemmal keratinization is found in the wall cells of trichilemmal cysts (Hashimoto et al. 1987). Mesenchymal condensation per se seems to be a characteristic feature of hair follicle tumors in general, but it might be absent in eccrine neoplasms (Rosen 1990).

A disturbance in regular morphogenesis can result from alterations of the cell surface, as shown by lectin histochemistry and by the altered expression of cell adhesion molecules and integrins (Kaufmann et al. 1990; Fenderson et al. 1990). Direct evidence for the involvement of glycoconjugates in morphogenesis has been obtained by studying the effect of milk oligosaccharides on preimplantation-stage mouse embryos. The appearance of stage-specific embryonic antigen 1 (SSEA-1, Le[x]) on the embryonic surface correlates approximately in time with the onset of compaction, i.e., the maximization of intercellular contacts and generation of polar distribution of microvilli by blastomeres. A multivalent Le[x] was able to decompact embryos in a dose-dependent manner. In vitro, migrating keratinocytes appear to express higher levels of β_1 integrin subunits than resting cells (Guo et al. 1990b). Monoclonal antibodies against β_1 integrin impaired the lateral aggregation of keratinocytes in vitro, whereas antibodies against β_4 prevented cell–matrix interactions, suggesting a correlation between the pattern of integrin expression on plasma membrane domains and epidermal assembly or morphogenesis (Marchisio et al. 1991). The possibility that cytoplasmic domains of adhesion molecules themselves act as signalling sites for the expression of other surface molecules or for clustering of preexisting surface molecules thus emerges (Anderson

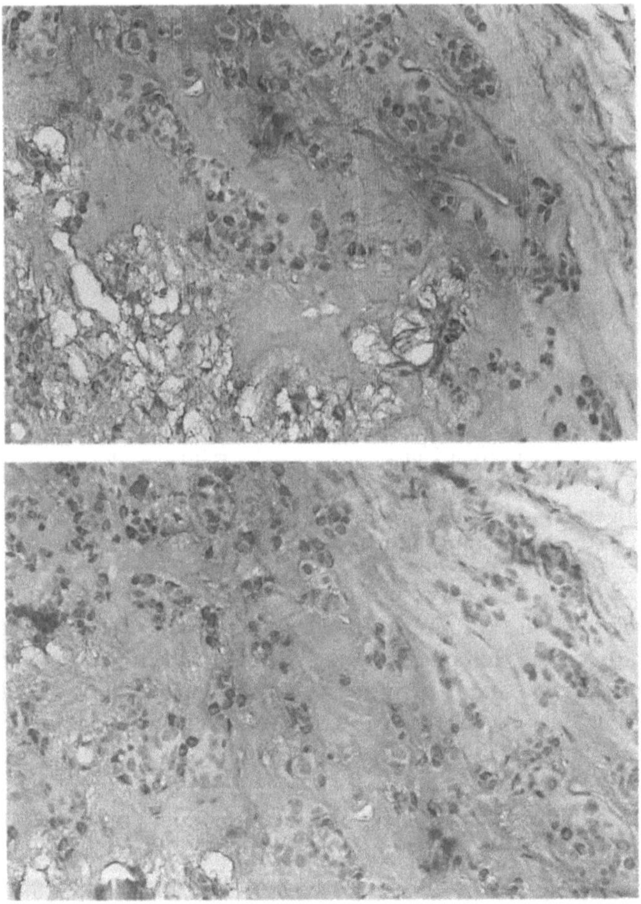

a

b

Fig. 5a,b. Chondroid hidradenoma showing a random pattern of different phenotypes (unlabeled peroxidase technique with amino-ethylcarbazol): **a** vimentin-positive cells (monoclonal V9[1]), **b** simple-type keratin-positive cells (monoclonal Cam 5.2). Original magnification ×250

1990). That would allow focal contacts to form between cells involved in differentiation.

It goes without saying that glycoconjugates play multiple roles in modulating cell functions by (1) providing signals for targeting molecules, (2) modifying protein structure and function, and (3) regulating the rheologic and dynamic properties of the plasma membrane. Each of the following factors is also working in skin disease: (1) overexpression of epidermal growth factor receptors by squamous cell carcinoma and psoriasis, (2) elevated levels and activities of protein kinase C, calmodulin, and phosphoinositol phosphate in psoriasis and phorbol ester-induced skin tumors, (3) elevated electrophoretic mobility and membrane fluidity of psoriatic

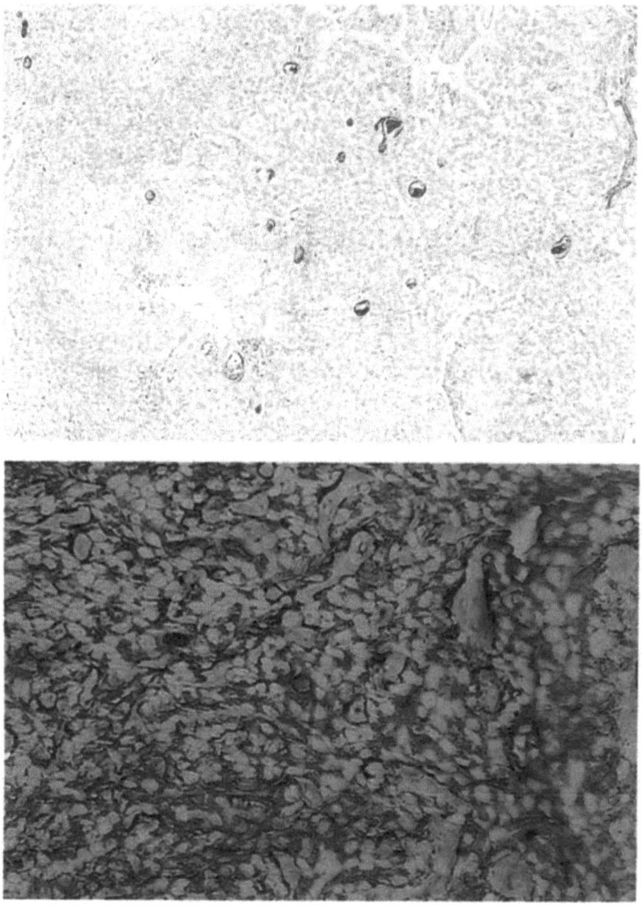

a

b

Fig. 6a,b. Dermal cylindroma with preluminal formations and lumina **a** positively stained with antibodies against lysozyme (unlabeled peroxidase technique with amino-ethylcarbazol and polclonal antilysozyme-DAKO); **b** double-stained with polyclonal antikeratin (Pankeratin-DAKO, peroxidase technique with amino-ethylcarbazole) and monoclonal antivimentin (V9[1], APAAP with fast blue BB salt). Original magnification **a** ×100, **b** ×250

keratinocytes (Chigira et al. 1990; Inohara 1990; Knopf and Wollina 1992; Wollina et al. 1989a). A change in cell surface composition, therefore, is common to all cases of a loss of epithelial homeostasis – in hyperproliferations *and* epithelial tumors. The consequences for cell biology, are very complex and far from being completely understood, but differential distribution of molecules on the cell surface and developing differential cell affinities will guide the morphogenetic process of epithelial skin tumors (see Steinberg 1986). Monoclonal antibodies against glycosylated epitopes of human milk fat globule membrane (MAM) have been found useful in the study of adnexal differentiation. Immunohistochemical evaluation of the distribution of MAM antigens among adnexal tumors of the skin demonstrated a loss of control of antigen expression in benign variants. In adnexal carcinomas the irregular presence of MAM antigens is even more evident and not as related to the tumor classification (Tsubura et al. 1987).

Uncoupling of Cytodifferentiation and Morphogenesis, Growth Factors

Morphogenesis and cytodifferentiation are two major events in the genesis of organs and tissues that normally take place inseparably. The presence of inductory factors has been assumed by embryologists since the last century, but it is only recently that experimental models have been developed indicating connective tissue signalling in adult skin which is capable of recreating the pattern of epithelial phenotypic expression and its mitotic activity (Mackenzie and Dabelsteen 1987; Hill and Mackenzie 1989). It became clear that local growth factors and the immune system play a pivotal role in the sophisticated regulation of morphogenesis (Ruben et al. 1989; Beresford 1990). Local growth factors of the cytokine and neuropeptide families might serve as illustratory examples (Table 3), though glycoconjugates in general and integrins in particular are essential "endogeneous" elements.

Epithelial morphogenesis can be determined by mesenchymal signals and, conversely, ectodermal factors contribute to the development of mesoderm. For instance, it was recently found that soluble peptides (tumor growth factor β-like peptides, activin, fibroblast growth factor) act as agents of mesoderm induction in *Xenopus*. In the absence of such peptide growth factors, cells of the equator of the blastula will form ectodermal skin only. Exposure of presumptive ectodermal cells to a single pure peptide can change their fate so that they form an array of mesodermal and neural tissues (see Tiedemann 1990). These findings throw light on the possible mechanisms of eccrine germ development as discussed above.

Recently, the keratinocyte growth factor (KGF) produced by stromal cells has been identified. In vitro experiments suggested that KGF is involved in morphogenetic events in several mammary carcinoma cell lines. Aaronson et al. (1990) identified markedly elevated *erbB-3* mRNA levels in these cells, which encodes a transmembrane receptor protein for KGF. There is some analogy to the overexpression of *erbB*/EGF receptor and *erbB-2* in epithelial malignancies.

There are a few exceptions to the rule of inseparable cytodifferentiation and morphogenesis: Salivary-type glands induced from mammary gland epithelium by salivary mesenchyme express lactose synthetase activity. Similarly, salivary-type glands induced from palate epithelium by salivary mesenchyme undergo palate-type cytodifferentiation (Mizuno and Yasugi 1990). An abnormal sequence of keratin expression was reported in the

Table 3. Selected growth factors and inhibitors for keratinocytes. Factors which can be produced by keratinocytes are marked by asterisks

Abbreviation		Importance for epithelial hyperplasia and tumors
1. Growth promotors[a]		
EGF*	epidermal growth factor	Psoriasis, basal cell carcinoma, squamous cell carcinoma, wound healing
TGF-α*	tumor growth factor	Psoriasis, squamous cell carcinoma
bFGF*	basic fibroblast growth factor	Psoriasis
KGF	keratinocyte growth factor	Mammary carcinoma
Amphiregulin		?
Insulin		Psoriasis
IGF-I	somatomedin C	Wound healing
IGF-II	insulin-like growth factor II	Wound healing, epidermal hyperproliferation
IL-1*	interleukin	Psoriasis
IL-6*	interleukin-6, interferon-β_2	Psoriasis, squamous cell carcinoma
IL-8*	interleukin-8	Psoriasis, phorbol ester-induced mouse skin hyperplasia
NGF*	nerve growth factor	UVB- and phorbol ester-induced tumorigenesis
VIP	vasoactive intestinal peptide	Psoriasis
2. Growth inhibitors[b]		
TGF-β1*	tumor growth factor	Psoriasis, squamous cell carcinoma
IFN-γ	interferon-γ	Psoriasis
aFGF*	basic fibroblast growth factor	Wound healing

[a] Increased or receptors overexpressed in pathological conditions.
[b] Levels either reduced or responses diminished in pathological conditions.

suprabasal epidermis covering dermatofibromas (Stolar et al. 1989). Another dermal tumor with secondary epithelial reactions is the acquired acral keratofibroma (Wollina and Schaarschmidt 1990b; Table 4). Both might serve as examples of the induction of cytodifferentiation in the absence of morphogenesis. As shown recently, pregerms and hair germ-like formations at the undersurface of the epidermis covering dermatofibromas exert a phentotypic pattern different from the outer hair root sheath (Wollina et al. 1991a). This is an example of morphogenesis without appropriate cytodifferentiation. It might be assumed that alterations in the cascade of growth factors and inhibitors, both epithelial and mesenchymal, may be responsible for this.

The regulation of cell division is a sophisticated event in normal growth. The majority of cells at any given time are in the resting phase G_0. Almost all of them retain the ability to divide. In malignancy, however, the ability to revert back to a normal resting state is impaired (for overview see Bhargava and Chandani 1988). In regenerative processes like healing of

Table 4. Epidermal immunoreactivity of acquired acral keratofibroma versus normal skin as an example of a changed epidermal phenotype due to mesenchymal tumors (from Wollina and Schaarschmidt 1990b)

Antibody	Acral keratofibroma	Normal skin
Anti-calmodulin (ACAM)	Basal cells, cytoplasmic Suprabasal cells, intercellular	Basal cells, cytoplasmic
A51-B/H4	Suprabasal cells, perinuclear	Basal cells, cytoplasmic
Ki67	Basal cells, reduced cytoplasmic intensity	Basal cells, cytoplasmic Parabasal cells, nuclear

Table 5. Immuno- and lectin staining of "hair germs" above dermatofibromas. The role of mesenchymal forces in morphogenesis and epidermal phenotype (from Wollina et al. 1991a)

Antibody	"Hair germs"	Normal epidermis
ConA	0	Suprabasal
PNA	0	Suprabasal
UEA I	0	Subcorneal
WGA	+	Vital epidermis
ACAM	suprabasal (in pre-germinal centers 0)	Basal
A51-B/H4	0	Basal
A53-B/A2	occasionally +	Only Merkel cells +
Ki67	0 (in large epithelial germinal centers suprabasal +)	Basal

epidermal wounds, the switch that starts the program of cell division is shut off when the wound is covered by a new skin. The resting state then is restored. In some benign hyperproliferative disorders like psoriasis, the switch stays on for a longer period. This is accompanied by distinct alterations of the cell surface by psoriatic keratinocytes, as indicated by lectin histochemistry (Mahrle 1982; Wollina 1988), expression of cell surface receptors, and secretion of growth factors and cytokines (for overview see Krueger et al. 1990).

In epithelial skin tumors, the switch gets "jammed" in the on position so that the cell is no longer dependent on the presence of mitogens. In basal cell carcinoma and squamous cell carcinoma significant epidermal growth factor (EGF)-receptor expression is evident (Lavrijsen et al. 1989). On the other hand, squamous carcinoma cell lines were found to be less sensitive to the growth inhibitory TGF-β, whereas TGF-α is induced by chemical carcinogens, leading to squamous cell carcinoma in vivo (Pittelkow et al.

1989). That overexpression of growth factor receptors alone preserves relatively controlled growth, but combination with a loss of growth inhibitors causes tumor enlargement, is reminiscent of the two-stage model of tumorigenesis. Many adnexal tumors are inherited (cylindroma, trichoepithelioma, etc.). It was postulated that genetically affected somatic cells express their second-stage aberrations in predetermined organs in certain distributions (Hashimoto and Kanzaki 1984). That throws light on the fact that any event which interferes with the complicated cascade of growth factors and inhibitors may activate somatic or epigenetic processes, leading to tumorigenesis.

The competence of cells to "inducers" is transient: Adult human epidermis is able to respond to mesenchymal tumor growth by formation of hair but not eccrine germs. Neuroectodermal tissues, however, show a greater plasticity in their phenotype: in Merkel cell carcinomas both squamous and eccrine differentiation was observed (Gould et al. 1988). Expression of neuroectodermal antigens not only occurs in neuroectodermal tumors but in eccrine neoplasms (Fig. 7).

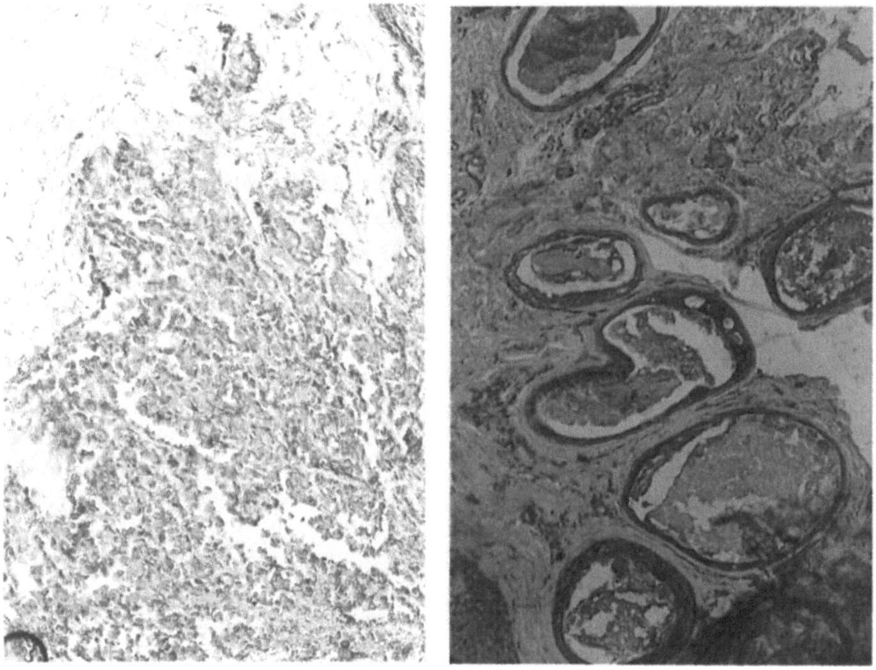

a b

Fig. 7a,b. Neuroectodermal antigen expression in adnexal tumors of skin. **a** Merkel cell carcinoma stained with monoclonal NKI/C-3 (APAAP with new fuchsin). **b** Syringoma with expression of neuroglandular antigen (monoclonal antibody LS59, unlabeled peroxidase technique with amino-ethylcarbazole). Original magnification **a** ×100, **b** ×250

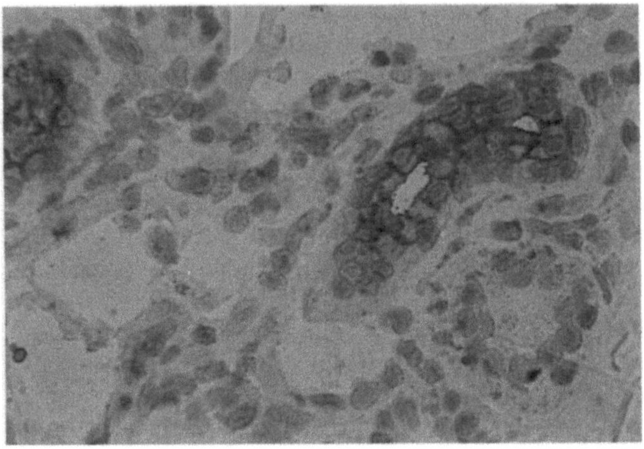

Fig. 8. Demonstration of immunoreactivity related to the receptor for vasoactive intestinal peptide in an eccrine dermal duct (cryostat section, unlabeled peroxidase technique with amino-ethylcarbazole and monoclonal antibody 109.10). Original magnification ×400

Neuropeptides are involved in the control of epithelial cell proliferation in the gastrointestinal mucosa (Goodland and Wright 1989). There is increasing evidence for neuropeptides acting as morphogens in human skin and related tumors (Wollina 1991c). In human skin, eccrine duct epithelium expresses receptors for the vasoactive intestinal peptide (VIP; Fig. 8) and keratinocyte growth is facilitated in vitro by VIP (Haegerstrand et al. 1989). Rapidly proliferating human HaCaT keratinocytes have a diminished growth capacity when cultured in absence of fetal calf serum. Recent experiments performed in collaboration with B. Bonnekoh and G. Mahrle at the Department of Dermatology in Cologne demonstrated that VIP is capable of partially restoring the growth capacity (Fig. 9; Wollina et al. 1992a,b).

A number of in vivo investigations suggest strongly that "neurohumoral factors" participate in epithelial growth regulation. Hyperplastic epidermis with precocious hair development was seen in opossum pups following partial neuralectomy (Jones and Munger 1987). In psoriasis, not only more dense innervation, but a higher level of neuropeptides in skin and more complex expression of neuropeptides by epidermal Merkel cells was noted (Eedy et al. 1991; Wollina and Mahrle 1992; Naukkarinen et al. 1989). Merot and Mooy (1989) observed a marked elevation of the number of epidermal Merkel cells in hypertrophic varieties of actinic keratoses vs nonhypertrophic keratoses (4.09 cells/mm epidermis vs 0.05 cells/mm epidermis) (Fig. 10). In granular cell tumors derived from neural tissue the epidermis is often hyperplastic with a considerable downward proliferation

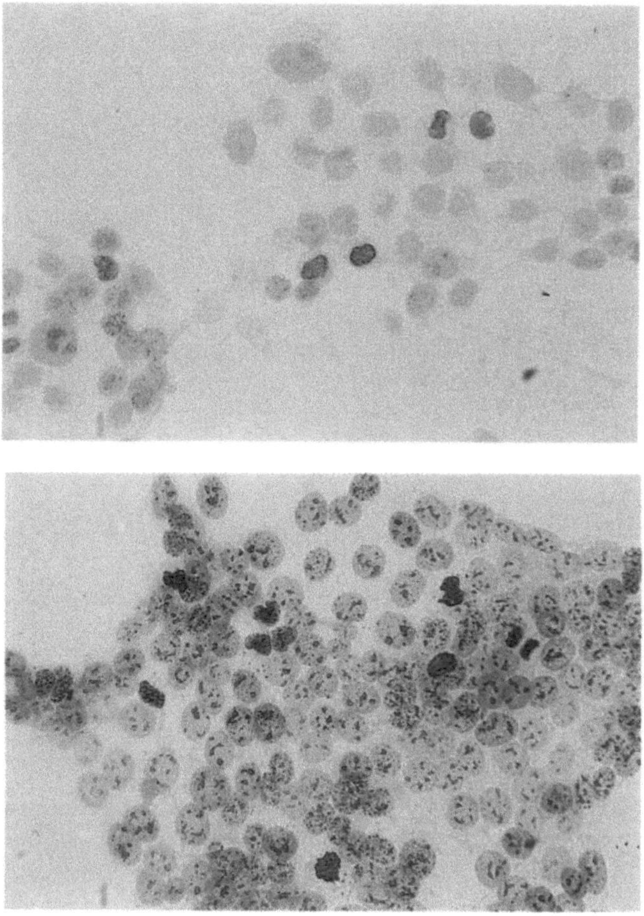

a

b

Fig. 9a,b. Vasoactive intestinal peptide (VIP) stimulates human keratinocyte growth. HaCaT keratinocytes were cultured in a medium depleted of fetal calf serum. Proliferative activity was detected by immunoperoxidase staining with amino ethylcarbazole and monoclonal antibody Ki67. **a** No VIP, **b** 10–11 *M* VIP. Note the marked increase in nuclear Ki67 reactivity. Original magnification ×400

and horn-pearl formation. In prurigo nodularis, an extreme variant of atopic dermatitis, the hyperkeratotic epidermis is acanthotic with papillomatosis and irregular downward proliferation. The number and size of cutaneous nerves is increased and the neural proliferation involves both axons and Schwann cells (Lever and Schaumburg-Lever 1990).

One can see that not only in *Xenopus* but in humans neuroectodermal and mesenchymal tissues contribute to epithelial morphogenesis, differ-

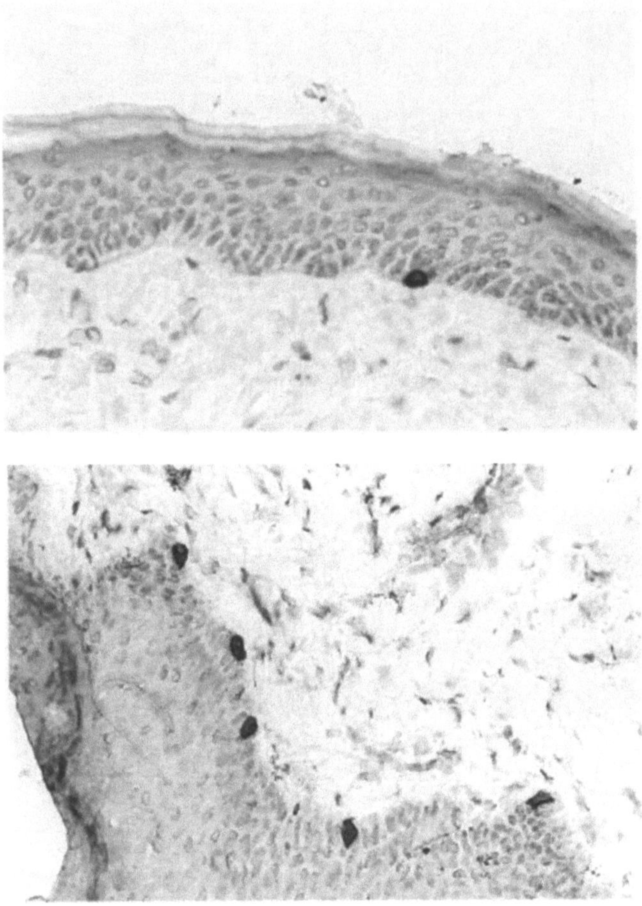

a

b

Fig. 10a,b. Distribution of epidermal Merkel cells in **a** normal skin and **b** above dermatofibroma (cryostat sections, unlabeled peroxidase technique with aminoethylcarbazole and monoclonal antibody Cam 5.2 against simple-type keratins). Original magnification ×250

entiation, and proliferative control. Cell surface qualities and the inducibility of cellular differentiation by soluble factors seem to be intimately connected. In epithelial skin tumors, these intermingled processes can potentiate each other, thus supporting autonomy of tumor cell growth.

Physiological and Tumor Cell Invasiveness

A central issue in developmental biology is the formation of spatial patterns and forms in the early embryo dependent on the migratory and invasive qualities of cells. The formation of complex tissues and organs like the skin *needs* cells to be physiologically invasive (Langerhans cells, melanocytes, lymphocytes), even after birth.

Invasiveness is supported by migratory activity and involves both release of enzymes (e.g., urokinase) and expression of surface receptors (Donaldson et al. 1987; Morioka et al. 1987; Poste and Greig 1986). Embryonic invasiveness in a chick gastrulation model demonstrated, however, that the primary determinant of the invasive behavior is a change in the cell surface carbohydrate determinants, and that there is no evidence for the participation of localized enzymatic activity (Sanders 1991). This is a major point of difference between physiological invasiveness and tumor cell invasiveness.

As shown by a number of in vitro experiments with different cell lines, invasiveness is not uniform in any tumor and seems only loosely linked to the chemotactic response (Albini et al. 1987). A substantial role of integrins has been proposed recently, since tumor cell lines with low and high metastasizing clones differ in their expression of selected adhesion molecules. It was demonstrated that integrins participate in attachment of tumor cells to extracellular matrix molecules like laminin or collagen type IV, proteolysis of basement membrane components by activation of proteases, and migration of tumor cells (Dedhar 1990).

Invasiveness of tumors is considered as a sign of malignancy. Tumor spread and formation of metastases have been attributed to urokinase, a trypsin-like serine protease (Bogenmann and Jones 1983). The tumor promotor 12-*O*-tetradecanoylphorbol-13-acetate (TPA) and EGF induced urokinase mRNA synthesis in murine keratinocytes (Rorth et al. 1990), but even in wound healing and benign tumors urokinase activity has been demonstrated. In a histochemical study on melanocytic nevi, single tumor cells invading the epidermis were labeled with polyclonal antiserum 20AS5 against urokinase (Wollina et al. 1989c). Though the melanocytic nevus is a neuroectodermal skin tumor, comparable mechanisms can account for transepidermal elimination of epithelial tumor cells and epidermal infiltration, too. On the other hand, urokinase reactivity was also evident among dermal duct epithelia of eccrine glands, in epithelial outgrowth of superficial wounds, and in psoriatic lesions (Wollina et al. 1991e; Grondahl-Hansen et al. 1988).

There is experimental evidence that plasminogen activators like urokinase also provide autocrine receptor-mediated growth promotion for epithelial tumor cell lines (Kirchheimer et al. 1987), thus providing support for tumor enlargement at different levels. In conclusion, local release of enzymes contributes to both morphogenesis and TCH but the mode of action is influenced by cell surface qualities (integrins, cell surface receptors) and the cellular microenvironment.

Transdifferentiation

Transdifferentiation is regarded as a subcategory of a diversity of reprogrammative phenomena. It means a switch in the phenotype of a cell that has acquired a stable working character not necessarily dependent on cell division (Beresford 1990).

Transdifferentiation is mediated or initiated by local factors. A proportion alterating factor (PAF) isolated from colonial hydroids increases transdifferentiation of isolated striated muscle of jellyfish into nerve cells, when applied shortly before or at the time of initiation of DNA synthesis (Schmid and Plickert 1990). In *Xenopus* embryos, factors related to the TGF-β superfamily have been partially purified (Tiedemann 1990). In other experimental models, adhesion molecules like laminin play a pivotal role (Ekblom 1989). The action of nerve factors like neuropeptides is another example of epigenetic modifications of cells (Bosco 1988; Wollina 1991a,b; Wollina and Mahrle 1992; Wollina et al. 1992a,b).

In amphibian skin, xanthophores can transdifferentiate into melanophores. In mammals, skeletal musles change their phenotype under extreme physical training from type II A fibres into type I. Arterial smooth muscle cells of the kidney can transdifferentiate into epitheloid endocrine cells, i.e., juxtaglomerular renin-secreting cells, under three conditions: (1) surgically restricted blood flow, (2) depletion of sodium by parotid-cannula drainage, and (3) sodium-deficient diet (Beresford 1990; Sugiyama and Komamine 1990; Bosco 1988).

Transdifferentiation also throws light onto the generation of epidermal Merkel cells. Recent investigations have provided a large body of evidence for the epithelial nature of Merkel cells (Gould et al. 1985; Moll et al. 1984). Vaigot et al. (1987) reported on their very low mitotic activity, but Merkel cells can be formed de novo in skin transplants (Moll et al. 1990). A role for neuroectodermal factors in the generation of Merkel cells was proposed (Mahrle et al. 1977). From this viewpoint, I suppose that epidermal Merkel cells are transdifferentiated from basal adnexal epithelia of skin (see Wollina 1990). There is a remarkable parallelism to the developmentally dependent cytokeratin 19 expression among neuroectodermal cells of other epithelia like human choroid plexus tissue (Miettinen et al. 1986), human and rodent retinal pigment epithelium (Kasper 1991), or human corneal epithelial cells (Kasper et al. 1988).

Direct transdifferentiation has implications for malignancy. Heterogeneity of the cellular phenotype might be a consequence of transdifferentiation factors, e.g., the coexpression of intermediate filaments by cylindromas or the development of the Merkel cell carcinoma of skin (Avesti et al. 1990; Heenan et al. 1990; see also Wollina 1990; Table 6; Fig. 6). It also has an impact on therapeutic strategies. Direct transdifferentiation bears the message that one can aim simultaneously at both

Table 6. Some arguments for an adnexal stem cell origin of Merkel cell carcinoma of skin (modified from Heenan et al. 1990; Wollina 1990)

- Frequent association with other forms of skin cancer (solar keratosis, lentigo maligna, squamous cell carcinoma)
- Similarity in epidemiological features with the common forms of human skin cancer
- Heterogeneity of differentiation with evidence of squamous and glandular phenotypes
- Similarity with other neuroendocrine tumors (oat cell carcinoma, neuroblastoma, pulmonary small cell anaplastic carcinoma), which arise from epithelial stem cells
- Coexpression of neuroendocrine and epithelial antigens
- Almost invariable dermal location

blocking proliferation and "treating" the malignant phenotype by modulation or blocking of local growth factors (see Beresford 1990).

Conclusions

Tumor classification serves to present reality in a simplified way that leads itself more readily to interpretation and explanation. Some aspects of complexicity have been discussed in this chapter. It was demonstrated that local and systemic, endogenous and exogenous factors contribute to TCH in epithelial skin tumors. A number of recently identified factors exert pleiotropic effects, making a simple determinism unreliable for the understanding of tumorigenesis. The process is rather linked to a breaking down of hierarchies in human biology. Remarkable progress in the field of tumor biology has been made possible by the introduction of more advanced techniques. Science proceeds by the experimental method. But the main question remains to be answered: How can we make sure that what we describe is correct, i.e., represents reality?

Acknowledgments. I gratefully acknowledge the inspiring discussions with my collaborators at the Department of Dermatology, Friedrich-Schiller-University Jena, Drs. Henning Schaarschmidt, Ute Henkel, and Professor Burkhard Knopf. I am grateful to Professor Gerd Klaus Steigleder and Professor Gustav Mahrle (Department of Dermatology, University of Cologne), who have generously supported my scientific interests and provided excellent working facilities at their Department. Parts of the work were supported by the Paul-Gerson-Unna-Stiftung, Deutscher Akademischer Austauschdienst (DAAD), and the Verein der Freunde und Förderer der Universitäts-Hautklinik Cologne.

References

Aaronson SA, Rubin JS, Finch PW, Wong J, Marchese C, Falco J, Taylor WG, Kraus MH (1990) Growth factor-regulated pathways in epithelial cell proliferation. Am Rev Respir Dis 142:S7–S10

Albini A, Iwamoto Y, Kleiman HK, Martin GR, Aaronson SA, Kozlowski JM, McEwan RN (1987) A rapid in vitro assay for quantitating the invasive potential of tumor cells. Cancer Res 47:3239–3245

Anderson H (1990) Adhesion molecules and animal development. Experientia 46:2–13

Avesti C, Grossin M, Toublanc M, Benjereb N, Bourgeois-Droin C, Delacretaz J, Belaich S, Bocquet L (1990) Association d'un carcinome neuro-endocrine cutané et d'une maladie de Bowen. Revue de la littérature à propos de quatre cas. Ann Pathol 10:86–98

Beresford WA (1990) Direct transdifferentiation: can cells change their phenotype without dividing? Cell Differ Dev 29:81–93

Bhargava PM, Chandani SA (1988) Regulation of cell division and malignant transformation. Biosci Rep 8:519–529

Bogenmann E, Jones PA (1983) Role of plasminogen in matrix breakdown by neoplastic cells. J Natl Cancer Inst 71:1177–1182

Bosco L (1988) Transdifferentiation of ocular tissues in larval Xenopus laevis. Differentiation 39:4–15

Chigira M, Noda K, Watanabe H (1990) Autonomy in tumor cell proliferation. Med Hypotheses 32:249–254

Cotsarelis G, Sun T-T, Lavker R (1990) Label-retaining cells reside in the bulge area of pilosebaceous unit: implications for follicular stem cells, hair cycle, and skin carcinogenesis. Cell 61:1329–1337

Dedhar S (1990) Integrins and tumor invasion. Bioessays 12:583–590

Donaldson DJ, Mahan JT, Smith GN Jr (1987) Newt epidermal cell migration in vivo and in vitro appears to involve Arg-Gly-Asp-Ser receptors. J Cell Sci 87:525–534

Eedy DJ, Johnston CF, Shaw C, Buchanan KD (1991) Neuropeptides in psoriasis: an immunocytochemical and radioimmunoassay study. J Invest Dermatol 96:434–438

Ekblom P (1989) Developmentally regulated conversion of mesenchyme to epithelium. FASEB J 3:2141–2150

El-Labban NG, Osorio-Herrera E (1986) Apoptotic bodies and abnormally dividing epithelial cells in squamous cell carcinoma. Histopathology 10:921–931

Fenderson BA, Eddy EM, Hakomori S (1990) Glycoconjugate expression during embryogenesis and its biological significance. Bioessays 12:173–179

Goodland RA, Wright NA (1989) Peptides and epithelial growth regulation. Experientia Suppl 56:180–191

Gould V, Moll R, Moll I, Lee I, Franke WW (1985) Neuroendocrine (Merkel) cells of the skin: hyperplasias, dysplasias, and neoplasms. Lab Invest 52:334–353

Gould E, Albores-Saavedra J, Dubner B, Smith W, Payne CM (1988) Eccrine and squamous differentiation in Merkel cell carcinoma: an immunohistochemical study. Am J Surg Pathol 12:768–772

Grondahl-Hansen J, Lund LR, Ralfkiaer E, Ottevanger V, Dano K (1988) Urokinase- and tissue type plasminogen activators in keratinocytes during wound epithelialization in vivo. J Invest Dermatol 90:790–795

Guo JF, Brown R, Rothwell CE, Bernstein IA (1990a) Levels of cytochrome P-450-mediated aryl hydrocarbon hydroxylase (AHH) are higher in differentiated than in germinative cutaneous keratinocytes. J Invest Dermatol 94:86–93

Guo M, Toda K, Grinnell F (1990b) Activation of human keratinocyte migration on type I collagen and fibronectin. J Cell Sci 96:197–205
Haegerstrand A, Jonzon B, Dalsgaard C-J, Nilsson J (1989) Vasoactive intestinal polypeptide stimulates cell proliferation and adenylate cyclase activity of cultured keratinocytes. Proc Natl Acad Sci USA 86:5993–5996
Hashimoto K, Kanzaki T (1984) Appendage tumors of the skin: histogenesis and ultrastructure. J Cutan Pathol 11:365–381
Hashimoto K, Gross BG, Lever WF (1966) The ultrastructure of human embryo skin: II. The formation of the intradermal portion of the eccrine sweat duct and of the secretory segment during the first half of embryonic life. J Invest Dermatol 46:513–529
Hashimoto K, Mehregan AH, Kumakiri M (1987) Tumors of skin appendages. Butterworth, Stoneham
Heenan PJ, Cole JM, Spagnolo DV (1990) Primary cutaneous neuroendocrine carcinoma (Merkel cell tumor). An adnexal epithelial neoplasm. Am J Dermatopathol 12:7–16
Hill MW, Mackenzie IC (1989) The influence of subepithelial connective tissues on epithelial proliferation in the adult mouse. Cell Tissue Res 255:179–182
Iki M (1990) Immunohistochemical studies on eccrine sweat apparatus neoplasms: 2. An immunohistochemical study on eccrine sweat apparatus neoplasms-direction of differentiation in eccrine sweat apparatus neoplasms. Skin Res 32:353–367
Inohara A (1990) Protein kinase C in psoriasis. Skin Res 32:339–344
Jones TE, Munger BL (1987) Neural modulation of cutaneous differentiation: epidermal hyperplasia and precocious hair development following partial neuralectomy in opossum pups. Neurosci Lett 79:6–10
Kasper M (1991) Heterogeneity in the immunolocalization of cytokeratin specific monoclonal antibodies in the rat eye: evaluation of unusual epithelial tissue entities. Histochemistry 95:613–620
Kasper M, Moll R, Stosiek P, Karsten U (1988) Patterns of cytokeratin and vimentin expression in the human eye. Histochemistry 89:369–377
Kaufmann R, Weber L, Klein CE (1990) Integrine – neue Rezeptormoleküle: Ihre Bedeutung für die Differenzierung, Regeneration und Immunantwort der Haut. Hautarzt 41:256–261
Kirchheimer JC, Wojta J, Christ G, Binder BR (1987) Proliferation of a human epidermal tumor cell line stimulated by urokinase. FASEB J 1:125–128
Klein CE, Steinmayer T, Mattes JM, Kaufmann R, Weber L (1990) Integrins of normal human epidermis: differential expression, synthesis and molecular structure. Br J Dermatol 123:171–178
Knopf B, Wollina U (1992) Electrophoretic mobilities of keratinocytes from normal skin and psoriatic lesions. Arch Dermatol Res 284:117–118
Krueger JG, Krane JF, Carter DM, Gottlieb AB (1990) Role of growth factors, cytokines, and their receptors in the pathogenesis of psoriasis. J Invest Dermatol 94:135s–140s
Lavrijsen AP, Tieben LM, Ponec M, van der Schroeff JG, van Muijen GN (1989) Expression of EGF receptor, involucrin, and cytokeratins in basal cell carcinomas and squamous cell carcinomas of the skin. Arch Dermatol Res 281:83–88
Lever WF, Schaumburg-Lever G (1990) Histopathology of the skin, 7th edn. Lippincott, Philadelphia
Mackenzie IC, Dabelsteen E (1987) Connective tissue influences on the expression of epithelial cell-surface antigens. Cell Tissue Res 248:137–141
Mahrle G (1982) Cell interactions and cell surface membranes in psoriasis. In: Farber EM, Cox AJ (eds) Psoriasis. Proceedings of the 3rd international symposium. Grune and Stratton, New York, pp 43–52

Mahrle G, Runne U, Orfanos CE (1977) Sensorische Innervation und autonome Kontrolle der menschlichen Epidermis. In: Lassmann G, Niebauer G, Jurecka W (eds) Wiener Symposium "Struktur und Pathologie des Hautnervensystems". Verband der wissenschaftlichen Gesellschaften Österreichs, Wien, pp VI/1–VI/7

Marchisio PC, Bondanza S, Cremona O, Cancedda R, De Luca M (1991) Polarized expression of integrin receptors (alpha 6 beta 4, alpha 2 beta 1, alpha 3 beta 1, and alpha v beta 5) and their relationship with the cytoskeleton and basement membrane matrix in cultured human keratinocytes. J Cell Biol 112:761–773

Mehregan AH (1985) The origin of the adnexal tumors of the skin: a viewpoint. J Cutan Pathol 12:459–467

Merk HF (1990) Die Haut als Signalorgan in der Entwicklung neuer Zytostatika und Antitumorstrategien. Z Hautkr 65:89–96

Merk H, Rumpf M, Bolsen K, Wirth H, Goerz G (1987a) Inducibility of arylhydrocarbon-hydroxylase activity in human hair follicles by topical application of liquor carbonis detergens (cool tar). Br J Dermatol 111:279–284

Merk H, Mukhtar H, Schutte B, Kaufmann I, Das M, Bickers DR (1987b) 7-Ethoxyresorufineethylase activity in human hair roots: a potential marker for toxifying species of cytochrome P-450 isoenzymes. Biochem Biophys Res Commun 148:755–760

Merot Y, Mooy A (1989) Merkel cell hyperplasia in hypertrophic varieties of actinic keratoses. Dermatologica 178:189–193

Miettinen M, Clark R, Virtanen I (1986) Intermediate filament proteins in choroid plexus and ependyma and their tumors. Am J Pathol 123:231–240

Mizuno T, Yasugi S (1990) Susceptibility of epithelia to directive influences of mesenchymes during organogenesis: uncoupling of morphogenesis and cytodifferentiation. Cell Differ Dev 31:151–159

Moll R, Moll I, Franke WW (1984) Identification of Merkel cells in human skin by specific cytokeratin antibodies: changes of cell density and distribution in fetal and adult plantar epidermis. Differentiation 28:136–154

Moll I, Lane AT, Franke WW, Moll R (1990) Intraepidermal formation of Merkel cells on xenografts of human fetal skin. J Invest Dermatol 94:359–364

Morioka S, Lazarus GS, Baird JL, Jensen PJ (1987) Migrating keratinocytes express urokinase-type plasminogen activator. J Invest Dermatol 88:418–423

Mukhtar H, Khan WA (1989) Cutaneous cytochrome P-450. Drug Metab Rev 20:657–673

Mukhtar H, Merk HF, Athar M (1989) Skin chemical carcinogenesis. Clin Dermatol 7:1–10

Nakhleh RE, Swanson PE, Wick MR (1990) Cutaneous adnexal carcinomas with divergent differentiation. Am J Dermatopathol 12:325–334

Naukkarinen A, Nickoloff BJ, Farber EM (1989) Quantification of cutaneous sensory nerves and their substance P content in psoriasis. J Invest Dermatol 92:126–129

Oriol R (1987) ABH and related tissues. Biochem Soc Trans 15:596–599

Pinkus H (1958) The concept of symbiosis applied to normal and abnormal growth in the human epidermis. Dermatologica 177:369–379

Pittelkow MR, Lindquist PB, Abraham RT, Graves-Deal R, Deryck R, Coffey RJ Jr (1989) Induction of transforming growth factor-alpha expression in human keratinocytes by phorbol esters. J Biol Chem 264:5164–5171

Poste G, Greig R (1986) The cell surface and cancer metastasis. In: Steinberg MS (ed) Developmental biology, vol 3. Plenum, New York, pp 15–31

Reiners JJ Jr, Cantu AR, Pavone A (1990) Modulation of constitutive cytochrome P-450 expression in vivo and in vitro in murine keratinocytes as a function of differentiation and extracellular Ca2+ concentration. Proc Natl Acad Sci USA 87:1825–1829

Rorth P, Nerlov C, Blasi F, Johnsen M (1990) Transcription factor PEA3 participates in the induction of urokinase plasminogen activator transcription in murine keratinocytes stimulated with epidermal growth factor of phorbol-ester. Nucleic Acids Res 18:5009–5017

Rosen LB (1990) A review and proposed new classification of benign acquired neoplasms with hair follicle differentiation. Am J Dermatopathol 12:496–516

Ruben LN, Clothier RH, Horton JD, Balls M (1989) Amphibian metamorphosis: an immunologic opportunity! Bioessays 10:8–12

Sanders EJ (1991) Embryonic cell invasiveness: an in vitro study of chick gastrulation. J Cell Sci 98:403–407

Schaarschmidt H, Wollina U (1990) Immunhistochemischer Nachweis von Calmodulin. Ein Beitrag zur histogenetischen Einordnung von ekkrinen Poromen und Klarzellakanthomen. Dermatol Monatsschr 176:363–370

Schmid V, Plickert G (1990) The proportion altering factor (PAF) and the in vitro transdifferentiation of isolated striated muscle of jellyfish into nerve cells. Differentiation 44:95–102

Stamp GW, Pignatelli M (1991) Distribution of beta 1, alpha 1, alpha 2 and alpha 3 integrin chains in basal cell carcinomas. J Pathol 163:307–313

Steinberg MS (1986) Cell surfaces in the control of growth and morphogenesis. In: Steinberg MS (ed) Developmental biology, vol 3. Plenum, New York, pp 1–13

Stolar A, Duvic M, Fuchs E (1989) Unusual patterns of keratin expression in the overlying epidermis of patients with dermatofibromas: biochemical alterations in the epidermis as a consequence of dermal tumors. J Invest Dermatol 93:728–738

Sugiyama M, Komamine A (1990) Transdifferentiation of quiescent parenchymatous cells into tracheary elements. Cell Differ Dev 31:77–87

Tiedemann H (1990) Cellular and molecular aspects of embryonic induction. Zool Sci 7:171–186

Tsubura A, Morii S, Ueda S, Sasaki M, Zotter S, Wätzig V, Mooi W, Hagemann P, Hilkens J, van den Tweel J, Meijer C, Hilgers J (1987) Immunohistochemical demonstration of MAM-3 and MAM-6 antigens in normal human skin appendages and their tumors. Arch Dermatol Res 279:550–557

Vaigot P, Pisani A, Darmon YM, Ortonne JP (1987) The majority of epidermal Merkel cells are non-proliferative: a quantitative immunofluorescence analysis. Acta Derm Venereol (Stockh) 67:517–541

Wiley LM, Kidder GM, Watson AJ (1990) Cell polarity and development of the first epithelium. Bioessays 12:67–73

Wollina U (1988) Abnorme Epidermiszelldifferenzierung bei Psoriasis vulgaris. Thesis, Friedrich-Schiller-University, Jena

Wollina U (1990) Immunohistochemical investigations in epidermal Merkel cells – a common phenotype with eccrine sweat gland epithelium. Acta Histochem 88:47–50

Wollina U (1991a) Human eccrine sweat gland. Expression of neuroglandular antigen and coexpression of intermediate filaments. Histol Histopathol 6:191–198

Wollina U (1991b) Ekkrine Schweißdrüsen – embryologische Aspekte und klinische Bezüge. Dermatol Monatsschr 177:1–6

Wollina U (1991c) Neuropeptide in der Dermatologie. Z Hautkrankh 66:1010–1017

Wollina U (1992) Histochemistry of the human hair follicle with consideration of anagen phases I to IV. Acta Histochem 92:171–178

Wollina U, Mahrle G (1992) Epidermal Merkel cells in psoriatic lesions – immunohistochemical investigations on frequency and neuropeptide expression. J Dermatol Sci 3:145–150

Wollina U, Schaarschmidt H (1990a) Chondroides Hidradenom. Immunhistologischer Nachweis von Zytokeratin und Calmodulin. Dermatol Monatsschr 176:173–178

Wollina U, Schaarschmidt H (1990b) Das erworbene akrale Fibrokeratom. Hautarzt 41:158–160
Wollina U, Klinger R, Wetzker R, Knopf B (1989a) Increase of epidermal calmodulin precedes the formation of a psoriatic lesion. Arch Dermatol Res 281:73–74
Wollina U, Klinger R, Wetzker R, Reissmann R, Knopf B (1989b) Immunohistological localization of calmodulin in normal and psoriatic epidermis. Arch Dermatol Res 280:497–498
Wollina U, Schaarschmidt H, Henkel U, Knopf B, Hipler C (1989c) Histochemische Untersuchungen zur transepidermalen Elimination von Nävuszellen. Z Hautkr 64:694–699
Wollina U, Schaarschmidt H, Knopf B, Feldrappe S (1990) Immunhistologische Untersuchungen zur Verteilung proliferativer Kompartimente in den Anhangsgebilden humaner adulter Haut. Z Mikrosk Anat Forsch 104:485–496
Wollina U, Henkel U, Schaarschmidt H, Knopf B (1991a) Histochemische Untersuchungen der Epidermisreaktion beim Dermatofibrom. Dermatol Monatsschr 177:111–115
Wollina U, Knopf B, Schaarschmidt H, Henkel U (1991b) Immunhistologische Lokalisation von Plasminogenaktivatoren in gesunder und pathologischer Epidermis. Dermatol Monatsschr 176:11–16
Wollina U, Schaarschmidt H, Berger U (1991c) Nävoide Bündelhaare. Hautarzt 42:189–191
Wollina U, Wevers A, Mahrle G (1991d) Localization of calmodulin in epidermis and skin glands. A comparative investigation in different vertebrate species. Acta Histochem 90:135–140
Wollina U, Henkel U, Schaarschmidt H, Knopf B, Hipler C (1991e) Human eccrine sweat glands – a histochemical approach. Anat Anz 173:155–159
Wollina U, Bonnekoh B, Klinger R, Wetzker R, Mahrle G (1992a) Vasoactive intestinal peptide (VIP) acting as a growth factor for human keratinocytes. Neuroendocrinol Lett 14:21–31
Wollina U, Bonnekoh B, Mahrle G (1992b) Vasoactive intestinal peptide (VIP) modulates the growth fraction of epithelial skin cells. Int J Oncol 1:17–24
Wyllie AH (1986) Commentary: what is apoptosis? Histopathology 10:995–998
Wyllie AH (1988) Apoptosis. ISI Atlas Sci Immunol 1:192–196
Wyllie AH, Kerr JFR, Currie AR (1980) Cell death: the significance of apoptosis. Int Rev Cytol 68:251–306

Keratinocyte Alterations in Skin Tumour Development

I.M. Leigh[1], P.E. Purkis[1], A. Markey[1,4], P. Collins[2], S. Neill[1,4], C. Proby[1], M. Glover[2], and E.B. Lane[3]

[1] ICRF Skin Tumour Laboratory, 56 Ashfield Street, London E1 2BL, UK
[2] Department of Dermatology, Royal London Hospital, London E1 1BB, UK
[3] CRC Laboratories, Department of Biochemistry, University of Dundee, Dundee DD1 4NN, UK
[4] Visiting clinical fellow

Introduction

Non-melanoma skin cancers (NMSC) comprise about a third of all cancers in the United States (Miller 1991). Basal cell carcinoma (BCC) occurs more frequently than squamous cell carcinoma (SCC), with particular risk factors for BCC being increasing age, susceptibility to sunburn, fair complexion, outdoor living, and fair hair and eyes (Gellin et al. 1965). SCC has additional risk factors of cigarette smoking and ultraviolet lamp exposure (Aubry and McGibbon 1985), previous X irradiation, and exposure to chemical carcinogens such as medicinal or environmental arsenic. The increasing incidence of NMSC probably reflects increased lifetime recreational sun-exposure (Diffey 1987; Urbach 1989). Therapeutic ultraviolet irradiation such as photochemotherapy with psoralen and long-wave ultraviolet light (PUVA) has also caused an increase in NMSC due to a combination of ultraviolet-induced mutation and photoimmunosuppression. The role of immune surveillance in the development of skin cancer is also emphasised by the finding that NMSC is increased in immunosuppressed renal transplant recipients. A study from Edinburgh demonstrated that 77% of 69 renal transplant patients with graft survival of more than 5 years had viral warts, 38% had keratoses, and 12% had skin cancers (Barr et al. 1989), markedly higher than expected. The ratio of SCC to BCC was a reversal of the ratio shown in the non-immunosuppressed population with, again, the majority of lesions found on sun-exposed sites. The presence of viral warts with suggestive histopathology (Blessing et al. 1989) in sun-exposed sites implicated ultraviolet radiation as a potentiating cofactor in virally mediated oncogenesis. These results were confirmed in a study at the Royal London Hospital (Glover et al. 1991a) in 190 renal transplant recipients, where overall 50% of patients had viral warts and 21% NMSC. These patients have provided samples for the current report.

Recent Results in Cancer Research, Vol. 128

The term VINIII (vulval intraepithelial neoplasia grade III) has been introduced to replace the older diagnoses of dysplastic conditions of the vulva including Bowen's disease, Bowenoid papulosis and erythroplasia of Queyrat. The role of human papillomavirus (HPV) in VIN is currently under investigation, but sequences for HPV 16 and 18 have been found within the lesions, particularly in younger patients (Eichenberg et al. 1983). The vulva itself is transitional between labia majora, phenotypically epidermal and the vestibule and vaginal epithelia, which are mucosal stratified squamous epithelia (S.M. Neill et al. 1993a). This junctional region seems to be the site of predilection for malignant transformation, possibly related to greater pluripotentiality of differentiation.

Keratinocyte Alterations in Structural Proteins During Differentiation

The basal cell compartment of human skin contains the generative compartment, although suprabasal cells can undergo a limited number of cell divisions on demand. During epidermal cell movement through the differentiating compartments, the keratinocytes undergo terminal differentiation and lose the ability to divide. A series of steps in this process involves changes in keratin synthesis and the production of precursors of the cornified envelope such as involucrin. There are also changes in membrane glycosylation with changes in blood group antigens and cell surface receptors for matrix proteins (integrins) and growth factors. The precise sequence and interaction of these different processes is poorly understood and their regulation a subject of current research. All of these processes may be altered by epidermal hyperproliferation in wound healing and skin diseases and during the development of skin malignancies.

Keratins in Skin Tumours

The expression of keratin intermediate filaments appears tightly linked with the tissue-specific and cell-specific pattern of differentiation of epithelial cells (Osborn and Weber 1982). Keratins (type I and type II intermediate filaments) form the major structural proteins of all epithelial cells and derive from a complex multigene family of more than 30 individual keratins, which polypeptides can be distinguished on the basis of their molecular weight and isolectric point on two-dimensional gel electrophoresis (Moll et al. 1982a). Intermediate filament type tends to be conserved during malignant transformation and therefore the intermediate filament expression of a tumour may be useful in identifying its histogenesis (Osborn et al. 1984). Tissue-specific expression depends on the coexpression of heterodimers of particular pairs of keratins containing one acidic and one basic keratin polypeptide (Eichner et al. 1986), which form the fundamental building blocks of the intermediate filament. Keratin pairs can be characteristic of simple epithelia (keratin 8 and 18) or of stratified squamous epithelia (keratin 5 and 14). The keratin profile in stratifying epithelia is complex, so suprabasal epidermal keratinocytes express differentiation-specific keratins 1 and 10, whereas non-cornifying stratified squamous epithelia such as genital and oral mucosa express keratins 4/13 and 6/16 pairs suprabasally. Thus the diversity of keratin expression in normal tissue raises the question of whether the phenotype of the epithelial cell is retained during malignant transformation and can thereby aid classification of tumours which are difficult to diagnose by routine histopathology such as adenocarcinomas or SCC. Data on the expression of keratins in epidermal tumours has depended upon a variety of detection systems involving one-dimensional gel electrophoresis, microdissection, two-dimensional gel electrophoresis, or immunocytochemistry (Moll et al. 1984a; Stoler et al. 1988; Kariniemi and Virtanen 1989). Gel electrophoresis fails to detect subtle changes in keratin expression by small subpopulations of cells in the tumour; also, hyperproliferative keratins 6 and 16 are induced in the epidermis overlying the BCC islands and this may cause these keratins to appear on gel electrophoresis. Immunohistochemistry using monoclonal antibodies allows the assessment of cell to cell expression of keratins within heterogeneous populations. A large range of monospecific monoclonal antibodies is now available, which has been well-characterised by two-dimensional gel immunoblotting. This panel can now be used to examine the in vivo expression of keratins in epidermal SCC and BCC (Habets et al. 1988; Thomas et al. 1984; Viac et al. 1982; Kariniemi et al. 1984; Robinson 1987). In previous studies, BCC have been found to express primarily the basal keratins 5 and 14 with additional expression of keratins 15 and 17 (Moll et al. 1982b). Keratin 15 appears to be a normal basal cell keratin, but keratin 17 is only found in adnexal basal epithelia and in the deep outer root sheath (Lane et al. 1991). Keratins 8 and 18 are not expressed in normal basal epidermis except in Merkel cells (Moll et al. 1984b). Some investigators have found keratins 8 and 18 in BCC and SCC, although this has been dependent on the detection systems (Markey et al. 1991). Keratins 1 and 10 have been found in SCC in differentiation-associated areas and even in some BCC. Since the comprehensive panel of antibodies has only recently become available, extensive studies have recently been performed of keratin expression in skin tumours of immunocompetent patients and immunosuppressed renal transplant recipients and vulval skin lesions.

Immunohistochemistry

Tumours are available from clinical studies, including: BCC and SCC from non-immunosuppressed patients (Markey et al. 1991); dysplastic warts and multiple skin tumours (both BCC and SCC) from a population study of

Table 1. Monospecific antibodies to keratin polypeptides

Keratin	Antibody	Source reference	Dilution
18	LE61	Lane 1982	1:5
	LE65	Lane 1982	
	RKK3	Virtanen et al. 1985	
	RGE53	Ramaekers et al. 1983	
	CK18.2	Broers et al. 1986	1:20
	RCK106	Ramaekers et al. 1987a	
	CK2	Debus et al. 1984	
	CK5	Debus et al. 1984	
	DC10	Lauerova et al. 1988	
19	LP2K	Stasiak et al. 1989	
	KM4.62	Gigi Leitner and Geiger 1986	
	BA16	Bartek et al. 1985	
	K19.2	Jahn et al. 1987	
8	LE41	Lane 1982	
	M20	Schaafsma et al. 1990b	
	LP3K	Lane et al. 1985	
	TROMA1(+7)	Kemler et al. 1981	
	Cam5.2(+7)	Makin et al. 1984	
7	RCK105	Ramaekers et al. 1987b	
	CK7	Tolle et al. 1985	1:5
	LP1K	Lane et al. 1985	
	LP5K	Lane et al. 1985	
14	LL001	Purkis et al. 1990	1:40
	LL002	Purkis et al. 1990	1:40
Basal	LH6/LH8	Purkis et al. 1990	1:5
5	2.1.D7	Purkis et al. 1990	
	RaK5	Purkis et al. 1990	1:10
10	LH1	Lane et al. 1985	1:5
	LH2	Lane et al. 1985	1:10
	RKSE60	Ramaekers et al. 1985	1:20
1	LL017	Leigh et al., in press	
	RaK1	Leigh et al., in press	
4	IC7	van de Muijen et al. 1986	
13	6B10	van de Muijen et al. 1986	
6	LL020	Lane et al., in prep	
	Ka12	Nagle gift	
16	LL025	Lane et al., in prep	
	LMM3	Gardner et al. 1988	
17	E3	Guelstein et al. 1988	
Polyspecific	AE1	Woodcock Mitchell et al. 1982 (keratins 10, 14, 15, 16, 19)	
	AE3	Woodcock Mitchell et al. 1982 (1, 2, 3, 4, 5, 6, 7, 8)	
	Ks8.12	Huszar et al. 1986 (13, 15 16)	
	PKK1	Virtanen et al. 1985 (8, 17, 18, 19)	
	PKK2	Virtanen et al. 1985 (16, 17, 19)	
	LP34	Lane et al. 1985 (5, 6, 18)	
	C46	Bartek et al. 1991 (7, 17)	

renal transplant patients (Glover et al. 1991b); and vulval condylomata (15 subjects), intraepithelial neoplasias (VIN-III) (15 subjects) and tumours (S.M. Neill et al. 1993b). These samples were biopsied in small representative samples; snap-frozen, 5-μm cryostat sections were cut and stained using a standard peroxidase, anti-peroxidase staining technique. Sections were incubated with primary antibodies for 60 min, and subsequently with peroxidase-conjugated rabbit anti-mouse antibody, and 3,3′-aminobenzidine was used as substrate. Sections were rinsed in tapwater, counterstained in Mayer's haematoxylin, dehydrated through graded alcohol, and mounted in DPX. The antibodies used, their dilutions and specificity are listed in Tables 1 and 2. Extensive work was performed using the large bank of keratin monoclonal antibodies in Table 1, which are monospecific and are available either through being produced in our own laboratories, through collaborative studies, or from commercial sources. From the total set of antibodies, a selected table (Table 2) documents the strongest, most reliable antibodies for individual keratins which we would recommend as a panel of monoclonal antibodies for pathological use in frozen tissue. Formalin

Table 2. Selected table of optimal antibodies for use and tissue reaction in skin and orogenital mucosa

Antibody	Keratin	Reaction with normal skin epithelia	Fixation
LL001	K14	Basal and suprabasal epidermis/mucosa excluding stratum granulosum.	Formalin
RaK5 (polyclonal)	K5	Basal and suprabasal epidermis/mucosa excluding stratum granulosum.	–
LL017 LH2	K1 K10	Suprabasal epidermis and high suprabasal orogenital mucosa.	– Formalin
Ka12 LL025	K6 K16	Sweat duct suprabasal cells. Suprabasal orogenital mucosa and suprabasal skin in hyperproliferation	–
LH8 LH6	Basal Basal	Basal cells: single layer in epidermis but multiple in orogenital mucosa	–
M20 RGE53	K8 K18	Sweat gland luminal epithelia and isolated Merkel cells in epidermis. All simple epithelia including heptocytes and gastointestinal epithelia.	– –
LP2K	K19	Sweat gland ducts and acini. Sebaceous glands. Stem cells in hair follicle.	–
E3	K17	Deep outer root sheath of hair follicle and appendageal basal cells.	–
RCK 105	K7	Sebaceous and sweat glands. Inner root sheath.	–

resistance is indicated in Table 2 but largely antibody reactivity is limited to frozen tissue.

Results

Results are summarised on Table 3, and will be reported in detail elsewhere. However, the following summarises the expression of keratin antigens in normal tissue and in the different tumour types.

Normal Skin and Genital Mucosa

Keratins 5 and 14. Antibodies LLOO1 and LLOO2 (Purkis et al. 1990), raised against the carboxy-terminal synthetic peptide to keratin 14, react with all living epidermal cells up to the granular cell layer. Monoclonal antibody 21D7 and polyclonal RaK5 to keratin 5 stain epibasal cells and basal cells but do not stain all living epidermal cells (Purkis et al. 1990). Basal cell markers LH6 and LH8 recognise confirmational epitopes within a basal cell monolayer (Purkis et al. 1990). The keratin target for these basal cell markers cannot be identified by immunoblotting, but the antigens used for development and the tissue distribution of the epitopes suggest that they involve keratins 5 and 14. They react with a single cell layer in normal epidermis and two or three cell layers in vaginal and vulval mucosa.

Keratins 1 and 10. Suprabasal epidermis reacts strongly from the epibasal cell layer throughout with antibodies (Lane et al. 1985). Genital mucosal sites show gradation of expression from skin in the labia majora, which shows epibasal reactivity, to the vagina, where there is no reactivity.

Keratins 6/16, 4/13. There is no expression of keratins 6 and 16 in normal skin except palm and sole skin, but they are found in mucosal sites of genital mucosa including the labia minora and vestibule of the vagina. Keratins 4 and 13 are not found in normal epidermis, but are found suprabasally in the labia minora, increasing to the vestibule and suprabasal vagina.

Simple Epithelial Keratins. Keratins 8 and 18 can be detected in basal keratinocytes of vagina and vestibule with RCK106 (Ramaekers et al. 1983) but not in normal epidermis or labia majora. Staining in skin is restricted to the luminal cells of the sweat glands and Merkel cells in the epidermis. Keratin 7 was not found in any epidermal or mucosal site except for the reaction of antibodies LP1K and LP5K with the inner root sheath of the deep hair follicle and the sebaceous glands and sweat glands (Lane et al. 1985). Keratin 19 reacts with the sweat gland, both secretory and ductal epithelia, and with the basal cell subpopulation in the outer root sheath below the insertion of the sebaceous gland (Stasiak et al. 1989).

Table 3. Results of keratin expression in skin and vulval lesions

Keratin	Wart	Dysplastic wart	Renal transplant squamous cell carcinoma	Squamous cell carcinoma	Basal cell carcinoma	Vulval wart	Vulval intraepithelial neoplasia grade III
5/14	++	+	++	++/−	+	++	++
1/10	SB	hSB	−	−	−	+SB	(+)hSB
6/16	SB	SB	−	−	Het[a]	++	++
17	SB	B/SB	+	+	++	SB	B/SB
19	−	−	(+)	(+)	+(4)	only found in vestibule	
7	−	−	−	(+)	+(3)	−	−
4/13	−	−	−	−	−	−	−
8/18	−	−	+	++(deep)	−	−	−

[a] Frequently induced in overlying epidermis, but only rarely expressed by small clusters of tumour cells. B, basal; SB, suprabasal; hSB, high suprabasal.

Tumours

Keratins 5 and 14. Antibodies LLOO1 and RAK5 stained all tumour cells in BCC. In SCC the expression of keratins 5 and 14 were disturbed with heterogeneity in poorly differentiated areas and also a loss of basal cell conformational epitopes. In warts keratins 5 and 14 were expressed normally, whereas in dysplastic lesions there was increased expression of basal cell conformational epitopes in epibasal and suprabasal cell layers. In vulval neoplasia there was patchy loss of basal cell epitopes in VINIII, but no loss of LLOO1.

Keratins 1 and 10. There was no expression of keratins 1 and 10 in BCC, but there was a delay or reduction in expression of keratins 1 and 10 in the SCC, particularly in the invasive areas. 1/10 expression was normal in suprabasal warts, but lost with increasing dysplasia in the renal transplant-associated lesions. Keratin 1/10 expression was also lost in the VINIII lesions, where late onset of expression was found which was patchy and irregular.

Keratins 6 and 16. Keratins 6 and 16 were not found very extensively in BCC, and only in occasional clusters of cells, but positive staining of the overlying epidermis was frequently seen. In SCC patchy expression of keratins 6 and 16 was found, and expression was also conserved in vulval condylomata and in vulval intraepithelial neoplasia.

Keratin 17. Keratin 17 was widely expressed by BCC and also by invasive SCC. There was variable expression of keratin 17 in basal dysplastic warts and microinvasive tumour, which suggested that the keratin 17 expression was closely correlated with malignant change. Similar changes were found in vulval and vaginal epithelia.

Simple Epithelial Keratins. There was variable expression of keratin 19 in BCC, particularly found in basal cells of the tumour islands in a small percentage of patients. However, this was increased to an extent in SCC, where widespread expression was found within the tumour cells. Keratins 8 and 18, which are characteristic of simple epithelia, were not found in the BCC, nor in dysplastic warts, or vulval and intraepithelial neoplasia condylomata. However, there is clear expression of simple epithelial keratins 8 and 18 in invasive islands of SCC in the dermis.

Discussion

There has long been the suggestion that keratin expression can be used to distinguish tumours of epithelial origin from other undifferentiated tumours such as sarcomas and lymphomas (Osborn et al. 1984; Gabbiani et al. 1981). All the tumours in this study retained expression of some keratins and most epidermal tumours retained expression of keratinocyte keratins. There was no aberrant expression of other intermediate filament proteins such as desmin or vimentin. Thus, broadly cross-reactive antibodies such as LP34 (Natrath et al. 1993) can be used to determine the tumour type as being a carcinoma of epithelial origin. However, epithelial keratin expression is very complex and tightly related to tissue differentiation, so it was of interest to examine the modulation of individual keratin polypeptides with different types of tumours. There appear to be important tumour-associated changes in keratin expression in skin tumours of different types. These include loss of differentiation-specific keratins and increased expression of simple epithelial keratins, particularly keratins 8 and 18, with increasing malignant transformation. The expression of keratin 17 in basal cells of dysplastic warts and early invasive islands suggests that this may also be a good marker for development of malignant transformation in squamous epithelia. Previous studies of SCC in skin have depended predominantly on biochemical techniques and on the use of cross-reactive monoclonal antibodies, which makes the interpretation somewhat difficult (Moll et al. 1984; Kariniemi and Virtanen 1989; Habets et al. 1988; Thomas et al. 1984; Viac et al. 1982; Kariniemi et al. 1984; Robinson 1987). However, they have failed to highlight the expression of simple epithelial keratins 8 and 18 as a characteristic of invasive SCC. Studies of SCC in other body sites, such as oesophagus, ectocervix and bladder, have also suggested that the expression of simple epithelial keratins was increased with increasing dysplasia (Smedts et al. 1990; Schaafsma et al. 1990a). Simple epithelial keratins may also be expressed in transformed keratinocytes in tissue culture, including SV40-transformed non-tumorogenic cell lines (Taylor-Papadimitrou et al. 1982). Although the function of intermediate filaments is not yet clear, replacement of the physical state of the cytoskeleton, from more rigid keratinocyte in type to a more plastic cytoskeleton such as in simple epithelia, may permit remodelling and migration to occur during tumour invasion.

There appears to be good correlation of alterations in keratin expression with other markers of epithelial differentiation, as loss of involucrin reactivity and basal cell integrin expression are found in the more invasive tumours. These areas have generally conserved ubiquitous basement membrane proteins such as type IV collagen and laminin but have lost keratinocyte-specific basement membrane proteins including type VII collagen. Conversely, in tumours which develop squamous differentiation such as in the lung SCC, acquisition of the keratinocyte keratin expression keratins 5 and 14 in particular is associated with expression of keratinocyte-associated type VII collagen in the basement membrane (Wetzels et al. 1991).

The expression of a distinctive keratin pattern in the BCC, with keratins 5, 14, 17, 19 being characteristic of this tumour, correlates well with a subgroup of basal cells in the outer root sheath forming the putative stem cell population (Lane et al. 1991). The expression of keratin 17 particularly led to the suggestion that BCC derives from the hair follicle (Moll et al. 1982). This may still be true, but the observations that keratin 17 can be found in hyperproliferative epidermis suprabasally and is expressed in warts and tumours of all varieties, including of the vulva, suggests that this cannot be used as an argument for tumour histogenesis. Overall, however the expression of keratin 17 in the basal cell layer does seem to correlate with epithelial instability and act as an early sign of transformation.

In summary, malignant transformation of epidermal keratinocytes is associated with disturbed expression of keratinocyte keratins 5 and 14 with early loss of conformational epitopes; loss of differentiation-associated keratins (1/10); the progressive induction of simple epithelial keratins with increasing malignancy; and the early expression of keratin 17. A panel of suitable monospecific antibodies has been defined to assess the pathological state of the malignant cells with specific markers to keratins 8, 17 and 18 being helpful in assessing the potential for invasion.

References

Aubry F, McGibbon B (1985) Risk-factors of squamous-cell carcinoma of the skin. A case-control study in the Montreal region. Cancer 55:907–911

Barr BB, Benton EC, McLaren K et al. (1989) Human papillomavirus infection and skin cancer in renal allograft recipients. Lancet i:124–129

Bartek J, Bartkova J, Taylor-Papadimitriou J, Rejthar A, Kovarik J, Lukas Z, Vojtesek B (1986) Differential expression of keratin 19 in normal human epithelial tissues revealed by monospecific monoclonal antibodies. Histochem J 18:565–575

Bartek J, Vojtsek B, Staskova Z, Bartkova J, Kerekes A, Refthan A, Kosarik J (1991) A series of 14 new monoclonal antibodies to keratins: Characterisation and value in diagnostic histopathology. J Pathol 164:215–224

Blessing K, McLaren KM, Benton EC et al. (1989) Histopathology of skin lesions in renal allograft recipients: an assessment of viral features and dysplasia. Histopathology 14:129–139

Broers JLV, Carney DN, Rot MK, Scaart G, Lane EB, Vooijs GP, Ramaeckers CS (1986) Intermediate filament proteins in classic and variant types of small cell carcinoma cell lines: a biochemical and immunochemical analysis using a panel of monoclonal and polyclonal antibodies. J Cell Sci 83:37–60

Debus E, Moll R, Franke WW, Weber K, Osborn M (1984) Immunohistochemical distinction of human carcinomas by cytokeratin typing with monoclonal antibodies. Am J Pathol 114:121–130

Diffey BL (1987) Analysis of the risk of skin cancer from sunlight and solaria in subjects living in Northern Europe. Photodermatology 4:118–126

Eichenberg H, Gissman L, Gross G, Grusenford-Conen EI, zur Hausen H (1983) Human papillomavirus 16 related DNA in genital Bowen's disease and in Bowenoid papulosis. Int J Cancer 32:563

Eichner R, Sun T-T, Aebi U (1986) The role of keratin subfamilies and keratin pairs in the formation of human epidermal intermediate filaments. J Cell Biol 102:1767–1777

Gabbiani G, Kapanci Y, Barazzone P, Franke WW (1981) Immunochemical identification of intermediate-sized filaments in human neoplastic cells. A diagnostic aid for the surgical pathologist. Am J Pathol 104:206–216
Gardner ID, Whitehead RH, Burgess AW (1986) Production and characterization of monoclonal antibodies reactive with subsets of epidermal cells. Pathology 18:314–320
Gellin GA, Kopf AW, Garfinkel L (1965) Basal cell epithelioma. Arch Dermatol 91:38–45
Gigi-Leitner O, Geiger B (1986) Antigenic Interrelationship between the 40-Kilodalton cytokeratin polypeptide and desmoplakins. Cell Motil Cytoskeleton 6:628–639
Glover MT, Kennedy LJ, Bodmer JG, Sachs JA, McCloskey DJ, Brown J, Leigh IM (1991a) HLA-associations in non-immunosuppressed patients and renal transplant recipients with epidermal tumours. Br J Dermatol 125 [Suppl 38]:34
Glover MT, Proby CM, Kwan J, Cerio R, Wright N, Leigh IM (1991b) Human Papilloma Virus and cutaneous malignancy in renal transplant recipients: clinicopathological correlation and cytokeratin expression. Br J Dermatol 125:477
Guelstein VI, Tchypysheva TA, Ermilova VD et al. (1988) Monoclonal antibody mapping of keratins 8 and 17 and of vimentin in normal human mammary gland, benign tumors, dysplasias and breast cancer. Int J Cancer 42:147–153
Habets JMW, Tank B, Vuzevski VD, Breve J, Stolz E, van Joost TH (1988) Absence of cytokeratin 8 and inconsistent expression of cytokeratins 7 and 19 in human basal cell carcinoma. Anticancer Res 8:611–616
Huszar M, Gigi-Leitner O, Moll R, Franke WW, Geiger B (1986) Monoclonal antibodies to various acidic (Type 1) cytokeratins of stratified epithelia. Selective markers for stratification and squamous cell carcinomas. Differentiation 31:141–143
Jahn L, Fouquet B, Rohe K, Franke WW (1987) Cytokeratins in certain endothelial and smooth muscle cells of two taxonomically distant vertebrate species, Xenopus Laevis and man. Differentiation 36:234–254
Kariniemi A-L, Virtanen I (1989) Altered keratin expression in benign and malignant skin diseases revealed with monoclonal antibodies. Am J Dermatopathol 11:202–208
Kariniemi AL, Holthofer H, Vartio T, Virtanen I (1984) Cellular differentiation of basal cell carcinoma studied with fluorescent lectins and cytokeratin antibodies. J Cutan Pathol 11:541–548
Kemler R, Brulet P, Schnebelen MT, Gaillard J, Jacob F (1981) Reactivity of monoclonal antibodies against intermediate filament proteins during embryonic development. J Embryol Exp Morphol 64:45–60
Lane EB (1982) Monoclonal antibodies provide specific intramolecular markers for the study of epithelial tonofilament organisation. J Cell Biol 92:665–673
Lane EB, Bartek J, Purkis PE, Leigh IM (1985) Keratin antigens in differentiating skin. Ann NY Acad Sci 455:241–258
Lane EB, Wilson CA, Hughes BA, Leigh IM (1991) Stem cells in hair follicle: cytoskeletal studies. Ann NY Acad Sci 642:197–213
Lauerova L, Kovarik J, Bartek J, Rejthar A, Vojtesek B (1988) Novel monoclonal antibodies defining epitope of human cytokeratin 18 molecule. Hybridoma 7:495–504
Makin C, Babrow LG, Bodmer WF (1984) Monoclonal antibody to cytokeratin for use in routine histopathology. J Clin Pathol 37:975–983
Markey AC, Lane EB, Churchill LJ, MacDonald DM, Leigh IM (1991) The expression of simple epithelial keratins 8 and 18 in epidermal neoplasia. J Invest Dermatol 97:763–770

Miller SJ (1991) Biology of basal cell carcinoma (part I). J Am Acad Dermatol 24:1–16
Moll R, Franke WW, Schiller DL, Geiger B, Krepler R (1982a) The catalog of human cytokeratins: patterns of expression in normal epithelia, tumours and cultured cells. Cell 31:11–24
Moll R, Franke WW, Volc-Platzer B, Kepler R (1982b) Different keratin polypeptides in epidermis and other epithelia of human skin: a specific cytokeratin of molecular weight 46 000 in epithelia of the pilosebaceous tract and basal cell epitheliomas. J Cell Biol 95:285–295
Moll R, Moll I, Franke WW (1984a) Differences of expression of cytokeratin polypeptides in various epithelial skin tumours. Arch Dermatol Res 276:349–363
Moll R, Moll I, Franke WW (1984b) Identification of Merkel cells in human skin by specific cytokeratin antibodies. Differentiation 28:136–154
Nathrath WBJ, Lane EB, Peat NP, Purkis PE (1993) Derivation, biochemical and immunohistochemical characterisation of the pan-epithelial anti-keratin monoclonal antibody LP34: staining of normal human tissues in alcohol-fixed, formalin fixed and unfixed frozen material (submitted)
Neill SM, Staughton RCD, Leigh IM, Lane EB (1993a) An immunohistochemical study of the cytokeratin profile in normal female genital epithelia (submitted)
Neill SM, Proby CM, Staughton RCD, Lane EB, Leigh IM (1993b) Expression of keratins in vulval condyloma acuminata and vulval intraepithelial neoplasia (submitted)
Osborn M, Weber K (1982) Intermediate filaments: cell-type specific markers in differentiation and pathology. Cell 31:303–306
Osborn M, Altmannsberger M, Debus E, Weber K (1984) Conventional and monoclonal antibodies to intermediate filament proteins in human tumour diagnosis, the transformed phenotype. In: Levine AJ, Van de Woude GF, Topp WC, Watson JD (eds) Cold Spring Harbor Laboratory, New York, pp 191–200
Purkis PE, Steel JB, Mackenzie IC, Nathrath WBJ, Leigh IM, Lane EB (1990) Basal cells in complex epithelia. J Cell Sci 97:39–50
Ramaekers FCS, Puts JJG, Moesker O, Kant A, Huysmans A, Haag PHK, Herman CJ, Vooijs GP (1983) Antibodies to intermediate filament proteins in the immunohistochemical identification of human tumours: an overview. Histochem J 15:691–713
Ramaekers FCS, Huysmans A, Schaart G, Mosker O, Vooijs P (1987a) Tissue distribution of keratin 7 as monitored by a monoclonal antibody. Exp Cell Res 170:235–249
Ramaekers FCS, Huysmans A,, Schaart G, Moesker O, Vooijs P (1987b) Tissue distribution of keratin 7 as monitored by a monoclonal antibody. Exp Cell Res 170:235–249
Robinson JK (1987) Expression of keratin proteins in deeply invasive basal and squamous cell carcinoma and immunohistochemical study. J Dermatol Surg Oncol 13:283–294
Schaafsma HE, Ramaekers FCS, van Muijen GNP, Leigh IM, Robben H, Huijsmans A, Ooms ECM, Reiter DJ (1990a) Distribution of cytokeratin polypeptides in human transitional carcinomas, with special emphasis on changing expression patterns during tumour progression. Am J Pathol 136:329–343
Schaafsma HE, Ramaekers FCS, van Muijen GNP, Lane EB, Leigh IM, Robben H, Huijsmans A, Ooms ECM, Ruiter DJ (1990b) Distribution of cytokeratin polypeptides in human transitional cell carcinoma with special emphasis on changing keratin patterns during tumour progression. Am J Pathol 136:329–343
Smedts F, Tamaekers FCS, Robben H, Pruszczynski M, van Muijen G, Lane B, Leigh I, Vooijs P (1990) Changing patterns of keratin expression during progression of cervical intraepithelial neoplasia. Am J Pathol 136:657–668

Stasiak PC, Purkis PE, Leigh IM, Lane EB (1989) Keratin 19. Predicted amino acid sequence and broad tissue distribution suggest it evolved from keratinocyte keratins. J Invest Dermatol 92:707–716

Stoler A, Kopan R, Duvic M, Fuchs E (1988) Use of monospecific antisera and mRNA probes to localize the major changes in keratin expression during normal and abnormal epidermal differentiation. J Cell Biol 107:427–446

Taylor-Papadimitrou J, Purkis PE, Lane EB, Mackay IA, Chang SE (1982) The effects of SV40 transformation on the cytoskeleton and behavioural properties of human keratinocytes. Cell Differ 11:169–180

Thomas P, Said JW, Nash G, Banks-Schlegel SP (1984) Profiles of keratin protein in basal and squamous cell carcinomas of the skin. Lab Invest 1:36–41

Tolle HG, Weber K, Osborn M (1985) Microinjection of monoclonal antibodies specific for one intermediate filament protein in cells containing multiple keratins allow insight into the composition of particular 10 nm filaments. Eur J Cell Biol 38:234–244

Urbach F (1989) Potential effects of altered solar radiation on human skin cancer. Photochem Photobiol 50:507–513

van Muijen GNP, Ruiter DJ, Franke WW, Achtstatter T, Haarsnoot WHB, Ponec M, Warnaar SO (1986) Cell type heterogeneity of cytokeratin expression in complex epithelia and carcinomas as demonstrated by monoclonal antibodies specific for cytokeratins nos. 4 and 13. Exp Cell Res 162:97–113

Viac J, Reano A, Thivolet J (1982) Cytokeratins in human basal and squamous cell carcinomas: biochemical, immunohistological findings and comparisons with normal epithelia. J Cutan Pathol 9:377–390

Virtanen I, Miettinen M, Lehto V-P, Kariniemi A-L, Paasivuo R (1985) Diagnostic applications of monoclonal antibodies to intermediate filaments. Ann NY Acad Sci 455:635–648

Wetzels RHW, Robben HCM, Leigh IM, Schaafsma HE, Vooijs GP, Ramaekers FCS (1991) Distribution patterns of type VII collagen in normal and malignant human tissues. Am J Pathol 139:451–459

Woodcock Mitchell J, Eichner R, Nelson WG, Sun T-T (1982) Immunolocalisation of keratin polypeptides in human epidermis using monoclonal antibodies. J Cell Biol 95:580–588

Cellular and Molecular Changes During Mouse Skin Tumor Progression

A.J.P. Klein-Szanto[1], B. Ruggeri[1], A. Bianchi[2], and C.J. Conti[2]

[1] Department of Pathology, Fox Chase Cancer Center, Philadelphia, PA 19111, USA
[2] Department of Carcinogenesis, The University of Texas, M.D. Anderson Cancer Center, Science Park, Smithville, TX 78957, USA

Introduction

The mouse skin models of chemical carcinogenesis have been extensively used to investigate the conversion of benign skin tumors (papillomas) to malignant squamous cell carcinomas (SCC). Less intense has been the use of these models for the study of tumor progression, which, as defined by Foulds (1975), does not necessarily include the conversion of benign into malignant tumors, but is a concept generally applied to define the gradual and sequential changes that take place in malignant tumors and that result in progressively more and more aggressive and life-threatening neoplasms. Although not fully exploited, the models of mouse skin carcinogenesis not only offer a very suitable in vivo system to study the biology of premalignant lesions and their possible transformation into completely malignant tumors, but also provide a gamut of malignant tumors of different biological potential that span from the nonmetastatic, slow-growing, well-differentiated SCC to the highly metastasizing, fast growing, poorly differentiated carcinomas that constitute an unusually relevant in vivo model of tumor progression (Klein-Szanto 1989).

The process of malignant conversion and the later gradual enhancement of malignancy constitute a continuum that could well be called tumor progression. Nevertheless, following the traditional terminology, we have divided the description of known changes into two separate sections, i.e., (1) papilloma-to-carcinoma conversion, and (2) tumor (carcinoma) progression.

Conversion of Papillomas to Carcinomas

The changes that result in the transformation of a skin papilloma into a SCC have been especially well studied in mice treated with the two-stage protocol

Recent Results in Cancer Research, Vol. 128

of chemical carcinogenesis using a polycyclic aromatic hydrocarbon such as 7,12-dimethylbenz(a)anthacene (DMBA) followed by repetitive application of a phorbol ester tumor promoter such as 12-*O*-tetradecanoylphorbol-13-acetate (TPA). The fact that this protocol results in the early formation of a large number of papillomas, some of which (approximately 1 in 4) convert to SCC, was observed by the pioneers in this field of chemical carcinogenesis (for review, see Burns et al. 1984). In this context, some investigators refer to "terminally benign" papillomas and a smaller fraction of premalignant papillomas that possess a definite potential for malignant transformation (Hennings et al. 1985; Reddy et al. 1987). In our laboratories we have observed that most papillomas show, sooner or later, premalignant or malignant changes, and that only the rate of transformation is variable, some reaching an early complete conversion to carcinoma, whereas others show a slower evolution that results in dysplastic changes but not in outright carcinoma (Aldaz et al. 1987, 1988, 1991; Aldaz and Conti 1989). It is probable that the main cause of this apparent paradox are the marked differences in the behavior of papillomas induced in different strains of mice. Papillomas in SENCAR mice are larger and more aggressive and progress more rapidly than papillomas in any other strain, including parental stock CD-1. Furthermore, I. Gimenez-Conti et al. (personal communication) have shown that an inbred mouse strain derived from the SENCAR (i.e., SSIN) (Fischer et al. 1987) has an enhanced susceptibility to phorbol ester promotion, but papillomas in this strain rarely convert to SCC. These results suggest that susceptibility and progression are regulated by different genetic mechanisms.

In addition to the histopathological alterations, i.e., formation of dysplastic foci in most papillomas, several molecular, biochemical, and chromosomal changes have been described in these tumors.

Changes in differentiation patterns, as detected by keratin changes, are very conspicuous during papilloma-to-carcinoma conversion. The proliferation-associated keratin K14, which is expressed in the basal layer of normal epidermis and nondysplastic or regular papillomas, continues to be present in the suprabasal layers of dysplastic papillomas. There is also a change of expression in differentiation-associated keratins. The keratin pair K1/K10, which is normally expressed in epidermis, is not detectable in large areas of advanced papillomas (Roop et al. 1988; Aldaz et al. 1988). The K1-negative area of the papilloma expresses K13, a differentiation-associated keratin expressed in internal epithelia but not in epidermis (Nischt et al. 1988; Gimenez-Conti et al. 1990). In later stages of papilloma development, some K1-negative areas of papilloma also start expressing the enzyme γ-glutamyl transpeptidase (GGT). GGT expression is a good marker of advanced dysplastic foci in papillomas and is also positive in most carcinomas (Klein-Szanto et al. 1983; Chiba et al. 1986, 1992; Aldaz et al. 1991). Although these changes in morphology and differentiation patterns were noted early, they are likely to be a consequence rather than the cause of conversion. Recent cytogenetic and molecular studies offer more direct evidence of the mechanism of premalignant and malignant progression of skin tumors. Chromosomal analysis of DMBA/TPA-induced mouse skin tumors demonstrated that aneuploid cells can be found in many papillomas during the first 20 weeks of treatment, and practically all benign tumors contained aneuploid cells in later stages (Conti et al. 1986; Aldaz et al. 1987). In addition, Aldaz et al. (1989) have shown that aneuploidy is due to nonrandom chromosomal duplication of chromosomes 6 and 7. Although H-*ras* mutations at codon 61 represent an initiating event (Quintanilla et al. 1986; Bizub et al. 1986; Brown et al. 1986) in a large majority of tumors induced with a two-stage carcinogenesis protocol using DMBA as initiator, recently Bianchi et al. (1990) have suggested that premalignant change could be associated with the nonrandom duplication of the chromosome bearing a mutated H-*ras* allele, thus resulting in a trisomy of chromosome 7 and overrepresentation of the mutated H-*ras* gene. Results of two different groups also indicate that increased copy number of the mutated Ha-*ras* gene may be related to the degree of anaplasia of the tumor (Buchmann et al. 1991; Bremmer and Balmain 1990; Bianchi et al. 1990). Similarly, loss of heterozygosity (LOH) at polymorphic markers of chromosome 7 has been detected in carcinomas, and has been proposed as a mechanism involving loss of a tumor suppressor gene in the progression of mouse skin tumors (Bremmer and Balmain 1990). Recently, Bianchi et al. (1991) have suggested that the putative gene would be linked to the *Hbb* locus in chromosome 7 F1-ter distal to H-*ras* locus, and that alterations at this locus may occur during malignant conversion of papillomas since some dysplastic papillomas show loss of heterozigosity on the distal portion of chromosome 7.

Mouse Skin Tumor (Carcinoma) Progression

It is generally accepted that skin SCC in mice derive from transformation of preexisting papillomas. This is especially true for the two-stage carcinogenesis protocol, but is not the case of the complete carcinogenesis protocol, in which many SCC seem to arise from non-papillomatous skin (Stenback 1980; Chiba et al. 1986) (See Fig. 1).

Histopathologically, SCC can be classified according to the degree of differentiation into four different types that are basically similar to the grades described by Broders for human squamous cell carcinomas (Broders 1932), i.e., SCC I, 75% or more of the tumor cells show some degree of keratinization; SCC II, 50%–75% of cells differentiate; SCC III, 10%–50% of cells show differentiation; and SCC IV, very little or no evidence of differentiation. Usually these grades are also accompanied by increased nuclear atypia, hyperchromatism, and irregularities of cell, size, shape, and staining affinity (Fig. 2).

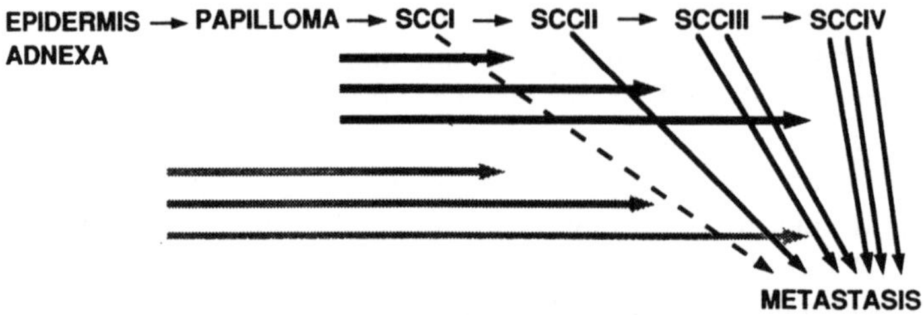

Fig. 1. Histopathological grading. Schematic representation of tumor progression in two stage carcinogenesis (*dark arrows*) and complete carcinogenesis (*lighter arrows*)

Once SCC are formed, they tend to follow a similar evolution irrespective of the carcinogenesis protocol used, i.e., earlier (25–42 weeks of treatment) there is a predominance of low-grade SCC, whereas after 42 weeks of treatment the higher grades (SCC II to IV) predominate (Fig. 3). Although these are general traits in all treatment protocols, SCC I is the predominant tumor type throughout the two-stage carcinogenesis experiments, whereas higher grades are more frequently observed in complete carcinogenesis protocols (Fig. 4) (Chiba et al. 1991). Three-stage carcinogenesis treatments show a higher incidence of SCC II–III than the two-stage protocol, but in general terms the tumor type distribution is similar to the two-stage treatment protocol.

The timecourse of the appearance of different tumor grades (Fig. 3), as well as the presence of intermediate types, in which a higher-grade tumor seems to arise from a lower-grade SCC, indicate a gradual progression from the lower grades to the higher SCC grades.

The biological differences between the different SCC types is not only morphological. In addition to the differences in degree of atypia and keratinization, the tumors show important differences in their malignant potential; whereas SCC I grow slowly and have a low metastatic potential, SCC of higher grade, especially SCC III and IV, grow fast and are very invasive and metastatic.

Cell lines derived from different types of SCC clearly show this tendency (Table 1) and confirm the in vivo observations. Biochemical and immunohistochemical studies have detected several changes that occur during tumor progression. The most clear-cut are a loss of keratin expression that eventually results in a subtype of SCC IV with no, or extremely low, expression of keratin that cannot be easily differentiated from a sarcoma and is aptly called spindle cell carcinoma (Klein-Szanto et al. 1989) (Fig. 5). Recent results seem to indicate that, in more advanced carcinoma, there is gradual loss of K13 concomitant with expression of K8 (F. Larcher et al., preliminary data). Other interesting changes recently noted in SCC III–IV are the decrease or absence of uvomorulin and Na^+,K^+-ATPase (B.R. Ruggeri and A. Klein-Szanto, preliminary data). Increased expression of

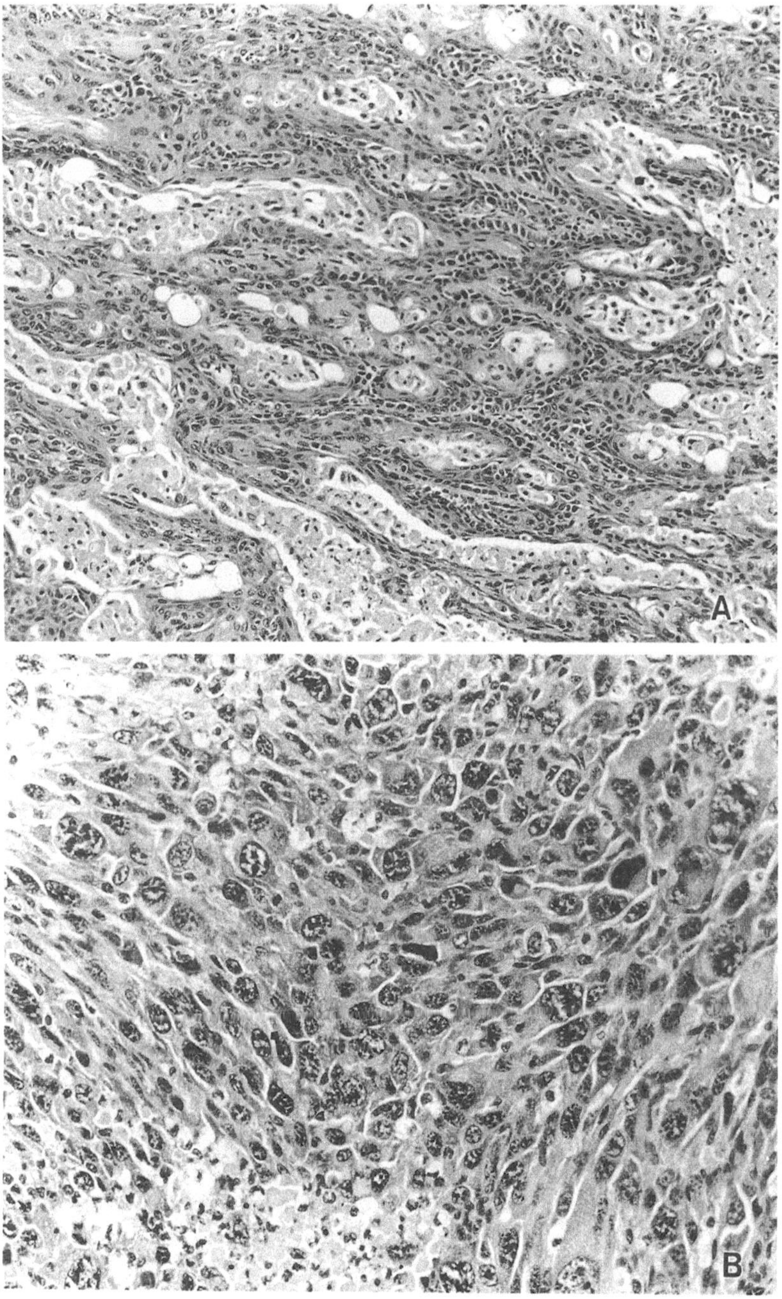

Fig. 2A,B. Representative examples of squamous cell carcinomas (SCC) of different grades. **A** SCC I, showing marked squamous differentiation, and formation of keratinized cells with moderate atypia (×100). **B** SCC III with marked nuclear atypia, but with clear epithelioid features (×370)

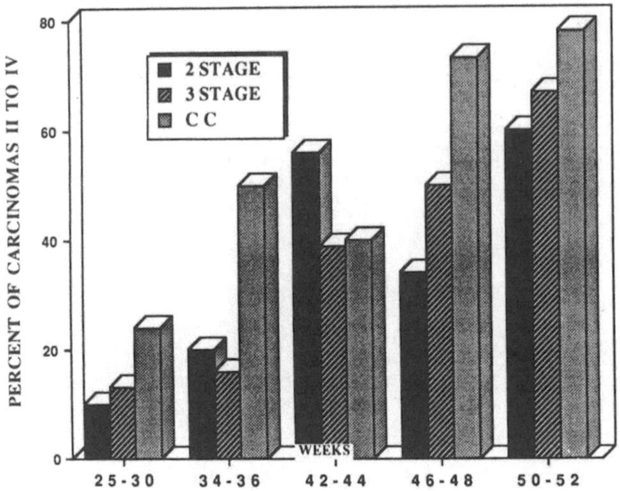

Fig. 3. Percent of higher-grade squamous cell carcinomas (SCC II to IV) during the latter half of the carcinogenesis experiments (weeks 25–52). Three protocols were used: two-stage carcinogenesis with DMBA-TPA; three-stage carcinogenesis with DMBA-TPA-MNNG; and complete carcinogenesis (*CC*) with DMBA (see Miller 1978)

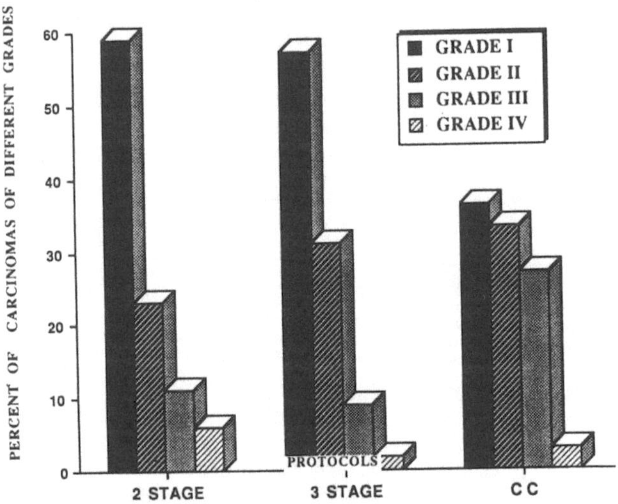

Fig. 4. Histopathological grading of squamous cell carcinomas produced by three different carcinogenesis protocols (see legend to Fig. 2)

Table 1. Histopathological grading and metastatic potential of cell line-derived tumors

	Histopathological grade	Metastatic ability[a]
FBI	SCC I	25
JWF-2	SCC I	0
CH72	SCC II	60
CH72-T1	SCC III	80
BB2	SCC IV	100
BB1	SCC IV	100
BB1-T1	SCC IV	100

[a] Expressed as percent of animals injected s.c. with 1×10^6 cells that developed spontaneous lung metastases at 10 weeks after inoculation.

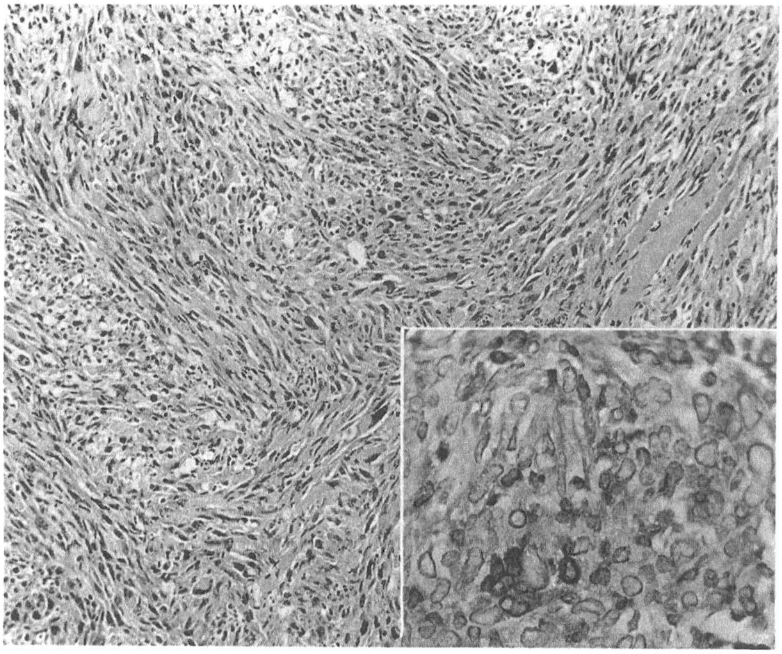

Fig. 5. Spindle cell carcinoma or SCC IV. Poorly differentiated tumor of fusiform cells (×100); immunohistochemical demonstration of keratin in some tumors cells confirms their epithelial derivation (*inset*, ×370)

metaloproteinases such as transin have also been described in metastasizing tumors (Matrisian et al. 1986).

Recently, we have shown an increased number of p53 abnormalities that include deletion and point mutations in high-grade SCC produced by a two-

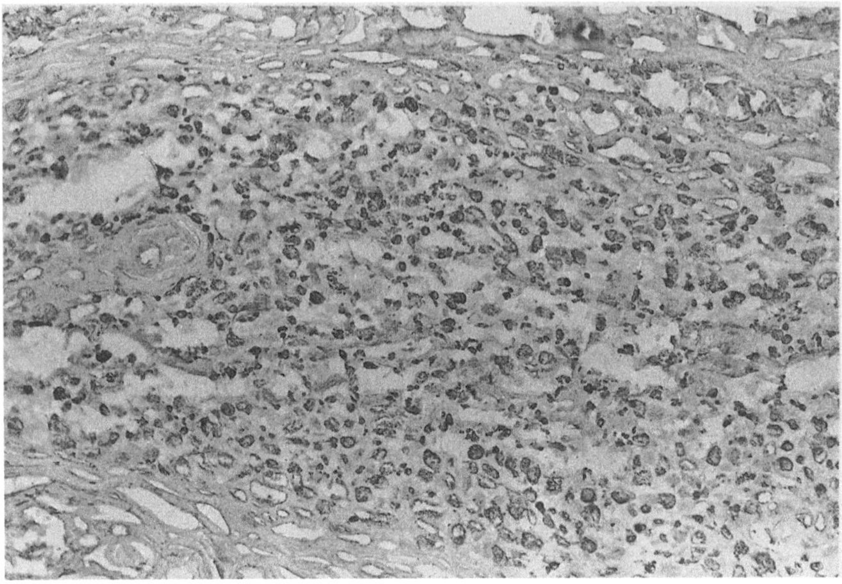

Fig. 6. Immunohistochemical demonstration of p53. Note positive nuclear stain in most nuclei of this SCC II (immunostain with pAb421, no counterstain, ×160)

stage carcinogenesis protocol (Ruggeri et al. 1992). From a total of 32 carcinomas analyzed by either immunoprecipitation or DNA sequencing, eight showed p53 abnormalities. Interestingly, neither papillomas nor early tumors showed p53 alterations. All SCC exhibiting changes were obtained from animals that had had between 48 and 60 weeks of treatment. Except for one SCC I, all the other tumors were SCC II–IV and showed immunohistochemically detectable p53 (Fig. 6). Interestingly, in animals exposed to complete carcinogenesis protocols, in which the incidence of SCC II–IV is higher than in two-stage carcinogenesis protocols, the number of tumors with p53 alterations seems to be even higher.

Although most of the evidence gathered indicates quite clearly that p53 changes occur late during mouse skin tumor progression, it is possible that the precise order of events is not the most important factor. As has been suggested in both human and laboratory animal tumors (Fearon and Vogelstein 1990; Ben David and Bernstein 1991), the accumulation of different sets of mutations are more important than the specific sequence in which they occur. In this context, it is noteworthy to mention that out of 25 premalignant lesions, we found only one, which was considered an exception, in which p53 could be detected by immunohistochemical methods (Fig. 7).

These changes in the p53 tumor suppressor gene appear approximately simultaneously with an increased dosage of the mutant H-*ras* allele, which

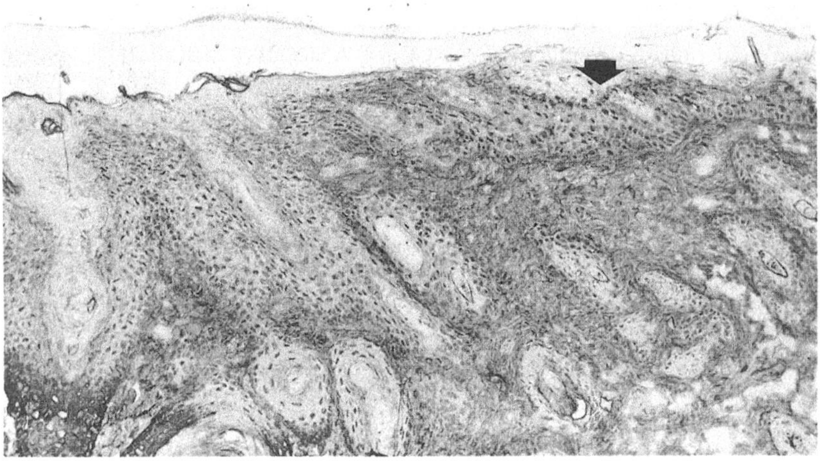

Fig. 7. Areas of atypical epidermal and follicular hyperplasia and carcinoma in situ (*arrowhead*) in the proximity of a SCC II. Note that most nuclei are positively stained (immunohistochemistry with the anti-p53 monoclonal antibody pAb421, no counterstain, (×50)

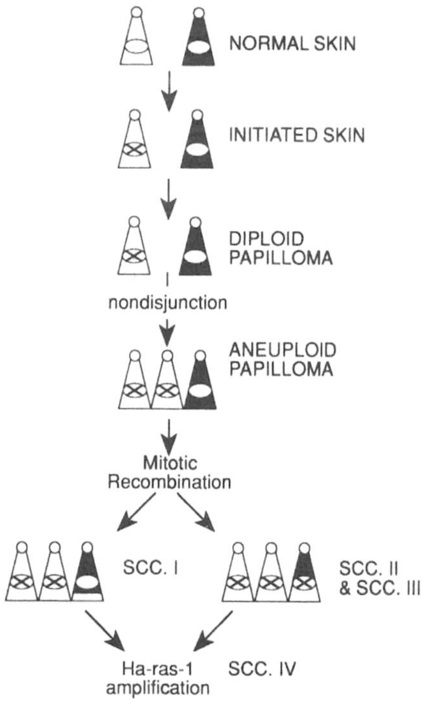

Fig. 8. Schematic representation of the normal/mutated composition of the H-*ras* gene at various stages of mouse skin tumor development. The locus with a *cross* represents the mutated allele

Table 2. Genetic changes in two-stage carcinogenesis

Normal epidermis and adnexa →Papilloma →SCC I →SCC II →SCC III →SCC IV

H-*ras*→ H-*ras* mutation→ Amplification→ Overrepresentation→ loss of normal allele

p53 | Late p53 mutation →

Other TCG →

↑ Loss of *pgr*
(putative suppressor gene in chromosome 7)

Chromosomal alterations

| Ts6 →

| Ts7 →

| Mitotic recombination chromasome 7 →

0 10 20 30 40 weeks

DMBA | TPA →

Initiation Promotion Progression

| → (Conversion) →

TCG, tumor suppressor genes

tends to be overrepresented in higher grade tumors, especially spindle cell carcinomas (SCC IV).

Several tumors presented the loss of a normal H-*ras* allele with two or three copies of the mutated gene. A few anaplastic tumors also showed amplification of the mutated H-*ras* gene. These results suggest that the number of copies of the mutated H-*ras* gene may be related to the degree of anaplasia of the tumors, with two copies in the well-differentiated tumors, three copies in the moderately differentiated tumors, and gene amplification (more than 10 copies) in the spindle cell carcinomas (Bianchi et al. 1990; Buchmann et al. 1991) (Fig. 8).

Conclusion

In conclusion, the gradual acquisition of advanced malignant features is accompanied by numerous genetic abnormalities, some of which can be ascribed to specific transitions in the biological behavior and morphological appearance of tumors (Table 2). These known changes in oncogenes and tumor suppressor genes are probably part of a larger picture in which other genes are also involved. The rapid developments in molecular oncology will certainly result in a more complete knowledge of the cascade of events that take place during tumor progression. The mouse skin carcinogenesis models are excellent systems to study these changes and will surely contribute to a better knowledge of animal and human tumor progression.

Acknowledgement. This work was supported in part by NiH grants CA 53713 and CA 44980.

References

Aldaz CM, Conti CJ (1989) The premalignant nature of mouse skin papillomas. Histopathological, cytogenetic and biochemical evidence. In: Conti C, Slaga T, Klein-Szanto AJP (eds) Carcinogenesis – a comprehensive survey, vol II. Skin tumors: experimental and clinical aspects. Raven, New York, pp 227–240

Aldaz CM, Conti CJ, Klein-Szanto AJP et al. (1987) Progressive dysplasia and aneuploidy are hallmarks of mouse skin papillomas: relevance to malignancy. Proc Natl Acad Sci USA 84:2029–2032

Aldaz CM, Conti CJ, Larcher F, Trono D, Roop DR, Chesner J, Whitehead T, Slaga TJ (1988) Sequential development of aneuploidy, keratin modifications, and γ-glutamyltransferase expression in mouse skin papillomas. Cancer Res 48:3253–3257

Aldaz CM, Trono D, Larcher F, Slaga TJ, Conti CJ (1989) Sequential trisomization of chromosomes 6 and 7 in mouse skin premalignant lesions. Mol Carcinog 2:22–26

Aldaz CM, Conti CJ, Chen A, Bianchi A, Walker SB, DiGiovanni J (1991) Promoter independence as a feature of most skin papillomas in SENCAR mice. Cancer Res 51:1045–1050

Ben-David Y, Bernstein A (1991) Friend virus-induced erythroleukemia and the multistage nature of cancer. Cell 66:831–834

Bianchi AB, Aldaz CM, Conti CJ (1990) Non-random duplication of the chromosome 7 bearing a mutated Ha-ras-1 allele in mouse skin tumors. Proc Natl Acad Sci USA 87:6902–6906

Bianchi AB, Navone NM, Aldaz CM, Conti CJ (1991) Overlapping loss of heterozygosity by mitotic recombination on mouse chromosome 7F1-ter in skin carcinogenesis. Proc Natl Acad Sci USA 88:7590–7594

Bizub D, Wood AW, Skalka AM (1986) Mutagenesis of the Ha-ras oncogene in mouse skin tumors induced by polycyclic aromatic hydrocarbons. Proc Natl Acad Sci USA 83:6048–6052

Bremmer R, Balmain A (1990) Genetic changes in skin tumour progression: correlation between presence of a mutant ras gene and loss of heterozygosity on mouse chromosome 7. Cell 61:407–417

Broders AC (1932) Practical points on the microscopic grading of carcinoma. NY J Med 32:667–684

Brown K, Quintanilla M, Ramsden M, Kerr IB, Young S, Balmain A (1986) V-ras genes from Harvey and Balb murine sarcoma viruses can act as initiators of two-stage mouse skin carcinogenesis. Cell 46:447–456

Buchmann A, Ruggeri B, Klein-Szanto AJP, Balmain A (1991) Progression of squamous carcinoma cells to spindle carcinomas of mouse skin is associated with an imbalance of H-ras alleles on chromosome 7. Cancer Res 51:4097–4101

Burns FJ, Albert RE, Altschuler B (1984) Cancer progression in mouse skin. In: Slaga TJ (ed) Mechanisms of tumor promotion: II. Tumor promotion and skin carcinogenesis. CRC Press, Boca Raton, pp 17–40

Chiba M, Maley MA, Klein-Szanto AJP (1986) Sequential study of GGT during complete and two stage skin carcinogenesis. Cancer Res 46:259–263
Chiba M, Aldaz CM, Conti CJ, Klein-Szanto AJP (1991) Metastatic potential of mouse skin carcinomas produced by different protocols of chemical carcinogenesis. Invasion Metastasis 11:287–296
Conti CJ, Aldaz CM, O'Connell J, Klein-Szanto AJP, Slaga TJ (1986) Aneuploidy, an early event in mouse skin tumor development. Carcinogenesis 7:1845–1848
Fearon ER, Vogelstein B (1990) A genetic model for colorectal tumorigenesis. Cell 61:759–767
Fischer SM, O'Connell JF, Conti CJ, Tacker K, Fries JW, Patrick K, Adams LM, Slaga TJ (1987) Characterization of an inbred strain of the SENCAR mouse that is highly sensitive to phorbol esters. Carcinogenesis 8:421–424
Foulds L (1975) Neoplasia of the skin. In: Foulds L (ed) Neoplastic development, vol 2. Academic, London, pp 17–107
Gimenez-Conti CI, Aldaz CM, Bianchi AB, Roop DR, Slaga TJ, Conti CJ (1990) Early expression of type I K13 in the progression of mouse skin papillomas. Carcinogenesis 11:1995–1999
Klein-Szanto AJP (1989) Pathology of human and experimental skin tumors. In: Conti CJ, Slaga TJ, Klein-Szanto A (eds) Skin tumors: experimental and clinical aspects. Raven, New York, pp 19–53
Klein-Szanto AJP, Nelson KG, Shah Y, Slaga TJ (1983) Simultaneous appearance of keratin modification and γ-glutamyltransferase activity as indicators of tumor progression in mouse skin papillomas. J Natl Cancer Inst 70:161–168
Klein-Szanto AJP, Larcher F, Bonfil RD, Conti CJ (1989) Multistage carcinogenesis protocols produce spindle cell carcinomas in the mouse skin. Carcinogenesis 10:2169–2172
Matrisian LM, Bowden GT, Krieg P, Furstenberger G, Briand J-P, Leroy P, Breathnach R (1986) An mRNA coding for the secreted protease transin is expressed more abundantly in malignant than benign tumors. Proc Natl Acad Sci USA 83:9413–9417
Nischt R, Roop DR, Mehrel T, Yuspa SH, Rentrop M, Winter H, Schweizer J (1988) Aberrant expression during two-stage mouse skin carcinogenesis of a type 147-kDA keratin K13, normally associated with terminal differentiation. Mol Carcinog 1:96–108
Quintanilla M, Brown K, Ramsden M, Balmain A (1986) Carcinogen-specific mutation and amplification of Ha-ras during mouse skin carcinogenesis. Nature 322:78–80
Reddy AL, Caldwell M, Fialkow PJ (1987) Studies of skin carcinogenesis in PGK mice: many promoter-independent papillomas and carcinomas do not develop from pre-existing promoter-dependent papillomas. Int J Cancer 39:261–265
Roop DR, Kreig TM, Mehrel T, Cheng CK, Yuspa SH (1988) Transcriptional control of high molecular weight keratin gene expression in multistage mouse skin carcinogenesis. Cancer Res 48:3245–3252
Ruggeri BR, Caamano J, Goodrow T, DiRado M, Bianchi A, Trono D, Conti CJ, Klein-Szanto AJP (1991) Alterations of the p53 tumor suppressor gene during mouse skin tumor progression. Cancer Res 51:6615–6621
Stenback F (1980) Characteristics of neoplastic progression and tumor behavior in skin carcinogenesis by different methods. Oncology 37:163–168

Influence of Aging and Malignant Transformation on Keratinocyte Gene Expression

M. Yaar, J. Arora, M. Garmyn, A. Gilani, and B.A. Gilchrest

USDA Human Nutrition Research Center on Aging, Tufts University, Department of Dermatology, Boston University School of Medicine, Boston, MA, USA

Incidence and Risk Factors

Skin cancer is the most common malignancy in humans (Yuspa 1987). Most skin cancers are strongly linked to UV exposure (Aubry and MacGibbon 1985; Stoll and Schwartz 1987; Streilein 1991), but other agents such as chemical carcinogens and immunosuppressants (Yuspa et al. 1980) may also contribute. In addition, age-specific skin cancer incidence rises exponentially during adulthood and available data suggest that advanced age itself, independent of exposure history, may be a risk factor (Lin et al. 1989).

Squamous cell carcinoma of the skin is a tumor of epidermal keratinocytes (Liberman and Lebovitz 1990). The overall annual incidence is 12.1 per 100000 white residents in the United States, but the incidence is much higher in the older adult population, particularly in the South and Southwest (Liberman and Lebovitz 1990; Weinstock 1989; Glass and Hoover 1989). Within this century there has been a marked increase in the proportion of the population that is elderly and, consequently, a substantial increase in the burden of dermatologic diseases associated with aging, particularly skin cancer (Weinstock 1989; Glass and Hoover 1989; Johnson 1989). Limited work has been done to elucidate the complex cellular and molecular events in aged skin that predispose it to malignant transformation in general, and to squamous cell carcinoma in particular (Gilchrest 1984).

Advancing age exponentially increases the risk of skin cancer and indeed of most human malignancies (Weinstock 1989; Glass and Hoover 1989). However, the biologic basis for this phenomenon is unknown. Age-associated decreases in cellular immune function (Streilein 1991; Sauder 1989) and the statistical likelihood of random unrepaired errors in cellular DNA over the lifespan (Yaar and Gilchrest 1988) have been suggested as contributing factors. A third possibility is that aging, through a differentiation-like process, is associated with programmed changes in the expression of certain genes

Recent Results in Cancer Research, Vol. 128

that facilitate the emergence of malignant clones of cells whose proliferation is not subject to normal regulatory mechanisms.

Molecular Mechanisms Implicated in Malignant Transformation

Studies in our laboratory, described below, address the hypothesis that there is a biologic progression from aging to photoaging to malignant transformation and that the high risk of skin cancer in old habitually sun-exposed (photoaged) skin is attributable in large part to changes in the expression of specific genes central to regulation of normal cell proliferation that, when abnormal, lead to malignant transformation. We further hypothesize that these changes might also be responsible in part for other universal age-associated changes in cell behavior, such as decreased proliferative capacity, but when compounded by further aberrations, perhaps mutations induced by UV irradiation, would permit uncontrolled cell growth, clinically manifest as skin cancer.

Recently, the concept of a common mechanism for the malignant transformation has been proposed. The discovery of genes whose mutation or deletion leads to malignant transformation has contributed greatly to our understanding of the molecular mechanisms of carcinogenesis.

The common denominator for cancer initiators (chemicals, viruses, radiation) is their mutagenic ability (Bishop 1985). The majority of the chemical carcinogens active in the skin have been found to bind covalently to DNA (Doll and Peto 1981; E. Miller 1978). The transformation of a cell from normal to malignant is typically a multistep process involving alterations in cellular genes due to point or frame-shift mutations, deletions, amplification, or gene rearrangement (Weinstein 1981; Land et al. 1983). Viruses give rise to tumors either by infecting the cell with all the genes responsible for the abnormal functions of the cell (Rassoulzadegan et al. 1982) or more commonly by providing some but not all of the functional changes required for tumor development. In the latter case, certain additional cellular changes, heritable or acquired during the lifespan, are required for the cell to give rise to a malignant tumor (Grunwald et al. 1982). In the skin, UV irradiation is a major environmental factor responsible for both initiation and promotion of skin cancer. UV irradiation is also known to adversely affect both systemic and cutaneous immunocompetence (Yaar and Gilchrest 1986).

Recent data suggest a critical role for cellular oncogenes and or tumor suppressor genes in malignant transformation (Sager 1989). These genes may represent the final common pathway by which many carcinogens act. The interaction of positive and negative signals to maintain homeostasis is a motif seen everywhere in biology. In cancer, where homeostasis is impaired, mutations of both oncogenes and tumor suppressor genes contribute to the malignant process.

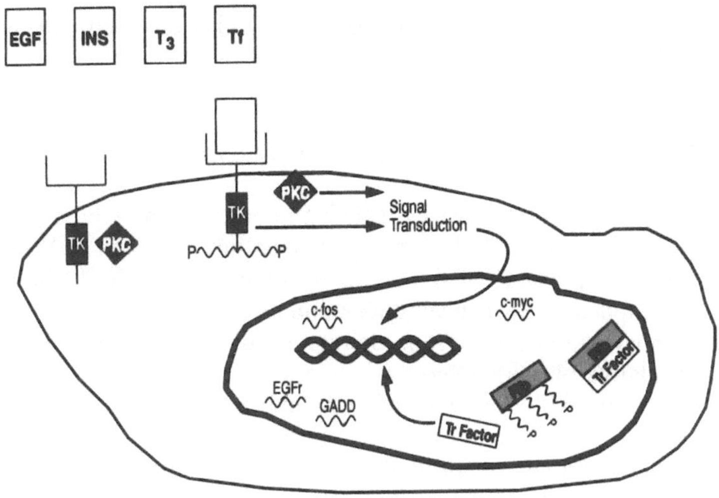

Fig. 1. Signal transduction pathway activation in keratinocytes. Growth factors (▮), by binding to their receptors, activate signal transduction pathways. Epidermal growth factor (*EGF*) activates tyrosine kinase (*TK*), which autophosphorylates EGF receptor (*EGFr*). Protein kinase C (*PKC* ◆) is activated. The signal is transduced to the nucleus and induces transcription of the protooncogenes c-*fos* and c-*myc*, and phosphorylation of retinoblastoma (*Rb*) protein with subsequent release of proliferation promoting transcription factors (*Tr Factor*). Also, EGF receptor mRNA is elvated. mRNA of the growth arrest-associated gene (*GADD*) is downregulated

The normal cellular oncogene homologs play a major role in normal growth and development. When under normal cellular control, they are called proto-oncogenes (Campisi et al. 1984; Studzinski et al. 1986; Lumpkin et al. 1986; Hunter 1984; Mushinski et al. 1983). Mutated, rearranged, amplified forms of these genes which have lost normal constraints on their activity have been found in numerous human and animal tumors, regardless of etiology. Oncogenes act in a dominant manner to produce cancer. Their protein products include growth factors, growth factor receptors, enzymes and proteins involved in intracellular signal transduction, and nuclear proteins presumed to regulate gene transcription (Mushinski et al. 1983; Feldman and Yaar 1991) (Fig. 1).

Genetic mechanisms of tumor suppression operate within the cell and control growth as well as terminal differentiation. Tumor suppressors have an essentially negative effect, blocking transformation and driving cells toward normality (Sager 1989). They produce cancer in a recessive fashion in that one normal allele of these genes is adequate to protect against malignancy and both alleles must be mutated or deleted before uncontrolled proliferation occurs.

Cancer is primarily a disease of late life, implying that during much of our lives we are protected against cancer through evolutionary anticancer mechanisms. Tumor suppressor genes may play a key role in this protection against cancer (Sager 1989).

Molecular Manifestations of Aging and Malignant Transformation

Cancer is a multistep process causing alterations in cellular genes along the lifespan. Because of the strong association between UV exposure and squamous carcinoma of the skin, we attempted to check the expression of genes implicated in cancer development in isolated benign and malignant keratinocytes, derived from donors of different ages, with and without cummulative photodamage.

To examine the influence of aging and photoaging on genes implicated in malignant transformation, keratinocytes derived from newborn, sun-protected, and sun-exposed skin at second or third passage were grown to 70%–90% confluence in serum-free medium supplemented with 10 μg/ml insulin, 10 μg/ml epidermal growth factor, 10^{-9} *M* triiodothyronine, 10 μg/ml transferrin, 1.4×10^{-6} *M* hydrocortisone, 10 μg/ml inositol, 10 μg/ml choline chloride, and 0.09 m*M* calcium. Cultures were provided fresh medium at 2–3-day intervals and 48 h prior to testing. At time 0, cultures were again provided fresh medium and harvested for northern blot analysis (Dean et al. 1983) immediately before and after 30 min, 2, 8, 16, 24, and 48 h (Yaar et al. 1991; Garmyn et al. 1991). Thirty micrograms of total cellular RNA was loaded in each lane, size separated and serially hybridized with radiolabeled complementary (c)DNA probes for the messenger (m)RNA species of interest. Even loading of the blots was confirmed by hybridization with glyceraldehyde phosphate dehydrogenase, a constitutively expressed gene (Yaar et al. 1990).

We chose to check the expression of three well studied proto-oncogenes, a putative tumor suppressor gene (*SPR1*) whose expression is prominent particularly during keratinocytes terminal differentiation, and a recently cloned gene (*GADD*) known to be expressed in nondifferentiated growth arrested keratinocytes. The protooncogenes examined were epidermal growth factor receptor (*EGFr*), c-*fos* and c-*myc* (Fig. 1). *EGFr* is the homolog of *erbB* and is critical for EGF binding and activation of intracellular signal transduction pathways (Sinkovics 1988). c-*fos* and c-*myc* code for two nuclear proteins first identified as causatively involved in mouse osteogenic sarcoma and Burkitt's lymphoma respectively. The c-*myc* mRNA species is induced in cells by mitogens and growth factors (Kelly et al. 1984) and its constitutive expression contributes to uncontrolled cellular proliferation (Kelly and Siebenlist 1985). Also, c-*myc* expression is suppressed during differentiation in a variety of cells (Gonda and Metcalf 1984; Lachman and Skoultchi 1984; Dean et al. 1986; Griep and Deluca 1986) and during terminal differentiation of keratinocytes (Griep and Deluca 1986). c-*fos* mRNA species are rapidly induced in a variety of cell types in response to both growth factors

Table 1. Influence of age and malignant transformation on keratinocyte gene expression

Gene	Time of change (h)	Induction from Baseline		
		Newborn	Adult	Squamous cell carcinoma
fos	0.5–1	++	+	++
myc	16	++	+	–
EGFr	48	++	+	–
GADD	16	+	++	–
SPR1	–[a]	+/–	+	–

[a] Constitutive expression

(Younus and Gilchrest 1991; Greenberg and Ziff 1984; Kruijer et al. 1984) and differentiation signals (Mitchell et al. 1985; Muller et al. 1985; Dotto et al. 1986).

The putative tumor suppressor gene codes for a small proline-rich protein, SPR1, and has been cloned from human epidermal keratinocytes (Kartasova et al. 1988; Kartasova and Van de Putte 1988). SPR1 protein has high proportion of the amino acids glutamine, lysine, serine, and threonine. Small nuclear proteins rich in these amino acids are known to be the products of tumor suppressor genes and to mediate DNA–protein interaction, and SPR1 may also fall into this category. The gene is induced in keratinocytes by lethal UV irradiation and terminal differentiation signals such as TPA and NQO 4- (Kartasova et al. 1987, 1988; Gibbs et al. 1990). Preliminary data from our laboratory suggest a high level of expression of *SPR1* accompanies growth arrest due to many factors.

The growth arrest associated gene *GADD* is known to be induced in proliferating fibroblasts and keratinocytes during growth factor deprivation (Fornace et al. 1988a,b, 1989) and following UV irradiation (M. Garmyn et al., in press). Its expression thus appears to be correlated with cellular distress.

In normal newborn keratinocytes and in squamous carcinoma cells, c-*fos* mRAN was hardly detectable prior to stimulation, but was rapidly and strongly induced after addition of growth factors. Adult sun-protected keratinocytes displayed a similar induction of c-*fos* mRNA, but the level of induction was less than in newborn keratinocytes (Table 1). However, adult sun-exposed keratinocytes expressed c-*fos* mRNA at a relatively high level prior to mitogenic stimulation, with hardly any further induction following addition of growth factors.

The c-*myc* mRNA level was easily detectable in all normal cultures 16 h after growth factor provision but hardly detectable in squamous carcinoma cells. c-*myc* mRNA levels were lower in keratinocytes from donors aged

40 years or older as compared to newborn or young adult donors (Table 1). One interpretation for the lower level of c-*myc* mRNA in squamous carcinoma cells 16 h after provision of growth factors is that the malignant cell type is more uniform and synchronized in behavior than the hererogeneous population of normal keratinocytes, as reported for other malignant cell lines (Bishop 1986), and thus c-*myc* mRNA is rapidly elevated by all cells and quickly returns to prestimulatory level. We therefore wanted to check the level of Myc protein in squamous carcinoma as compared to newborn keratinocytes. Cells were cultured and stimulated with growth factors as above and processed for western blot analysis using mouse monoclonal antibody against human Myc. The 62-kDa Myc protein level was higher in squamous carcinoma cells than in newborn keratinocytes at all times. Myc protein levels in young versus old adults need to be determined.

In newborn and adult keratinocytes but not in squamous carcinoma cells, *EGFr* mRNA was induced within 2 h and again within 48 h after stimulation. It was prominently induced in newborn cells but less in adult keratinocytes. In contrast, in squamous carcinoma cells *EGFr* mRNA level was low and there was no change in the level throughout the 48 h (Table 1).

After stimulation, the initially high *GADD* mRNA level observed 48 h after the last medium change was downregulated in all cells. *GADD* was undetectable in newborn cells between 4 and 8 h, but in contrast expression persisted in adult cells. *GADD* mRNA level was strongly induced in adult keratinocytes within 14 h, but in newborn keratinocytes within 24 h and in squamous carcinoma cells only within 48 h after growth factor provision (Table 1).

SPR1 mRNA was weakly expressed in newborn cells, was mildly expressed in adult cells, and was not expressed in squamous carcinoma cells (Table 1).

Our data suggest that the well-known rapid proliferation rate of newborn cells and slower proliferation of adult cells is reflected at the molecular level by higher and lower c-*myc* mRNA levels, respectively, and the rapid proliferative rate of squamous carcinoma cells is reflected by higher levels of Myc protein at all times. This is especially of note because during stimulation cell number and density are comparable and the cells are supplemented with the same concentration of mitogens. As well, *GADD*, a genetic marker signalling perceived lack of growth factors, is induced earlier in adult cells and later in newborn and squamous carcinoma cells, suggesting less dependence of the newborn and malignant cells on outside growth signals, possibly consistent with the known autocrine growth factor production of newborn cells (Sauder et al. 1988; Clemmons 1983; Stanulis-Praeger and Gilchrest 1986) and the continuous autocrine stimulation of malignant cells (Sager 1989; Sinkovics 1988) which is the result of over-expression of oncogenes or under-expression of tumor suppressor genes. The early perceived growth factor deprivation by adult cells may thus possibly be related to their failure to produce autocrine growth factors (Sauder et al. 1988).

One example of the diminished dependence of squamous carcinoma cells on outside stimuli for growth is their lack of *EGFr* mRNA response to stimulation with EGF, in contrast to that of normal keratinocytes. One possible explanation is that the squamous carcinoma cell line SCC 12F used in our experiments, like the extensively studied vulvar squamous carcinoma A431 (Merlino et al. 1984), either has far more receptors on the surface than normal cells or has receptors which are constitutively activated, independent of the presence or absence of their ligand.

Of particular interest is the lack of expression of the growth arrest-associated gene *SPR1*, postulated to be a growth repressing nuclear protein (Dotto et al. 1986; Kartasova et al. 1988; Kartasova and Van de Putte 1988), in squamous carcinoma cells. Immunohistochemical staining of normal skin cross-sections reveals abundant SPR1 protein in the nonproliferative, terminally differentiated stratum granulosum and stratum spinosum of the epidermis. Its absence in squamous carcinoma cells may thus directly contribute to their uncontrolled proliferation.

Our studies suggest that aging is associated with loss of cellular sensitivity to or awareness of external signals as manifested by less induction of EGF receptor, c-*fos* and c-*myc* mRNA following growth factor stimulation as compared to newborn cells and earlier induction of growth arrest and/or distress associated genes, such as *SPR1* and *GADD*. Of particular interest is c-*fos* mRNA regulation. Since this gene is rapidly induced by a variety of outside stimuli and its protein product works in concert with other nuclear proteins to modulate expression of target genes, its induction may be a crucial signal for the cell for its proper response to a variety of outside stimuli. c-*fos* mRNA induction is less in adult than in newborn cells, in agreement with loss of cellular sensitivity to outside stimulation, but interestingly its control seems to be different in sun-exposed cells. Our studies suggest that in these cells the c-*fos* level is constitutively elevated and there is only minimal induction following outside stimuli. At least as far as c-*fos* regulation is concerned, photoaging differs from physiologic aging.

Conclusion

In conclusion, we have shown profound differences in cellular response to outside signals between newborn and adult keratinocytes and between squamous carcinoma cells and normal keratinocytes. The findings are consistent with age-associated loss of sensitivity to external signals and an earlier greater perceived requirement for growth factors. The response of squamous carcinoma cells to growth stimuli is consistent with proliferation largely independent of external signals. Whether these molecular changes represent cumulative random genetic damage or a programmed aging process cannot be determined. Nevertheless, our data correlate with the well-known differences in biologic responsiveness between newborn, adult, and squamous carcinoma cells. Thus, our findings represent a beginning from which more comprehensive understanding of the relationship between cutaneous aging and malignancy will evolve.

Acknowledgements. This work was supported by grants from the National Institute on Aging (AG00354 and AG07114) and by the USDA Agricultural Research Service.

References

Aubry F, MacGibbon B (1985) Risk factors of squamous cell carcinoma of the skin. Cancer 55:907–911

Bishop JM (1985) Viral oncogenes. Cell 42:23–38

Bishop JM (1986) The pathobiology of proto-oncogenes. Int Symp Princess Takamatsu Cancer Res Fund 17:3–9

Campisi J, Gray HE, Pardee AB, Dean M, Sonenshein GE (1984) Cell-cycle control of c-myc but not c-ras expression is lost following chemical transformation. Cell 36:241–247

Clemmons DR (1983) Age dependent production of a competence factor by human fibroblasts. J Cell Physiol 114:61–67

Dean M, Kent RB, Sonenshein GE (1983) Transcriptional activation of immunoglobulin alpha heavy chain genes by translocation of the c-myc oncogene. Nature 305:443–446

Dean M, Levine R, Campisi J (1986) C-myc regulation during retinoic acid induced differentiation of F-9 cells is post-transcriptional and associated with growth arrest. Mol Cell Biol 6:518–524

Doll R, Peto R (1981) The causes of cancer. Quantitative estimates of avoidable risks of cancer in the United States today. J Natl Cancer Inst 66:1191–1308

Dotto GP, Gilman MZ, Maruyama M, Weinberg RA (1986) C-myc and c-fos expression in differentiating mouse primary keratinocytes. EMBO J 5 11:2853–2857

Feldman SR, Yaar M (1991) Oncogenes: the growth control genes. Arch Dermatol 127:707–711

Fornace AJ Jr, Alamo I Jr, Hollander MC (1988a) DNA damage-inducible transcripts in mammalian cells. Proc Natl Acad Sci USA 85:8800–8804

Fornace AJ Jr, Alamo I Jr, Hollander MC, Lamoreaux E (1988b) Ubiquitin mRNA is a major stress induced transcript in mammalian cells. Nucleic Acids Res 17:1215–1230

Fornace AJ Jr, Nebert DW, Hollander MC, Luethy JD, Papathanasiou M, Fargnoli J, Holbrook NJ (1989) Mammalian genes coordinately regulated by growth arrest signals and DNA-damaging agents. Mol Cell Biol 9:4196–4203

Garmyn M, Yaar M, Howrigan P, Gilchrest BA (1991) Influence of aging on gene expression in cultured human keratinocytes. J Invest Dermatol 96:618

Garmyn M, Yaar M, Holbrook N, Gilchrest BA. Immediate and delayed molecular response of human keratinocytes to solar-simulated irradiation. Lab Invest (in press)

Gibbs S, Lohman F, Teubel W, Putte Van de P, Backendorf C (1990) Characterization of the human SPR2 promoter: induction after UV irradiation or TPA treatment and regulation during differentiation of cultured primary keratinocytes. Nucleic Acids Res 18:4401–4407

Gilchrest BA (1984) Skin and aging processes. CRC Press, Boca Raton
Glass AG, Hoover RN (1989) The emerging epidemic of melanoma and squamous cell skin cancer. JAMA 262:2097–2100
Gonda T, Metcalf D (1984) Expression of myb, myc, and fos proto-oncogenes during the differentiation of a murine myeloid leukemia. Nature 310:249–351
Greenberg ME, Ziff EB (1984) Stimulation of 3T3 cells induces transcription of the c-fos proto-oncogene. Nature 311:433–438
Griep AE, Deluca HF (1986) Decreased expression of c-myc is an early event in retinoic acid induced differentiation of F-9 teratocarcinoma cells. Proc Natl Acad Sci USA 83:5539–5543
Grunwald DJ, Dale B, Dudley J, Lamph W, Sugden B, Ozanne B, Risser R (1982) Loss of viral gene expression and retention of tumorigenicity by Abelson lymphoma cells. J Virol 43:92–103
Hunter T (1984) Oncogenes and proto-oncogenes: how do they differ? J Natl Cancer Inst 73:773–786
Johnson MLT (1989) Aging of the United States population: the dermatologic implications. Clin Geriatr Med 41–51
Kartasova T, Van de Putte P (1988) Isolation, characterization, and UV-stimulated expression of two families of genes encoding polypeptides of related structure in human epidermal keratinocytes. Mol Cell Biol 8:2195–2203
Kartasova T, Cornelisseu BJC, Belt P, Putte Van de P (1987) Effects of UV, 4-NQ0 and TPA on gene expression in cultured human epidermal keratinocytes. Nucleic Acids Res 15:5945–5962
Kartasova T, Van Muijen GNP, Van Pelt-Herschap H, Van de Putte P (1988) Novel protein in human epidermal keratinocytes: regulation of expression during differentiation. Mol Cell Biol 8:2204–2210
Kelly K, Siebenlist U (1985) The role of c-myc in the proliferation of normal and neoplastic cells. J Clin Immunol 5:65–77
Kelly K, Cochran BH, Stiles CD, Leder P (1984) Cell specific regulation of the c-myc changes during differentiation of mouse leukemia cells. Nature 310:592–594
Kruijer W, Cooper JA, Hunter T, Verma IM (1984) PDGF induces rapid but transient expression of the c-fos gene. Nature 312:711–716
Lachman HM, Skoultchi AI (1984) Expression of c-myc changes during differentiation of mouse leukemia cells. Nature 310:592–594
Land H, Parada LF, Weinberg RA (1983) Cellular oncogenes and multistep carcinogenesis. Science 222:771–778
Liberman MW, Lebovitz RM (1990) Neoplasia. In: Kissane JM (ed) Anderson's pathology. Mosby, St Louis, pp 566–614
Lin AN, Carter DM, Balin AK (1989) Skin cancer in the elderly. Clin Geriatr Med 161–170
Lumpkin CK, Knepper JE, Butel JS, Smith JR, Periera-Smith OM (1986) Mitogenic effects of the proto-oncogene and oncogene forms of c-H-ras DNA in human diploid fibroblasts. Mol Cell Biol 6:2990–2993
Merlino GT, Xu YH, Ishii S, Clark AJL, Semba K, Toyoshima K, Tamamoto T, Pastan I (1984) Amplification and enhanced expression of the epidermal growth factor receptor gene in A431 human carcinoma cells. Science 224:417–419
Miller AD, Curran T, Verma IM (1984) C-fos protein can induce cellular transformation: a novel mechanism of activation of a cellular oncogene. Cell 36:51–60
Miller EC (1978) Some current prospectives on chemical carcinogenesis in humans and experimental animals: presidential address. Cancer Res 38:1479–1496
Mitchell RL, Zokas L, Schreiber RD, Verma IM (1985) Rapid induction of the expression of the proto-oncogene c-fos during human monocytic differentiation. Cell 40:209–217

Muller R, Curran T, Muller D, Guilbert L (1985) Induction of c-fos during myelomonocytic differentiation and macrophage proliferation. Nature 314:546–548
Mushinski JF, Potter M, Bauer SR, Reddy EP (1983) DNA rearrangement and altered RNA expression of the c-myb oncogene in mouse plasmacytoid lymphosarcomas. Science 220:795–798
Rassoulzadegan M, Cowie A, Carr A, Glaichenhaus N, Kamen R, Cuzin F (1982) The roles of individual polyoma virus early proteins in oncogenic transformation. Nature 300:713–718
Sager R (1989) Tumor suppressor genes: the puzzle and the promise. Science. 246:1406–1412
Sauder DN (1989) Effect of age on epidermal immune function. Clin Geriatr Med 149–160
Sauder DN, Stanulis-Praeger BM, Gilchrest BA (1988) Autocrine growth stimulation of human keratinocytes by epidermal derived thymocyte-activating factor: implications for skin aging. Arch Dermatol. Res 280:71–76
Sinkovics JG (1988) Oncogenes and growth factors. Crit Rev Immunol 8:217–298
Stanulis-Praeger BM, Gilchrest BA (1986) Growth factor responsiveness declines during adulthood for human skin derived cells. Mech Ageing Dev 35:185–198
Stoll HL Jr, Schwartz RA (1987) Squamous cell carcinoma. In: Fitzpatrick TB, Eisen AZ, Wolff K, Freedberg IM, Austen KF (eds) Dermatology in general medicine. McGraw-Hill, New York, pp 746–758
Streilein JW (1991) Immunogenetic factors in skin cancer. N Engl J Med 325:884–886
Studzinski GP, Brelvi ZS, Feldman SC, Watt RA (1986) Participation of c-myc protein in DNA synthesis of human cells. Science 234:467–470
Weinstein IB (1981) Current concepts and controversies in chemical carcinogenesis. J Supramol Struct Cell Biochem 17:99–120
Weinstock MA (1989) The epidemic of squamous cell carcinoma. JAMA 262:2138–2140
Yaar M, Gilchrest BA (1986) Bullous Pemphigoid: model for aging. Clin Dermatol 135–145
Yaar M, Gilchrest BA (1988) Cellular and molecular mechanisms of cutaneous aging. J Dermatol Surg Oncol 16:915–922
Yaar M, Peacocke M, Cohen MS, Gilchrest BA (1990) Dissociation of protooncogene induction from growth response. J Cell Physiol 145:39–45
Yaar M, Gilani A, Garmyn M, Gilchrest BA (1991) Keratinocyte gene activation following growth or differentiation signals. Clin Res 39:148
Younus J, Gilchrest BA (1991) Molecular events in human keratinocyte differentiation. J Invest Dermatol 96:618
Yuspa SH (1987) Carcinogenesis: chemical. In: Fitzpatrick TB, Eisen AZ, Wolff K, Freedberg IM, Austen KF (eds) Dermatology in general medicine. McGraw-Hill, New York, pp 722–729
Yuspa SH, Lichti U, Morgan D, Hennings H (1980) Chemical carcinogenesis studies in mouse epidermal cell cultures. Curr Prob Dermatol 10:171–191

Molecular Mechanisms of Skin Carcinogenesis Induced by Chemicals and Ionizing Radiation

G.T. Bowden[1], M.A. Nelson[1], J.P. Levy[1], J. Finch[1], and P. Krieg[2]

[1] Department of Radiation Oncology, University of Arizona Medical School, Tucson, AZ 85724, USA
[2] Institute for Virus Research, German Cancer Research Center, W-6900 Heidelberg, Fed. Rep. of Germany

Introduction

The progression of target stem cells through a premalignant to a malignant state during either chemical or radiation carcinogenesis is accompanied by a variety of biochemical, cytological, and morphological changes. These phenotypic alterations result in turn from either qualitative alterations in the encoded gene product or changes in the level of expression of the cellular gene. There are three classes of cellular genes that are known to be altered during carcinogenesis and are thought to play a functional role in tumor formation. One of these classes are the cellular protooncogenes (Bishop 1983; Land et al. 1983; Bowden 1985) that are activated by mutation and encode for products that are involved in growth factor signal transduction. Another class are the tumor suppressor genes (Klein 1987) whose products are involved in regulating cellular growth, differentiation, and senescence. During tumor formation these tumor suppressor genes are inactivated, presumably through mutational events. The third class of genes are effector genes (Zarbl et al. 1991) that are regulated by the oncogenes or the tumor suppressor genes and whose altered expression plays a role in induction or maintainence of various tumor phenotypes. Both chemical carcinogens and ionizing radiation are known to induce the types of activating mutations seen in oncogenes and the inactivating mutations observed in tumor suppressor genes. These mutations can lead to structural changes in encoded gene products or loss of normal control of expression of these genes. An important unanswered question is whether these carcinogens directly induce the mutations found in these critical genes or whether the carcinogens are indirectly involved, perhaps in selection for cells containing spontaneously induced target gene mutations.

The mouse skin model of multistage carcinogenesis is an ideal system to identify critical gene alterations during chemical and radiation induction of skin tumors. The process of malignant tumor formation in this model can be

Recent Results in Cancer Research, Vol. 128

subdivided into distinct operational stages including initiation, promotion, and progression (Boutwell 1974; Scribner and Suss 1978). A single subcarcinogenic dose of a chemical carcinogen or ionizing radiation can be delivered to the epidermis and no tumors will be observed unless the epidermis is treated repeatedly with a phorbol ester or okadaic acid tumor promoter. The majority of the skin tumors generated from initiation and promotion are benign papillomas. In the third stage of tumor progression, the papillomas are converted to malignant squamous cell carcinomas by the action of agents including some of the initiating agents (Hennings et al. 1983), certain peroxides (O'Connell et al. 1986) and ionizing radiation (Jaffe et al. 1987). There are also epidermal cell cultures that represent each of the stages in the formation of malignant squamous cell carcinomas (SCCs). Therefore, questions can be asked with this model concerning the nature and timing of gene alterations, and chemical carcinogenesis protocols can be compared to ionizing radiation protocols in terms of these gene alterations. In addition, potential functional roles for altered gene expression in tumor formation can be evaluated using mammalian expression vectors and the various epidermal cell cultures that represent the stages in tumor formation.

Over the last 6–7 years a number of laboratories have used this multistage model to study protooncogene activation (Balmain and Pragnell 1985; Balmain et al. 1984; Quintanilla et al. 1986; Bizub et al. 1986; Bonham et al. 1989) and differential gene expression (Toftgard et al. 1985; Pelling et al. 1986; Melber et al. 1986; Matrisian et al. 1986; Krieg et al. 1987, 1988; Bowden et al. 1987a,b; Ostrowski et al. 1989) of tumor-associated genes. Here, we summarize our results in which we compared and contrasted cellular gene alterations found in mouse skin tumors induced by chemical carcinogens and ionizing radiation. In addition, we have presented preliminary results related to the detection of epidermal cells with Harvey *ras* mutations soon after chemical carcinogen initiation of the mouse skin and our studies of gene activation by the nonphorbol ester tumor promoter, okadaic acid.

Detection of Transforming Genes in Chemically Initiated Mouse Skin Tumors and Initiated Epidermis

A number of laboratories including our own have detected the presence of activated Harvey (Ha)-*ras* oncogenes in chemically initiated benign and malignant mouse skin tumors (Balmain and Pragnell 1985; Bonham et al. 1989). Most recently we have reported the presence of dominant transforming activity in skin tumors initiated by the carcinogen, ethyl carbamate or urethane (Bonham et al. 1989). Urethane has been reported to be a pure initiator of mouse skin tumors, and this initiator requires metabolic activation to yield an ultimate carcinogenic form, most likely an epoxide (Mirvish 1968; Dahl et al. 1978; Miller and Miller 1983). Using the NIH 3T3 focus assay, dominant transforming activity was detected in DNA isolated from SCCs initiated with urethane and promoted with the phorbol ester 12-*O*-tetradecanoylphorbol-13 acetate (TPA). Amplified and rearranged copies of the c-Ha-*ras* gene were detected in DNA isolated from transformant cell lines, indicating that an activated Ha-*ras* gene had been transfered to the NIH 3T3 recipient cells. Analysis of $p21^{ras}$ from the transformant cell lines suggested that the activating *ras* mutation was present in codon 61. An A to T transversion mutation was detected at the second position of the Ha-*ras* oncogene in the NIH 3T3 transformants. This mutation created a new *Xba* 1 site in the cellular Ha-*ras* gene and this restriction fragment length polymorphism was used to demonstrate this mutation in the primary papillomas and SCCs initiated with urethane and promoted with TPA. Southern blot analysis showed *Xba* 1 polymorphisms in codon 61 of primary mouse skin tumors all of which were initiated with urethane. Published results (You et al. 1989) concerning urethane-induced lung tumors in A/J mice showed evidence for consistent activation of the Kirsten (Ki)-*ras* gene by the same A to T transversion mutation at codon 61. In addition, vinyl carbamate, a proximate carcinogen that is a probable intermediate metabolite of urethane, produced mouse hepatomas with the same codon 61 A to T transversion mutation in the Ha-*ras* gene (Wiseman et al. 1986). Therefore, three different mouse tumor types induced with urethane or its metabolite contained a high frequency (though not exclusively) of *ras* gene activation by the same A to T transversion mutation at the 61st codon. The idea of direct interaction of tumor initiator active metabolites with specific target bases in the *ras* protooncogene cannot be directly related to what is known about the major DNA adduct formed with urethane or vinyl carbamate. Initially, following administration of urethane or vinyl carbamate, 7-(2-oxoethyl) guanine was the only major adduct identified in rat liver (Scherer et al. 1980). Subsequently, a second minor adduct, 1,N^6-ethenodeoxyadenosine, has been identified in rodent liver DNA following administration of vinyl chloride (Eberle et al. 1989). It has been shown that incorporation of 1,N^6-etheno-adenine into a polynucleotide when replicated in an in vitro system gives rise to an A to T tranversion mutation (Singer 1982). It is interesting to speculate that 1,N^6-ethenodeoxyadenosine is a minor adduct produced in mouse skin from urethane initiation that gives rise to the A to T tranversion mutation in the Ha-*ras* gene.

The exact timing of mutational activation of the Ha-*ras* protooncogene relative to the application of the chemical initiator to the skin is not known. We have developed a sensitive mutation-specific polymerase chain reaction (PCR) amplification technique (MSPA) based on a published procedure by Ehlen and Dubeau (1989) to experimentally address the timing of Ha-*ras* activation. The MSPA assay is based on the rationale that a DNA primer with a 3′-end complementary to a specific point mutation allows chain elongation only of mutant DNA sequences during PCR reactions. The MSPA PCR reaction is carried out using ^{32}P end-labeled downstream primer to enhance the sensitivity of the assay. With this sensitive technique we asked whether mutated *ras* oncogenes could be detected in the epidermis of mice initiated with carcinogens prior to the development of premalignant lesions. In these experiments we used carcinogens which we knew initiated skin tumors that contained Ha-*ras* oncogenes with 61st codon A to T mutations. These carcinogens were 7,12-dimethyl-benz(a)anthracene (DMBA) and urethane. Epidermal DNA was isolated from mice 1 week after initiation with DMBA or urethane and subjected to MSPA analysis for the presence of 61st codon Ha-*ras* mutant alleles. Initiated epidermis but not acetone-treated epidermis demonstrated 1 week after carcinogen treatment the presence of Ha-*ras* genes with 61st codon A to T mutations. By operational definition, initiated mice will not develop either benign or malignant skin tumors unless they are treated with a tumor promoter such as a phorbol ester. To observe the first benign papilloma the initiated mice must be promoted for at least 5–6 weeks. Ninety percent of papillomas initiated by either DMBA or urethane and promoted with TPA contain an activated Ha-*ras* oncogene with the same mutation as seen in the epidermal cells 1 week after initiation. Thus epidermal cells with an activated Ha-*ras* oncogene can exist in the skin prior to the appearance of benign tumors. Our finding that mutant Ha-*ras* genes can be detected in epidermal tissue 1 week after carcinogen treatment is consistent with the findings of Kumar et al. (1990) These investigators found both mutated Ha-*ras* and Ki-*ras* genes in rat mammary glands 2 weeks after carcinogen treatment and 2 months before the onset of neoplasia.

Detection of Distinct Non-*ras* Transforming Genes in Ionizing Radiation-Initiated Mouse Skin Tumors

Besides studying chemical carcinogen-initiated mouse skin tumors, we have focused on ionizing radiation-initiated, TPA-promoted skin tumors and dominant transforming genes. We found that ionizing radiation can act as a weak initiator of malignant skin tumors (i.e., SCCs) when initiation is followed by TPA promotion (Jaffe and Bowden 1986, 1987). In addition, we observed that ionizing radiation was capable of inducing basal cell carcinomas (BCCs), a tumor histology not seen with chemical agents in the mouse skin system. We have also observed that fractionated doses of accelerated electrons were effective in the third stage of tumor progression (Jaffe et al. 1987). DNAs from mouse skin tumors initiated with ionizing radiation, including papillomas, SCCs, BCCs, and pilomatrixomas, demonstrated dominant transforming activity by the production of transformed foci in the mouse recipient line, NIH 3T3 (Jaffe and Bowden 1989). Dominant transforming activity was not found in DNA from normal epidermis or from the corresponding liver.

The NIH 3T3 transformants induced with SCC DNAs grew in soft agar and formed tumors in nude mice. Southern blot analyses of primary NIH

3T3 transformant DNAs carrying transforming genes from radiation-initiated SCCs indicated that the oncogenes responsible for transformation of the recipient cells were not Ha-*ras*, Ki-*ras*, or N-*ras*, nor were they *erbB*, *B-lym*, *met*, *neu*, or *raf*. The transforming genes transfered by DNA from four SCCs were further characterized by determining their sensitivity to digestion with a series of restriction enzymes. The results of these experiments indicated that were at least three different transforming genes present in four SCCs initiated with ionizing radiation.

Our data suggest that the target gene(s) for oncogenic activation are different for chemical carcinogens and ionizing radiation. Support for this finding has been presented by Borek et al. (1987) as well as by Krolewski and Little (1989). These workers have also detected distinct non-*ras* transforming genes in ionizing radiation-transformed rodent cells in culture. It is perhaps not surprising that activation of the *ras* protooncogene was not identified with radiation-initiated mouse skin tumors as was consistently observed with chemically intiated mouse skin tumors. The *ras* family of oncogenes is activated by point mutations, and the chemical initiating agents or their metabolites are known to be relatively efficient point mutagens. In contrast, ionizing radiation is a relatively weak point mutagen and instead induces larger genomic alterations (Goodhead 1984; Rauth 1987).

Differential Gene Expression During Mouse Skin Carcinogenesis

In addition to studying transforming genes in chemically and radiation induced mouse skin tumors, we have identified and characterized cellular genes whose expression is altered during tumor development (Melber et al. 1986; Bowden et al. 1989). To achieve this goal, we have used differential screening of cDNA libraries that were made from polyA$^+$ RNA isolated from SCCs induced by DMBA initiation and TPA promotion. The libraries were screened using complementary cDNA probes made from RNA isolated from normal epidermis and SCCs. We isolated six cDNAs (*mal1* to *mal6*) that identified distinct RNA transcripts that were overexpressed at different stages of skin tumor formation. To investigate a potential role of the *mal* genes in the process of skin carcinogenesis, we asked whether there was a correlation between the stage of tumor development and the level of expression of different mal genes. In addition, we sequenced the cDNAs for the *mal* genes and searched data bases for homology or identity with known genes.

Our work to date has focused on the *mal1* to *mal4* genes. The *mal1* gene was found to be overexpressed in both benign and malignant skin tumors compared to normal epidermis (Bowden et al. 1989). Sequencing of the *mal1* cDNA has revealed extensive sequence homology to a family of low molecular weight, hydrophobic, ligand-binding proteins. This family includes a differentiation-associated protein in adipocytes (adipocyte lipid-binding protein) and cellular retinol-binding protein (CRBP) (Demmer et al. 1987).

These low molecular weight, cytosolic, nonenzymatic proteins form a multigene family of proteins presumably derived from a common ancestral gene. These proteins bind fatty acids or retinoids and are presumed to function in some aspect of intracellular lipid metabolism. Some of them play a functional role in proliferation and differentiation. Recent studies suggest a role for CRBP in carcinogenesis (Gates and Rees 1985; Yanogita et al. 1986; Wahlberg et al. 1988). Several workers have shown that SCCs of the head and neck contained increased levels of CRBP compared to normal tissue. Since retinol inhibits terminal differentiation of keratinocytes, it has been suggested that increased CRBP levels in SCCs may cause decreased terminal differentiation in these tumors.

We have found that the *mal2* gene transcripts are overexpressed in both benign and malignant skin tumors. Our expression data have shown that there is a higher steady-state level of *mal2* transcripts in benign papillomas that are autonomous (i.e., no longer require promoter treatment) than in papillomas that are dependent on continued promoter treatment. Sequencing of a *mal2* cDNA and a *mal2* genomic clone has recently revealed identity with the sequence for a mouse hyperproliferative keratin, K-6 (Finch et al. 1991). The expression pattern of the *mal2* gene is consistent with its enhanced expression under conditions of hyperproliferation. As an example, we found the *mal2* gene to be induced in adult epidermis that has been treated with both tumor promoters and a non-tumor promoting hyperplastic agent.

The *mal3* cDNA used in probing of northerns has revealed multiple hybridizing bands. The intensity and pattern of these *mal3*-related transcripts changed during tumor development. A ubiquitin-coding region probe (Finch et al. 1990) detected five transcripts. Oligonucleotides were designed for unique parts of three mouse ubiquitin gene transcripts. The overexpressed transcripts at 2.4, 2.8 and 6.4 kilo bases (kb) were detected by an oligonucleotide specific for a mouse UbC polyubiquitin clone. A 1.2-kb UbB overexpressed transcript was detected by an oligonucleotide for a mouse four-unit polyubiquitin and a 0.7-kb overexpressed transcript was recognized by an oligonucleotide for the mouse ubiquitin carboxyl-extension protein of 52 amino acids. All three subfamilies of transcripts were induced in mouse skin by the hyperproliferative agent ethylphenyl propiolate (EPP) and by the tumor promoting agent 12-*O*-tetradecanoylphorbol-13 acetate (TPA). Heat shock of cultured keratinocytes induced both the 6.4- and 7.8-kb transcripts recognized by the UbC polyubiquitin oligonucleotide. Consistent with the overexpression of the ubiquitin transcripts, the level of free ubiquitin protein, as determined by western analysis, was elevated in the tumors and proliferating epidermis compared to normal epidermis. These results indicated that overexpression of ubiquitin genes in both benign and malignant skin tumors compared to resting epidermis could be related to a sustained state of proliferation and stress in the tumors compared to normal, resting tissue.

The *mal4* cDNA detected a 1.9-kb transcript overexpressed in SCCs compared to papillomas and normal epidermis. Sequencing of a full-length *mal4* cDNA revealed identity with the mouse β-actin cDNA (Ostrowski et al. 1989). Southern analysis of DNAs from normal epidermis, papillomas, and SCCs showed no evidence for amplification or rearrangement of the β-actin gene during tumor progression. The RNA–RNA hybrid protection assay was used to screen for the expression of mutated β-actin(s) in mouse skin tumors. No evidence for a mutation was obtained in benign and malignant skin tumors that were examined. We found approximately equal amounts of β-actin protein detected by two-dimensional gel electrophoresis and extracted from normal epidermis, papillomas, or SCCs. These results indicated that overexpression of β-actin message in SCCs did not result in an increased steady-state level of β-actin protein. This would indicate that translational or posttranslational mechanisms may be functioning to maintain a relatively constant cellular concentration of actin in the presence of high levels of β-actin-specific RNA. It is possible that in SCCs there is increased synthesis of β-actin protein but that there is increased degradation of β-actin protein such that the steady-state level of protein is not altered. An increased turnover of actin has been reported in cultured fibroblasts from individuals susceptible to dominantly inherited cancer (Antecol et al. 1986). Because these predisposed fibroblasts show reduced and disorganized microfilaments, features that have been associated with increased motility of tumor cells in culture and increased metastatic potential in vivo, it is clear that alterations in the properties or metabolism of actins can have profound effects on cellular phenotypes.

Expression Pattern of the Transin Gene During Mouse Skin Tumor Promotion and Progression

The rodent transin gene encodes an oncogene and growth factor-inducible protein that has been shown to be a rodent homolog (Matrisian et al. 1986) of an extracellular matrix-degrading metalloproteinase known as stromelysin (Chin et al. 1985). Stomelysin is known to degrade a number of extracellular matrix proteins including laminin, fibronectin, proteoglycans, gelatins, and to some extent collagen types III, IV, and V. The rat transin or stromelysin cDNA was originally cloned because of its selective expression in polyoma virus-transformed rat fibroblasts and lack of expression in untransformed parental cells (Matrisian et al. 1985). Later studies indicated that stromelysin was present in cell lines transformed by a number of different oncogenes. These results prompted us to study the expression pattern of the stromelysin gene in mouse skin tumors produced by various carcinogen protocols (Matrisian et al. 1986).

When RNA was isolated from tumors resulting from DMBA initiation and TPA promotion, stromelysin transcripts were detectable in 73% of the SCCs, but only 6% of the papillomas expressed low levels of stromelysin. Similar results were obtained with tumors initiated by *N*-methyl-*N*-nitroso-*N*′-nitro-guanidine (MNNG) and promoted with TPA. When mice were treated with repeated applications of MNNG, a protocol which produces SCCs with a high probability of invading and metastasizing, 100% of the primary tumors expressed very high levels of stromelysin message (Ostrowski et al. 1988). This overexpression of transin or stromelysin in invasive malignant tumors could play a functional role in tumor cell invasion because the encoded protein degrades proteins found in the basement membrane separating the epidermis from the dermis, and this membrane must be transversed by the malignant tumor cells for invasion and metastasis to occur.

Since we observed in the mouse skin that ionizing radiation enhances the progression of chemically initiated papillomas to malignant SCCs (Jaffe et al. 1987), we decided to develop a cell culture model to study radiation-induced malignant progression. A squamous papilloma-producing cell line called 308 (Strickland et al. 1988) which has an activated Ha-*ras* oncogene has been used to model the benign tumor state. The 308 cells were irradiated with 10 Gy of X-rays and surviving cell clones were assessed for their ability to form SCCs in athymic nude mice. One malignantly progressed clone called 308 10 Gy 5 has been further characterized in terms of gene expression. One gene for which we have evidence supporting its role in malignant progression and in particular tumor cell invasion through basement membrane is the stromelysin gene. This collagenase gene encodes for a protease that degrades proteins found in basement membrane. Therefore, we have measured the steady-state levels of stromelysin message in both parental 308 cells and the malignant variant cell line 308 10 Gy 5. The variant cells showed measurable expression of the stromelysin gene but in the parental 308 cells there was no detectable expression. A potential reason for the upregulated expression of the stromelysin gene in the 308 10 Gy 5 variant cells could be alterations in either the *cis*-regulatory elements of the gene or changes in the levels of specific *trans*-regulatory proteins or mutations in tumor suppressor genes. To begin to study the *cis* and *trans* regulation of the gene we have cloned approximately 1.6 kb of 5′-flanking region of the mouse stromelysin gene. 850 base pairs (bp) of the promoter region of the gene were cloned into a chloramphenicol (CAT) reporter expression vector. Transient transfection of the mouse stromelysin promoter regulating the CAT reporter gene was carried out using the parental 308 cells and the 308 10 Gy 5 malignant variant cells lines. Constitutive expression of the CAT gene was found using the stromelysin gene promoter in the 308 10 Gy 5 variant cells but no constitutive activity of the promoter was found in the parental 308 cells. These results indicated that there was a *cis* element in the 850 bp of the mouse stromelysin 5′-flanking region that was responsible for the constitutive overexpression of the stromelysin gene in the 308 10 Gy 5 malignant variant cell line compared to the benign parental 308 cells. The exact identity of this *cis* element is presently being pursued. Sequencing of the 5′-flanking region of the stromelysin gene has revealed the presence of a number of consensus *cis* regulatory elements including a TPA-responsive element (TRE) that binds the AP1 transactivating complex and a PEA-3 site bound by the protooncogene, c-*ets*, and a CACCC box bound by *Sp-1*. We therefore investigated whether there was upregulated expression of other cellular genes known to contain TREs in the malignant variant cells compared to the parental 308 cells. We found evidence for upregulated expression of the metallothionein IIA, c-*fos* and c-*jun* genes in the 308 10 Gy 5 cells when compared to the parental 308 cells. All three of these genes are known to contain TREs or other TPA responsive elements.

In addition to finding constitutive expression of the stromelysin gene in malignant skin tumors, we have also observed transient induced expression of the gene in both phorbol ester (Krieg et al. 1988) treated and okadaic acid treated normal mouse epidermis and in cultured mouse keratinocytes (Holladay et al. 1991). We have shown that the phorbol esters TPA and 12-*O*-retinyl-phorbol-13-acetate (RPA) transiently induced the expression of the transin or stromelysin gene in adult mouse epidermis with a peak stimulation between 12 and 18 h. This induction did not appear to be associated with a hyperproliferative response since the weak or nonpromoting agent ethyl phenylpropriolate did not induce the expression of the transin gene. In addition to the phorbol esters we have investigated the effects of a nonphorbol ester tumor promoter, okadaic acid, on gene expression in mouse keratinocytes. Okadaic acid is a potent and relatively specific inhibitor of phosphatases I and IIA (Chin et al. 1985; Bialojan 1988) and treatment with this compound could lead to an apparent activation of protein kinases. Adult mice were treated topically with okadaic acid and the steady-state levels of various gene transcripts in the skin were determined at different times after treatment. Okadaic acid induced the expression of the nuclear protooncogene c-*fos* in a biphasic manner. The initial induction peaked 6 h after treatment and the second induction peaked at 48–72 h. The steady-state level of expression of the nuclear protooncogene c-*jun* in untreated skin was relatively high, and okadaic acid induced a slight increase of c-*jun* expression from 12 to 48 h after treatment. In comparison to the induction by TPA, okadaic acid induced the expression of transin or stromelysin and plasminogen activator (PA) type urokinase, two secondary response genes which contain *cis* regulatory elements that are TPA responsive, with delayed kinetics.

In the mouse papilloma cell line 308, okadaic acid induced dramatically higher steady-state levels of early response genes c-*jun* and c-*fos* than equimolar doses of TPA, and the okadaic acid-induced expression was sustained over a longer period of time. The secondary response genes for transin and PA-urokinase were induced to similar levels by TPA and okadaic acid in 308 cells. However, the induction of each of these genes by okadaic acid was delayed in comparison to induction by TPA. The existence of different patterns of induced expression of early and secondary response genes by okadaic acid and TPA suggests that these tumor promoters affect gene expression in mouse keratinocytes through different signal transduction pathways.

Our studies reported above confirm other reported work in which it has been shown that okadaic acid can transcriptionally regulate both immediate-early and secondary response genes in mammalian cells (Thevenin et al. 1991). Okadaic acid has been shown to transactivate the human collagenase promoter through an AP-1 response element and another element upstream of the AP-1 binding site. We have shown that both TPA and okadaic acid transactivate an isolated TPA response element (TRE) when placed in front of the thymidine kinase heterologous promoter in a chloramphenicol acetyl transferase (CAT) reporter plasmid and electroporated into the benign papilloma mouse keratinocyte cell line 308. In contrast, we found that okadaic acid but not TPA can transactivate a novel mutant TRE sequence, GGAGTCA. This is the reverse complement of the sequence TGACTCC. In addition, the similar sequence TGAGTCC is okadoic acid, but not TPA *trans*-activated. We call the consensus of these two sequences, TGA(c/g)TCC, the okadaic acid response element (ORE). By deletion and site-directed mutagenesis analysis we have found that the rat JE immediate-early gene promoter (Timmers et al. 1990) was okadaic acid, but not TPA inducible through the enhancer element TGACTCC. Deletion analysis of the human collagnease gene promoter revealed that the region between −73 and −137 (containing the sequence GGAGTCA) was responsible for the additional transcritional activity above that of the TRE at −73 to −67. We have discovered that the ORE is transactivated by binding of a transcription factor complex that contained both Jun and Fos proteins. We have also found that in malignant murine tumor cells Jun and Fos constitutively bind to and activate transcription through the ORE element. Binding of transcription factors to the element was shown to be dependent upon phosphorylation. A computer homology search showed that the ORE was found in the ε- but not α-, β-, or γ- globin gene promoters (Gong et al. 1990). This element has been shown to be footprinted in human erythroleukemia K562 cells. The signal transduction pathway involving the ORE cis element which is transiently induced in the benign murine keratinocytes, 308, by OA appeared to be autoinduced in the malignant keratinocytes, PDV and in the human erythroleukemia cells, K562.

Conclusion

The multistage model of mouse skin carcinogenesis has been a very useful model of carcinogenesis in which both biological and molecular events related to tumorigenesis have been studied. This model has been subdivided into at least three operational stages (i.e., initiation, promotion, and progression). Initiation is thought to involve permanent genetic alterations, promotion may involve clonal expansion of initiated cells to give rise to a benign tumor, and progression may result from multiple genomic alterations that bring about the phenotypic changes seen in malignancy. Chemical carcinogens have been shown to be very effective in their ability to initiate the process of carcinogenesis. In contrast, ionizing radiation was found to be a relatively weak initiator of malignant squamous cell carcinomas (Jaffe and Bowden 1986, 1987). In addition, a unique histology of skin tumor observed in mice treated with ionizing radiation was basal cell carcinoma (Jaffe and Bowden 1987), a tumor not normally observed with chemical carcinogens in the skin of mice. Besides demonstrating a weak initiating effect of ionizing radiation, we have shown that 1-MeV electrons in fractionated doses were effective in enhancing the conversion of chemically initiated benign papillomas to malignant squamous cell carcinomas (Jaffe et al. 1987). The biological potential of ionizing radiation as a carcinogen in this mouse skin system and the known genomic alterations induced by ionzing radiation tend to suggest that ionizing radiation acts as a weak initiating agent because point mutations are not efficiently induced by this type of radiation. Instead we have found that ionizing radiation functions more efficiently in a third stage of tumor progression which could involve larger genomic alterations more efficiently induced by ionizing radiation. In support of our finding are data from O'Connell's laboratory (O'Connell et al. 1986) showing that free radical-generating chemical peroxides are also effective in enhancing malignant conversion of benign papillomas. These data are consistent with the hypothesis that free radicals play a role in malignant progression.

Our data related to transforming genes in chemical- and radiation-initiated mouse skin tumors suggest that the target gene(s) for oncogenic activation are different for these two types of initiators. Support for our finding has been provided by other researchers investigating in vitro transformation of mouse C3H 10T 1/2 cells by chemicals and radiation (Borek et al. 1987; Krolewski and Little 1989). It is perhaps not surprising that activation of the Ha-*ras* oncogene was not identified in radiation-initiated mouse skin tumors as was consistently observed with chemically initiated mouse skin tumors. The *ras* family of oncogenes is activated by point mutations and chemical initiating agents or their active metabolites are known to be relatively efficient point mutagens. In contrast, ionizing radiation is a relatively weak point mutagen and instead induces larger genomic alterations. Our finding of at least three different transforming genes in four radiation-initiated malignant skin tumors supports the hypothesis that direct activation of transforming genes may not be occurring in radiation carcinogenesis. The presence of multiple transforming genes in these radiation-initiated tumors is likely to result from secondary DNA damage due to ionizing radiation direct effects on some cellular genes that regulate DNA replication or genomic stability.

Ionizing radiation has been shown to be effective in the third stage of skin tumor progression. This has been demonstrated both in the whole animal as well as in cultured benign papilloma cells. Though the underlying genetic alterations responsible for progression from a benign to malignant state are not known, we have observed the upregulated expression of a cellular gene that encodes for a secreted metalloproteinase, stromelysin, that degrades basement membrane. We have hypothesized that the overexpression of this gene product plays a functional role in tumor cell invasion. We have demonstrated that the overexpression of the stromelysin gene in a radiation-induced malignant variant cell line could be mediated at the transcritional level through a certain *cis* regulatory element(s) that we know is within 850 bp of the transcriptional start site. A candidate *cis* element that may be involved in this overexpression is a TRE (TPA responsive element). We know that a TRE is in the 5′-flanking region of the mouse stromelysin gene. In support of the potential role of the TRE in the regulated overexpression of the stromelysin gene is the fact that we found coordinate overexpression of other cellular genes that are known to contain TREs in the radiation-induced malignant variant cell line. Perhaps the altered expression of the genes with TREs is mediated through constitutive qualitative or quantitative changes in the AP-1 *trans*activating complex known to transactive the TRE. How ionizing radiation might mediate such a constitutive effect on AP-1 activity is not clear but this possibility is being explored.

We have observed that the mouse stromelysin gene can be regulated at the transcriptional level by the two tumor promoters, TPA (Krieg et al. 1988) and okadaic acid (Holladay et al. 1991), in mouse keratinocytes. Both tumor promoters could mediate the transcriptional activation of stromelysin gene through an AP-1-binding TPA *cis*-regulatory element (i.e., TRE) present in the 5′-promoter region of the gene. We have shown that okadaic acid can activate transcription through a distinct AP-1 related but non-TPA induced enhancer element in addition to the well-characterized TRE. An okadaic acid responsive element was functionally mapped in the rat JE gene promoter and by deletion analysis in the human collagenase promoter. This element can be isolated and placed in front of the TK CAT reporter plasmid and it behaved as an okadaic acid- but not TPA-inducible enhancer. This same sequence, termed the ORE, binds a distinct transcription complex involving both Jun and Fos. Binding and transcriptional activation through the ORE is transiently induced by OA in benign tumor keratinocytes and constitatively active in a malignant murine keratinocyte cell line and in a human leukemia cell line.

Our concept of the role of stromelysin in tumor progression is summarized as follows. Initiation of mouse skin with chemical carcinogens results in the activation of the Ha-*ras* oncogene in a small population of epidermal cells. These cells with the activated *ras* oncogene are thought to be "initiated" cells that undergo clonal expansion under the influence of a tumor promoter to give rise to a benign papilloma. Repeated treatment with the tumor promoter also results in repeated, transient elevations in stromelysin. Papillomas can be classified by their behavior after withdraw from tumor promoter treatment. "Dependent" papillomas are dependent on continuous promoter treatment or they will regress, whereas "autonomous" papillomas are no longer dependent on promoter treatment. Since a small percentage of papillomas contain stromelysin transcripts, we speculate that these tumors may have been "autonomous" and premalignant. Stromelysin expression may be constitutive in these premalignant tumors and no longer dependent on tumor promoter treatment. Conversion to malignant tumors is usually accompanied by constitutive expression of stromelysin. The reason for the constitutive expression of stromelysin in malignant SCCs is not because of either amplification or gross rearrangement of the stromelysin gene. Since the tumors with the greatest probability of becoming invasive and metastatic have the greatest probability of expressing high levels of stromelysin, we speculate that this enzyme plays a causal role in promoting invasion through basement membrane barriers. Experiments being conducted in our laboratory are testing the hypothesis that the overexpression of the stromelysin gene is both necessary and sufficient for progression of benign papilloma cells to malignant tumor cells and the hypothesis that the overexpression of this gene is necessary but not sufficient for progression.

Acknowledgements. This work was supported in part by USPHS Grants CA-40584 and CA-42239 awarded to G.T.B. The authors also acknowledge the expert secretarial assistance of Ms. Robin Dyer.

References

Antecol MH, Darveau A, Sonenberg N, Mukherjee BB (1986) Altered biochemical properties of actin in normal skin fibroblasts from individuals predisposed to dominantly inherited cancers. Cancer Res 462:1867–1873

Balmain A, Pragnell IB (1985) Mouse skin carcinomas induced in vivo by chemical carcinogens have a transforming Harvey-ras oncogene. Nature 303:72–74

Balmain A, Ramsden M, Bowden GT, Smith J (1984) Activation of the mouse cellular Harvey-ras gene in chemically induced benign skin papilloams. Nature 307:658–660

Biajolan C, Takai A (1988) Inhibitory effect of a marine sponge toxin, okadaic acid, on protein phosphatases. Biochem J 256:283–290

Bishop JM (1983) Cellular oncogens and retroviruses. Annu Rev Biochem 52:301–352

Bizub D, Wood AW, Skalka AM (1986) Mutagenesis of the Ha-ras oncogene in mouse skin tumors induced by polycyclic aromatic hydrocarbons. Proc Natl Acad Sci USA 83:6048–6052

Bonham K, Embry T, Gibson D, Jaffe DR, Roberts RA, Cress AE, Bowden GT (1989) Activation of the cellular Harvey ras gene in mouse skin tumors initiated with urethane. Mol Carcinog 2:34–39

Borek C, Ong A, Mason H (1987) Distinctive transforming genes in x-ray transformed mammalian cells. Proc Natl Acad Sci USA 84:794–798

Boutwell RK (1974) The function and mechanisms of promoters of carcinogenesis. Crit Rev Toxicol 2:419–443

Bowden GT (1985) A National Institutes of Health workshop report: chemical carcinogenesis and the oncogenes – a chemical pathology study section workshop. Cancer Res 45:914–918

Bowden GT, Furstenberger G, Krieg P, Matrisian LM, Breathnach R (1987a) Gene activation during multistep skin carcinogenesis. In: Zur Hausen H, Schlenhofer JR (eds) Accomplishments in oncology, vol 2. Lippincott, Philadelphia, pp 106–116

Bowden GT, Jaffe DR, Krieg P (1987b) Gene activation during multistage carcinogenesis in mouse skin. In: Colburn NH (ed) Genes and signal transduction in multistage carcinogenesis. Dekker, New York, pp 191–206

Bowden GT, Jaffe DR, Krieg P, Bonham K, Ostrowski L (1989) Differential gene expression in skin tumors initiated by ionizing radiation or chemical carcinogens. In: Slaga TJ, Klein-Szanto AJP, Boutwell RK, Stevenson DE, Spitzer HL, D'Motto B (eds) Skin carcinogenesis mechanisms and human relevance, vol 298. Liss, New York, pp 147–164

Chin JR, Murphy G, Werb Z (1985) Stromelysin, a connective tissue-degrading metalloendopeptidase secreted by stimulated rabbit synovial fibroblasts in parallel with collagenase. J Biol Chem 260:12367–12376

Dahl GA, Miller JA, Miller EC (1978) Vinyl carbamate as a promutagen and a more carcinogenic analog of ethyl carbamate. Cancer Res 38:3793–3804

Demmer LA, Birkenmeier EH, Sweetser DA, Levin MS, Zollman S, Sparkes RS, Mohandas T, Lusis AJ, Gordon JI (1987) The cellular retinol binding protein II gene. J Biol Chem 262:2458–2467

Eberle G, Barbin A, Laib RJ, Ciroussel F, Thomale J, Bautsch H, Rajewsky MF (1989) 1,N^6-etheno-2′-deoxyadenosine and 3,N^4-etheno-2′-deoxycytidine detected by monoclonal antibodies in lung and liver DNA of rats exposed to vinyl chloride. Carcinogenesis 10:209–212

Ehlen T, Dubeau L (1989) Detection of ras point mutations by polymerase chain reaction using mutation-specific inosine containing oligonucleotide primers. Biochem Biophys Res Commun 160:441–447

Finch JS, Bonham K, Krieg P, Bowden GT (1990) Murine polyubiquitin mRNA sequence. Nucleic Acids Res 18:1907

Finch J, Andrews K, Krieg P, Furstenberger G, Slaga T, Ootsuyama A, Tanooka H, Bowden GT (1991) Identification of a cloned sequence activated during multistage carcinogenesis in mouse skin. Carcinogenesis 12:1519–1522

Gates RE, Rees RS (1985) Altered vitamin A-binding proteins in carcinoma of the head and neck. Cancer 56:2598–2604

Gong QH, Stern J, Dean A (1990) Transcriptional role of a conserved GAT A-1 site in the human ε-globin gene promoter. Mol Cell Biol 11:2558–2566

Goodhead DT (1984) Deductions from cellular studies of inactivation, mutagenesis and transformation. In: Boice JD Jr, Fraumeni JF Jr (eds) Radiation carcinogenesis: epidemiology and biological significance. Raven, New York, pp 369–385

Hennings H, Shores R, Weick ML, Spangler EF, Tarone R, Yuspa SH (1983) Malignant conversion of mouse skin tumor is increased by tumor initiators and unaffected by tumor promoters. Nature 304:67–69

Holladay K, Fujiki H, Bowden GT (1991) Okadaic acid induces the expression of both early and secondary response genes in keratinocytes. Mol Carinog (in press)

Jaffe DR, Bowden GT (1986) Ionizing radiation as an initiator in the mouse two-stage model of skin tumor formation. Radiat Res 106:156–165

Jaffe DR, Bowden GT (1987) Ionizing radiation as an initiator: effects of proliferation and promotion time on tumor incidence in mice. Cancer Res 47:6692–6696

Jaffe DR, Bowden GT (1989) Detection of distinct transforming genes in x-ray induced tumors. Carcinogenesis 10:2243–2247

Jaffe DR, Williamson JF, Bowden GT (1987) Ionizing radiation enhances malignant progression of mouse skin tumors. Carcinogenesis 8:1753–1755

Klein F (1987) The approaching era of the tumor suppressor genes. Science 238:1539–1545

Krieg P, Melber K, Furstenberger G, Bowden GT (1987) In vivo and in vitro expression pattern of genes activated during multistage carcinogenesis in the mouse skin. UCLA Symp Mol Cell Biol 58:267–274

Krieg P, Finch J, Furstenberger G, Melber K, Matrisian L, Bowden GT (1988) Tumor promoters induce a transient expression of tumor-associated genes in both basal and differentiated cells of the mouse epidermis. Carcinogenesis 9:95–100

Krolewski B, Little JB (1989) Molecular analysis DNA isolated from the different stages of x-ray-induced transformation in vitro. Mol Carcinog 1:27–33

Kumar R, Sukumar S, Barbacid M (1990) Activation of ras oncogenes proceeding the onset of neoplasia. Science 248:1101–1104

Land H, Parada LF, Weinberg RA (1983) Cellular oncogenes and multi-step carcinogenesis. Science 222:711–717

Matrisian LM, Glaichenhaus N, Gesnel MC, Breathnach R (1985) Epidermal growth factor and oncogenes induce transcription of the same cellular mRNA in rat fibroblasts. EMBO J 4:1435–1440

Matrisian LM, Bowden GT, Krieg P, Furstenberger G, Briand JP, Leroy P, Breathnach R (1986) The mRNA coding for the secreted protease transin is expressed more abundantly in malignant than in benign tumors. Proc Natl Acad Sci USA 83:9413–9417

Melber K, Krieg P, Furstenberger G, Marks F (1986) Molecular cloning of sequences activated during multi-stage carcinogenesis in mouse skin. Carcinogenesis 7:317–322

Miller JA, Miller EC (1983) The metabolic activation and nucleic acid adducts of naturally-occurring carcinogens: recent results with ethyl carbamate and the spice flavors safrole and estragole. Br J Can 48:1–15

Mirvish SS (1968) The carcinogenic action and metabolism of urethan and N-hydroxyurethan. Adv Cancer Res 11:1–42

Nishiwaki S, Fujiki H, Suganuma M, Ojika M, Yamada K, Sugimura T (1990) Photoaffinity labeling of protein phosphatase 2A, the receptor for a tumor promoter okadaic acid, b[27-^{3}H] methyl 7-0-(4-azidobenzoyl) okadaate. Biochem Biophys Res Commun 170:1359–1364

O'Connell JF, Klein-Szanto AJP, DiGiovanni DM, Fries JW, Slaga TJ (1986) Enhanced malignant progression of mouse skin tumors by the free-radical generator benzoyl peroxide. Cancer Res 46:1863–1866

Ostrowski LE, Finch J, Krieg P, Matrisian L, Patskan G, O'Connell JR, Phillips J, Slaga TJ, Breathnach R, Bowden GT (1988) Expression pattern of a gene for a secreted metalloproteinase during late stages of tumor progression. Mol Carcinog 1:13–19

Ostrowski LE, Krieg P, Finch J, Cress AE, Nagle RB, Bowden GT (1989) Expression of β-actin during progression of mouse skin tumors. Carcinogenesis 10:1439–1444

Pelling JC, Ernst SM, Strawhecker JM, Johnson JA, Nairn RS, Slaga TJ (1986) Elevated expression of Ha-ras is an early event in two-stage skin carcinogenesis in SENCAR mice. Carcinogenesis 7:1599–1602

Quintanilla M, Brown K, Ramsden M, Balmain A (1986) Carcinogen-specific mutation and amplifications of Ha-ras during mouse skin carcinogenesis. Nature 322:78–80

Rauth MR (1987) Radiation carcinogenesis. In: Tannock IF, Hill RP (eds) The basic science of oncology. Pergamon, New York, pp 117–118

Scherer E, Steward AP, Emmelot P (1980) Formation of precancerous islands in the rat liver and modification of DNA by ethyl carbamate: implications for its metabolism. In: Holmstead B, Lauwerys M, Robertfroid M (eds) Mechanisms of toxicity and hazard evaluation. Elsevier/North Holland, New York, pp 249–254

Scribner JD, Suss R (1978) Tumor initiation and promotion. Int Rev Exp Pathol 18:137–198

Singer B (1982) Mutagenesis from a chemical perspective: nucleic acid reactions, repair, translation and transcription. Basic Life Sci 20:1–42

Strickland JE, Greenhalgh DA, Koceva-Chyla A, Hennings H, Restrepo C, Balaschak M, Yuspa SH (1988) Development of murine epidermal cell lines which contain an activated ras Ha oncogene and form papillomas in skin grafts on athymic nude mouse hosts. Cancer Res 48:165–169

Thevenin C, Kim SJ, Kehr JH (1991) Inhibition of protein phosphatases by okadaic acid induces AP1 in human T cells. JBC 266:9363–9366

Timmers HTH, Pronk GJ, Bos JL, van der Eb AJ (1990) Analysis of the rat JE gene promoter identifies an AP-1 binding site essential for basal expression but not for TPA induction. Nucleic Acid Res 18:23–34

Toftgard R, Roop DR, Yuspa SH (1985) Proto-oncogene expression during two-stage carcinogenesis in mouse skin. Carcinogenesis 6:655–657

Wahlberg P, Fex G, Biorklund A, Trope C, Willen P (1988) Quantitation and localization of cellular retinol-binding protein in squamous cell carcinoma of the cervix uteri and the oral cavity. Int J Cancer 41:771–776

Wiseman RW, Stowers SJ, Miller EC, Anderson MW, Miller JA (1986) Activating mutations of the c-Ha-ras protooncogene in the chemically induced hepatomas of the male B6C3 F1 mouse. Proc Natl Acad Sci USA 83:5825–5829

Yanogita T, Komizawa S, Kuwano M (1986) Cellular retinol binding proteins in head and neck tumors and their adjacent tissues. Cancer 58:2251–2255

You M, Candrian U, Maronpot RR, Stoner GD, Anderson MW (1989) Activation of the Ki-ras protooncogene in spontaneously occurring and chemically induced lung tumors of the strain A mouse. Proc Natl Acad Sci USA 86:3070–3074

Zarbl H, Kho CJ, Boylan MO, Van Amsterdam J, Sullivan RC, Hoemann CD, Afshani VL (1991) Functional in vitro assay for the isolation of cell transformation effector and suppressor genes. Environ Health Perspect 93:83–89

Threshold-like Dose Response of Mouse Skin Cancer Induction by Repeated Beta Irradiation and its Relevance to Radiation-Induced Human Skin Cancer

H. Tanooka and A. Ootsuyama

Radiobiology Division, National Cancer Center Research Institute, Tsukiji, Tokyo 104, Japan

Introduction

"Repeated irradiation gives rise to a unique threshold-type dose response in skin tumor induction." This statement is the main subject of this paper. Although information on radiation-induced tumors has been accumulated from experimental data (Upton et al. 1986), most has come from experiments using a single exposure or a few fractionated exposures to radiation. Estimation of radiation risk for humans is mainly based upon data obtained from cases of single exposure: very few data are available on the dose–response relationship of tumor incidence to continuous or repeated exposures to radiation. However, such data are necessary for evaluating the risk of continuous exposure of humans to environmental radiation.

This report summarizes experimental results obtained in our laboratory during the past 20 years, showing that repeated local beta irradiation of the skin of mice had a threshold dose for tumor induction. A brief summary of our results was presented at the symposium on "Radiation Carcinogenesis in the Whole Body System" held in Tokyo in 1990 (Tanooka and Ootsuyama 1991).

Recently, Hecker (1990) and Hecker and Rippmann (1988, 1990) reported the threshold dose for chemical tumor promoters repeatedly applied after a single dose of a tumor-initiating chemical. Comparison of their results with ours suggests that repeatedly applied ionizing radiation may act as a promoter in carninogenesis.

Carcinogenic Effect of Beta Radiation of Mouse Skin

The beta ray source used in our experiments was a 2 cm diameter disk applicator on which 40 mCi $^{90}Sr-^{90}Y$ was initially loaded (maximum beta ray energy, 2.24 Mev; dose rate, 2.28 Gy/min at the surface in February, 1985; with 20% decrease at 0.4 mm depth from the surface). Female ICR or

Recent Results in Cancer Research, Vol. 128

Table 1. Carcinogenic effects of beta rays (β) in mouse skin (summarized from data in Hoshino et al. 1968; Hoshino and Tanooka 1975; and Ootsuyama and Tanooka 1987)

Treatment	Malignant tumor
β^{a}	–
$4NQO^{b}$	–
β^{c} + $4NQO^{b}$	+
β^{d} + (interval 11–408 days) $4NQO^{b}$	+
$4NQO^{b}$ + β^{c}	+
β^{e} + TPA^{f}	$-^{i}$
$DMBA^{g}$ + TPA^{f}	$(+)^{j}$
$DMBA^{g}$	$-^{i}$
$DMBA^{g}$ + β $repeat^{h}$	Lower tumor incidence than with repeated β alone

[a] 5.8–174 Gy, single dose at surface.
[b] 2 mg in 20 fractions, painted 3×/week.
[c] 6.8–34 Gy.
[d] 27 Gy.
[e] 24 Gy.
[f] 5 μg/treatment, painted 3×/week for 210 days.
[g] 100 μg, single dose.
[h] 4.7 Gy per exposure, repeated 3×/week for 210 days.
[i] Papillomas were produced at the same level as with TPA alone.
[j] Papillomas were produced at high frequency.

C3H/He mice were fixed in a holder and areas of the backs of individual mice 2 cm in diameter were irradiated individually. Results obtained are summarized in Table 1.

Tumors in the mouse skin were not induced within 300 days after a single exposure to irradiation with doses of 5.8–174 Gy in our system. In contrast, adnexal tumors developed frequently in rat skin after single-dose beta irradiation, with a peak incidence at a dose of 30 Gy (Albert et al. 1961). This difference in the tumor induction sensitivities of mouse and rat skin was explained by the difference of the hair follicle structure by Albert et al. (1972). Beta irradiation caused unscheduled DNA synthesis in a dose-dependent manner in mouse skin, indicating dose-dependent formation of excisable DNA damage (Ootsuyama and Tanooka 1986).

A latent carcinogenic effect remained after single beta irradiation of mouse skin with 27 Gy and could be expressed by application of a chemical carcinogen, 4-nitroquinoline-1-oxide (4NQO), at a subcarcinogenic dose (2 mg in 20 divided doses, 3 times weekly) (Hoshino et al. 1968). The tumors produced were benign and malignant tumors, i.e., papillomas and squamous cell carcinomas, respectively. 4NQO applied before beta irradiation also induced tumors, indicating that the actions of the two agents could be reversed. Therefore, this effect is interpreted as representing "summation" of divided carcinogenic effects (Druckrey and Küpfmüller 1948), or "summation" of carcinogenic effects of multiple unrelated carcinogens (Nakahara and Fukuoka 1960).

Furthermore, the additive tumorigenic effects of beta irradiation and 4NQO were similar when the interval between beta irradiation and subsequent 4NQO treatment was extended from 11 to 408 days (Hoshino and Tanooka 1975), indicating the persistence of the latent tumorigenic effect of beta irradiation for the lifespan of mice. A similar absence of effect of the interval between irradiation with the beta rays and painting croton oil on mouse skin has been reported (Shubik et al. 1953). Although the molecular nature of the latent effect is not clear, it must involve a genetic change in DNA such as mutation, gene deletion, or gene rearrangement.

A single beta irradiation with 24 Gy followed by repeated treatments with the chemical promoter 12-*O*-tetradecanoylphorbol-13-acetate (TPA) (5 µg/treatment, 3 times per week) caused only a slight increase of papillomas over that with TPA alone, while replacement of beta rays by 7,12-dimethylbenz[a]anthracene (DMBA) followed by TPA treatment as a positive control resulted in many papillomas, indicating weak tumor-initiating activity of beta rays (Ootsuyama and Tanooka 1987).

Repeated Local Irradiation

Since single beta irradiation was ineffective in inducing tumors, it was then repeated 3 times a week until the appearance of tumors or death of mice. The results obtained in our experiments (Ootsuyama and Tanooka 1988, 1989, 1991) are summarized in Fig. 1, in which the cumulative tumor incidences calculated by the Kaplan–Meier method are plotted against the time of irradiation. Irradiations at 2.5–11.8 Gy per exposure resulted in almost identical time courses of tumor incidence (dose saturation effect). There was a latent period of about 200 days before the appearance of tumors in this dose range. However, once tumors started to appear, the cumulative tumor incidence rapidly increased with time and finally reached 100% within 500 days. Tumors included skin tumors (squamous cell carcinomas, basal cell carcinomas, and fibrosarcomas of the skin) and bone tumors (osteosarcomas). Approximately the same number of carcinomas were produced as sarcomas for all doses used. Repeated irradiation was, therefore, effective in inducing tumors in our mouse system. This effect of repeated irradiation seemed to be independent of the radiation dose in a certain dose range, but dependent on the frequency of repeat.

Repeated irradiation did not change immunological parameters of the mice, such as the proliferative response of lymphocytes to mytogens, the

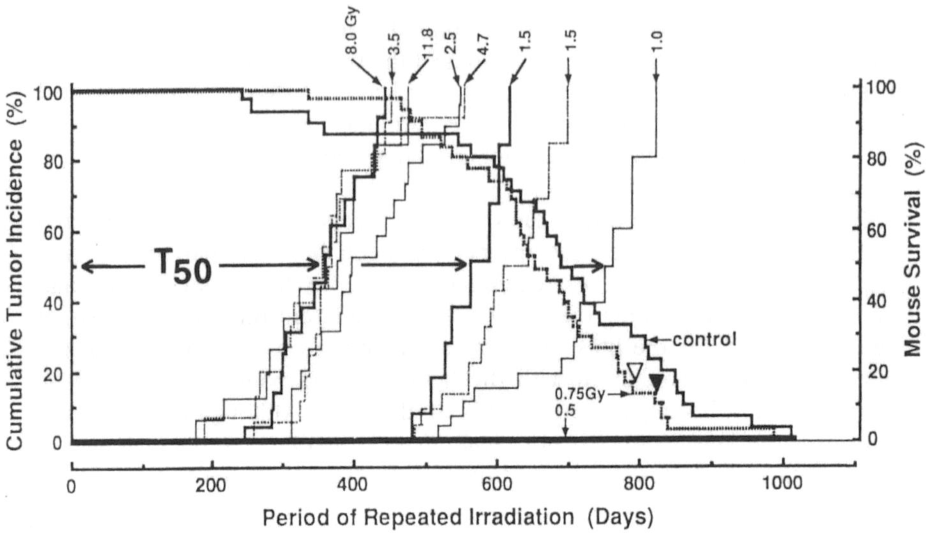

Fig. 1. Cumulative incidences of total tumors in mice with time during repeated beta irradiation. Number of mice in each group, 15–50. (Summarized from data in Ootsuyama and Tanooka 1988, 1989, 1991 and unpublished data)

mixed lymphocyte reaction, the killer T-cell activity, or the natural killer cell activity (Sado, Ootsuyama and Tanooka, unpublished), indicating that the immunological status of the whole body of the mice was not affected by repeated local beta irradiation.

A test of clonality of these tumors produced by repeated doses of 3 Gy in C3H/He *Pgk-1*^{a}/*Pgk-1*^{b} mice with X-chromosome inactivation cellular mosaicism (Tanooka 1988) showed that all the tumors were monoclonal (unpublished). It is interesting that although many cells must be affected by repeated irradiation, a clone of only one cell develops into a tumor. Repeated irradiation was, therefore, effective in inducing tumors in our mouse system, although a single dose of up to 175 Gy was ineffective.

The enhancing effect of repeated treatment on tumor induction was observed in other earlier experiments using ionizing radiation and UV. Repeated irradiation with soft X-rays is effective for inducing mouse skin tumors (Epstein 1972). The optimum treatment for inducing mouse thymic lymphomas was four repeated whole body X-irradiations with a sublethal dose, rather than single dose (Kaplan and Brown 1952). Fission neutrons also have the greatest tumor-inducing effect at low dose rates in a certain dose range (Ullrich et al. 1979). Repeated UV irradiation induces 100% incidence of skin tumors (Blum 1955). Chemical carcinogens or promoters are also effective when given repeatedly.

On the basis of available information, the underlying mechanism of this effect of repeated treatment is considered to be that repeated DNA damage is favorable for induction of error-prone repair of DNA, although this has not been proved in mammalian cells. At the tissue level, injured cells are replaced by uninjured cells, and this repopulation is enhanced by repeated treatment, which is thought to increase the chance of error. The tissue misrepair hypothesis for radiation carcinogenesis was recently presented by Kondo (1991). This error-prone mechanism is distinct from error-free repair, which operates more efficiently by dividing a dose or by reducing the dose rate.

The overall effect of repeated irradiation is thought to be expressed by a combination of the antagonistic effects of these two mechanisms, not only at the cellular level but also at the tissue level. The error-prone mechanism seems to predominate over the error-free repair mechanism when the radiation dose per treatment exceeds a certain level.

Threshold Response

Reduction of the radiation dose per exposure below 2.5 Gy resulted in an abrupt delay of tumor emergence (Fig. 1). At 1.5 Gy, this delay was about 200 days, although the final incidence was still 100%. At 0.75 Gy, tumors did not appear nearly until the end of the lifespan of mice, where one squamous cell carcinoma and one ostersarcoma were found after 800 days in the five surviving mice (Ootsuyama and Tanooka 1991). At 0.5 Gy, no tumor appeared during the whole lifespan of 50 mice (A. Ootsuyama and H. Tanooka, in preparation). The time–survival plot for mice irradiated repeatedly at 0.5 Gy or 0.75 Gy did not differ from that of unirradiated controls. Although absolute zero effectiveness at these doses cannot be concluded from this number of mice, the results at least show that the dose–response relationship on repeated irradiations is not linear, but is all-or-none (threshold response).

A similar threshold response has been observed in experiments with a chemical tumor promoter and UV. Hecker and Rippmann (1990) applied various concentrations of a tumor-promoter, 3-*O*-tetradecanoylingenol (3-TI), repeatedly to the skin of NMRI mice (×2 per week) after a single dose of the tumor initiator DMBA. Fig. 2a, cited from the paper of Hecker and Rippmann (1990), shows a log–log plot of the time required for 50% incidence of tumors (papillomas) against the dose of the promoter applied per treatment. This time increased sharply on reducing the dose of the promoter, and they observed essentially no tumors at doses of below 2.5 nmol 3-TI. Similar results have been observed with other promoters, i.e., TPA (Hecker and Rippmann 1988) and teleocidin (Hecker 1990). In contrast, repeated application of a solitary carcinogen, DMBA, did not result in a threshold-type response of tumor production. Hecker and Rippman (1990) proposed that the action of DMBA could be expressed as dose/exposure ×50% tumor incidence time (T_{50}) = constant. This rela-

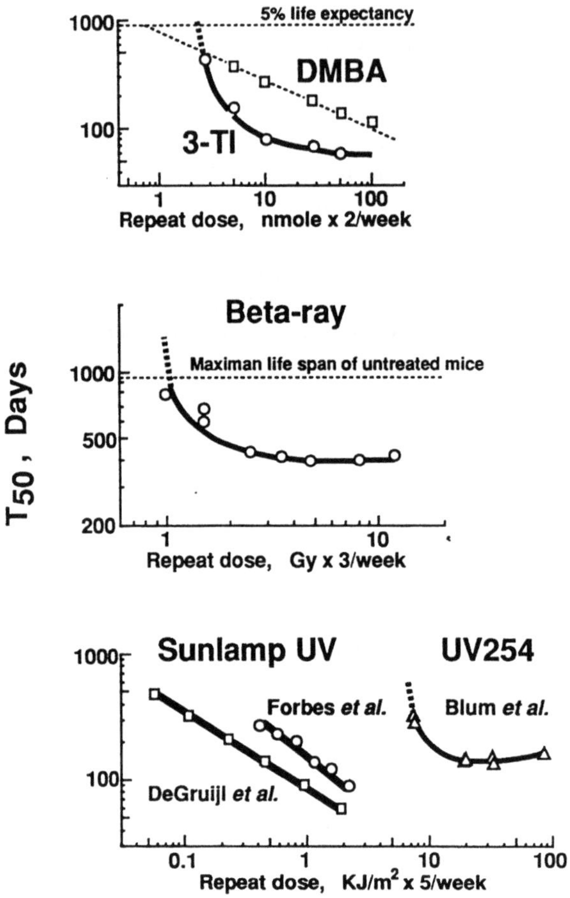

Fig. 2. Comparison of the times required for 50% skin tumor incidence (T_{50}) by various carcinogenic agents in mice on repeated treatment plotted against the dose per exposure on a log–log scale. *Top*, Repeated treatment with 3-TI (2×/week) after a single dose of DMBA (○) and repeated treatment with DMBA (2×/week) (□) (from Hecker and Rippmann 1990). *Middle*, Repeated beta irradiation (3×/week). (rearranged from data from Ootsuyama and Tanooka 1991). *Bottom*, Repeated UV_{254} and sunlamp UV irradiations (5×/week) (rearranged from data from Blum et al. 1941; Forbes et al. 1981; De Gruijl et al. 1983)

tion essentially represents the idea of Druckrey and Küpfmüller (1948), "summation" of the divided carcinogenic effects of a carcinogen.

On the other hand, a log–log plot of our results on the 50% incidence of malignant skin tumors against the dose per exposure on repeated beta irradiation gave a similar curve to that for repeated treatment with the chemical promoter 3-TI after a single application of DMBA (Fig. 2b). This figure indicates that beta rays may act as a promoter when applied repeatedly.

Furthermore, we reanalyzed data obtained for skin tumor induction in mice by repeated irradiation with UV with a peak wavelength of 254 nm,

UV_{254} (Blum et al. 1941), and 313 nm, UV_{313}, or sunlamp UV (Forbes et al. 1981; De Gruijl et al. 1983). These results are shown on a log–log scale in Fig. 2c. The curve representing the relationship between the dose per exposure and the 50% tumor incidence time for UV_{254} resembled that for beta rays or the chemical promoter, whereas the straight line for sunlamp UV resembled that for DMBA.

Is Radiation an Initiator or Promoter?

Comparison of Fig. 2a, 2b, and 2c indicates that beta rays and UV_{254} act like chemical promoters, when applied repeatedly. On the other hand, ionizing radiation and UV have been considered to act as initiators or solitary carcinogens, since they produce tumors by themselves. Ionizing radiation produces various types of DNA damage such as strand breaks and base modifications. UV irradiation produces various types of photoproducts of DNA. After error-free repair of these DNA damages, the remaining damage may serve as an inducer of error, including insertion of mismatch error into newly transcribed DNA (mutation), enhacement of gene rearrangement, and gene deletion, leading to loss of gene function or, if the altered gene is a suppressor gene, activation of other gene functions. These processes occur at the cellular level. Furthermore, cell-to-cell interaction is involved at the tissue level in the whole body. Cell death itself induces new cellular functions through stimulation of repopulation of cells in the injured tissue. Repeated irradiation may have a promoting action by causing repeated tissue injury and its healing. In fact, in the skin, chemical tumor promoters are known to be irritants.

Sunlamp UV irradiation has much less cytocidal effect than UV_{254} irradiation, but is much more effective than the latter in tumor induction (Fig. 2c). The high tumor induction efficiency of sunlamp UV-irradiation has been attributed to its high penetration into deep tissue of the skin. However, its effects may also be attributable to its mild cytocidal action, causing genetic damage without much cytocidal effect. The nonthreshold type action of sunlamp UV in inducing tumors may also be due to this mild cytocidal action.

We think that repeated ionizing radiation and UV_{254} act as promoters by causing repeated tissue injury. We also think that the effect of repeated irradiation is enhanced if error-free repair is blocked in conditions such as error-free repair deficiency disease of the host, or repeated exposure to high linear energy transfer (LET) radiation, which creates irreparable DNA damage. Furthermore, we think that the threshold-like response in tumor induction appears clearer on partial body irradiation than on whole body irradiation, because this repeat-injury and repeat-recovery process is greater on partial body irradiation. Suppression of cancer cells may be more efficient when the surrounding tissue is uninjured in partial body irradiation, and this suppression is thought to be released in a threshold-like manner when the radiation dose exceeds the threshold dose.

In summary, ionizing radiation acts either as a tumor initiator or promoter depending on the mode of its application.

Relevance to Human Skin Cancer

It seems that human skin, like mouse skin, is resistant to ionizing radiation in tumor induction. The rat skin tumors produced at high frequency by a single dose of beta irradiation are adnexal tumors. As this type of tumor is rare in human skin, as in mouse skin, data for mice seem more applicable to humans than those for rats.

After a single exposure of humans to A-bomb radiation in Nagasaki (major component, gamma rays), skin tumors developed very slowly in a dose-dependent manner with an increasing incidence even 40 years after the exposure (Sadamori et al. 1989). Almost all tumors produced were of epithelial origin and appeared in the skin of the head and neck, suggesting the summation of the carcinogenic effect of A-bomb radiation with that of sunlight or the promotion of ionizing radiation effect by sunlight.

Repeated local irradiation with soft X-rays had been applied in treatment of noncancerous human diseases in Japan, such as trichophytia and angioma, and has resulted in development of cancers as a late effect of the treatment. The records of the National Cancer Center Hospital on the distribution of the latent periods (Ishihara et al. 1981) are summarized in Fig. 3, together those for A-bomb cases. Most of the cancers produced were squamous cell carcinomas (88%). The peak incidence was seen between 10 and 20 years after treatment. The latent periods are considerably shorter than those after a single exposure to the A-bomb. Although the radiation dose for medical treatment was much higher than that on A-bomb exposure, the accelerated tumor appearance cannot be explained only by the high total dose, since a single high dose kills cells. The accelerated tumor formation is thought to have been due to repeated irradiation. These figures are consistent with the results in experiments on mice.

The findings that the repeated irradiation enhances tumor induction and that there is a threshold dose for induction of tumors provide important clues for estimation of cancer risk of humans who are exposed to radiation professionally or who are exposed chronically to a low level of radiation from the environment. It is expected that linear extrapolation of human risk from data obtained at high doses of radiation will give an overestimate of the risk. This problem requires assessment.

Conclusion

There seems to be a threshold for the response of tumor induction in the whole body system. This threshold can be observed more clearly on repeated

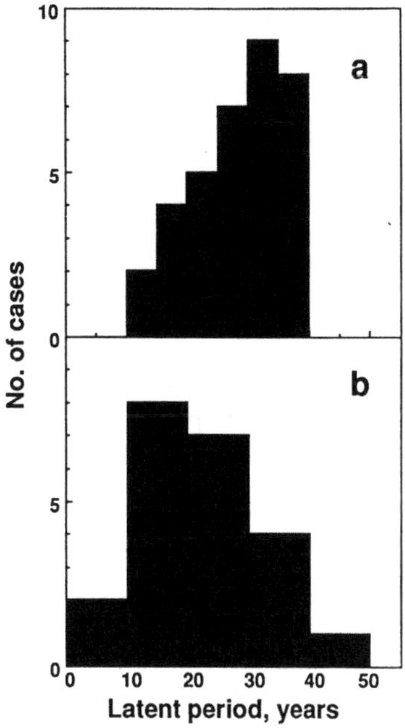

Fig. 3a,b. Latent periods for human skin cancers after irradiation. **a** Single whole-body exposure to A-bomb radiation in Nagasaki; estimated dose, 0–5 Gy. **b** Repeated local irradiation with soft X-rays; estimated total surface dose, 10–100 Gy. (Rearranged from data from Sadamori et al. 1989; Ishihara et al. 1981)

irradiation of local tissues. The molecular mechanism of the threshold is considered to involve a balance between error-free repair and error-prone repair at the cellular and tissue levels. There is probably a threshold dose for tumor induction in human skin and other organs.

Acknowledgements. We thank Dr. R.J.M. Fry and Dr. N. Munakata for useful suggestions. Our series of studies described here was supported by grants-in-aid for cancer research from the Ministry of Health and Welfare, by the Ministry of Education, Science and Culture of Japan, and by grants from the Nissan Science Foundation and the Adult Disease Clinic Memorial Foundation, Tokyo.

References

Albert RE, Newman W, Altshuler B (1961) The dose-response relationships of beta-ray-induced skin tumors in the rat. Radiat Res 15:410–430

Albert RE, Burns FJ, Bennett P (1972) Radiation-induced hair-follicle damage and tumor formation in mouse and rat skin. J Natl Cancer Inst 49:1131–1137

Blum HF (1955) Ultraviolet radiation and cancer. In: Hollaender A (ed) Radiation biology, vol 2. McGraw-Hill, New York, pp 529–559

Blum HF, Kirby-Smith JS, Grady HG (1941) Quantitative induction of tumors in mice with ultraviolet radiation. J Natl Cancer Inst 2:259–268

De Gruijl FR, Van der Meer JB, Van der Leun JC (1983) Dose-time dependency of tumor formation by chronic UV exposure. Photochem Photobiol 37:53–62

Druckrey H, Küpfmüller KZ (1948) Quantitative Analyse der Krebsentstehung. Z Naturforsch 3b:254–266

Epstein JH (1972) Examination of the carcinogenic and cocarcinogenic effects of grenz radiation. Cancer Res 32:2625–2629

Forbes PD, Blum HF, Davies RE (1981) Photocarcinogenesis in hairless mice: dose-response and the influence of dose-delivery. Photochem Photobiol 34:361–365

Hecker E, Rippmann F, Fujiki H (1990) Threshold doses for teleocidin and other environmental promoters for mouse skin (abstr). 16–21 Jan 1990, J Cancer Res Clin Oncol [Suppl] 116:1074

Hecker E, Rippmann F (1988) Quantitative determination of experimental threshold doses ("no-effect levels") for environmental promoters in the initiation/promotion protocol on skin of NMRI-mice. Naunyn Schmiedebergs Arch Pharmacol 338:R11 (abstr)

Hecker E, Rippmann F (1990) Outline of a descriptive general theory of environmental chemical cancerogenesis – experimental threshold doses for tumor promoters. In: Kappas A (ed) Mechanisms of environmental mutagenesis-carcinogenesis. Plenum, New York, pp 167–173

Hoshino H, Tanooka H (1975) Interval effect of beta-irradiation and subsequent 4-nitroquinoline 1-oxide painting on skin tumor induction in mice. Cancer Res 35:3663–3666

Hoshino H, Tanooka H, Fukuoka F (1968) Summation of carcinogenic effect of 4-nitroquinoline 1-oxide and β-rays. Gann (Jpn J Cancer Res) 59:43–49

Ishihara K, Hayasaka K, Kameya T (1981) Radiation-induced keratosis. Gan no Rinsho (Cancer Clinics) 27:937–941 (in Japanese)

Kaplan HS, Brown MB (1952) Further observations on inhibition of lymphoid tumor development by shielding and partial-body irradiation of mice. J Natl Cancer Inst 12:427–436

Kondo S (1991) Tissue misrepair hypothesis for radiation carcinogenesis. International Symposium on radiation carcinogenesis in the whole body system, Tokyo. J Radiat Res 32 [Suppl 2]:1–13

Nakahara W, Fukuoka F (1960) Summation of carcinogenic effects of chemically unrelated carcinogens, 4-nitroquinoline 1-oxide and 20-methylcholanthrene. Gann (Jpn J Cancer Res) 51:125–137

Ootsuyama A, Tanooka H (1986) Unscheduled DNA synthesis after β-irradiation of mouse skin in situ. Mutat Res 166:183–185

Ootsuyama A, Tanooka H (1987) The tumor-initiating and -promoting effects of ionizing radiations in mouse skin. Jpn J Cancer Res 78:1203–1206

Ootsuyama A, Tanooka H (1988) One hundred percent tumor induction in mouse skin after repeated β irradiation in a limited dose range. Radiat Res 115:488–494

Ootsuyama A, Tanooka H (1989) Induction of osteosarcomas in mouse lumbar vertebrae by repeated external β-irradiation. Cancer Res 49:1562–1564

Ootsuyama A, Tanooka H (1991) Threshold-like dose of local β irradiation repeated throughout the life span of mice for induction of skin and bone tumors. Radiat Res 125:98–101

Sadamori N, Mine M, Hori M (1989) Skin cancer among atom bomb survivors. Lancet i:1267

Shubik P, Goldfarb AR, Ritchie AC (1953) Latent carcinogenic action of beta-irradiation on mouse epidermis. Nature 171:934–935

Tanooka H (1988) Monoclonal growth of cancer cells: experimental evidence. Jpn J Cancer Res 79:657–665
Tanooka H, Ootsuyama A (1991) Radiation carcinogenesis in mouse skin and its threshold-like response. International symposium on radiation carcinogenesis in the whole body system, Tokyo. J Radiat Res 32 [Suppl 2]:195–201
Ullrich RL, Jernigan MC, Adams LM (1979) Neutron carcinogenesis. Dose and dose-rate effects in BALB/c mice. Radiat Res 72:487–498
Upton AC, Albert RE, Burns FJ, Shore RE (eds) (1986) Radiation carcinogenesis. Elsevier, New York

Note added to proof:

Two papers, mentioned in this article "in preparation" or "unpublished", and a related paper were added.

Ootsuyama A, Tanooka H (1992) Clonal origin of skin and bone tumors produced by repeated beta-irradiation in mosaic cell mice. Jpn J Cancer Res 83:964–967
Ootsuyama A, Tanooka H (1993) Effect of inhibitor of tumor promotion, α-difluoromethylornithine, on tumor induction by repeated beta irradiation in mice. Jpn J Cancer Res 84:34–36
Ootsuyama A, Tanooka H (1993) Zero tumor incidence in mice after repeated lifetime exposures to 0.5 Gy of beta radiation. Radiat Res (in press)

Environmental Risk Factors for Skin Cancer

F. Urbach

Temple Medical Practices, 220 Commerce Drive, Fort Washington, PA 19034, USA

Introduction

That chronic exposure to environmental agents can lead to the development of skin cancer in humans has been known for more than 200 years, since Percival Pott described scrotal cancer in chimney sweeps in 1775. Today, the evidence is convincing that the vast majority of skin cancers are due to chronic repeated exposure to solar ultraviolet (UV) radiation. Skin cancers are most prevalent on light complexioned, easily sunburning individuals, and in those who receive the most solar exposure, whether because of occupational or deliberate social reasons. Furthermore, non-melanoma skin cancers occur primarily on sunlight-exposed sites. The recent significant decrease in stratospheric ozone, which increases transmitted short-wavelength UV radiation, has the potential of significantly increasing skin cancer incidence in the future. The dose–response relationships and epidemiologic features of UV-induced skin cancers will be discussed here. Other environmental causes for skin cancer development are exposure to chemicals (polycyclic hydrocarbons derived from the incomplete combustion or distillation of coal or petroleum; inorganic arsenic and photosensitizing agents such as psoralens). In the past, occupational or therapeutic exposure to ionizing radiation has caused skin cancer. Finally, there is some evidence that intense, chronic infrared radiation can enhance the development of skin cancer.

Ultraviolet Radiation

Introduction

The high-energy, short-wavelength portion of the solar electromagnetic spectrum (wavelengths shorter than 320 nm) is potentially very detrimental

Recent Results in Cancer Research, Vol. 128

to living cells and tissues. A low concentration of ozone, formed in the stratosphere, absorbs most of the photons of this UV radiation and thus prevents most of them from reaching earth. However, even in the presence of this ozone layer, which varies in thickness at various latitudes and at various seasons, a biologically significant amount of UV radiation reaches the surface of the earth.

The major effects on humans of UV radiation in the UV-B (320-280 nm) range are on the skin and on the eyes. Acute effects consist of "sunburn," an inflammatory response of the tissues which may be no more than mild redness, or slight stinging of the eyes, or may develop into the equivalent of second degree (blistering) "burns." The acute effects of single overdoses of UV-B are transient, heal without scarring; and lead to adaptive changes of skin thickening and pigmentation, which afford some degree of protection. The only established positive (beneficial) effect of UV-B in humans is the production of vitamin D precursors in the skin, which are absorbed into the bloodstream and prevent rickets, a serious vitamin deficiency disease. It should be recognized that most work has been on the harmful effects of UV-B, and relatively little attention has been given to possible beneficial effects.

Repeated UV-B exposure, prolonged over many years, can result in chronic degenerative changes in the skin, characterized by skin "aging" and the development of premalignant and malignant skin lesions. The skin cancers can be broadly divided into two types: nonmelanoma skin cancers (NMSC) and malignant melanoma (which will not be discussed here).

There is excellent, although circumstantial evidence that NMSC is primarily due to repeated exposure of the skin to UV radiation (Blum 1959). The major arguments in favor of such a causal role of UVR in NMSC are:

- The most frequent location of NMSC is on the exposed sites (head, neck, arms, hands).
- Pigmented races, who sunburn much less readily than people with white skin, have much less NMSC, and when it does occur, it does not affect the sun-exposed areas.
- Among white skinned people who spend more time outdoors and who live in areas of greater UV exposure (near the equator and in tropical and semitropical areas) the risk of NMSC is much greater.
- Genetic diseases resulting in greater sensitivity to solar UV radiation are associated with premature NMSC development (xeroderma pigmentosum, albinism).
- Skin cancers of the NMSC type can be readily induced in the skin of experimental animals, and the upper wavelength limit for this is near 320 nm, similar to the spectral range producing sunburn in man.

Exposure to UV radiation occurs from both natural and artificial sources. The sun is the principal natural source. The known effects of UV radiation on man may be beneficial, or detrimental, depending on a number of circumstances.

Artificial UV sources are widely used in industry and, because of the germicidal properties of certain portions of the UV spectrum, they are also used in hospitals, biological laboratories, and schools. UV radiation is extensively used for therapeutic purposes, in the prevention of vitamin D deficiency and for treatment of skin diseases. Artificial UV sources are available as consumer products for cosmetic purposes.

The migration of people between areas of different UV radiation exposure, whether for occupational or recreational reasons, gives rise to unforseen exposures.

UV radiation can be classified into UV-A, UV-B, and UV-C regions. Wavelengths in the UV-C region (200–280 nm) cause unpleasant but usually not serious effects on skin and eyes. Although UV-C is very efficiently absorbed by nucleic acids, the overlying dead layers of skin absorb the radiation to such a degree that there is only mild erythema and, usually, no late sequelae, even after repeated exposures. Since solar UV radiation below 290 nm is effectively absorbed by stratospheric ozone, no such radiation reaches living organisms from natural sources.

Most observed biological effects of UV-B radiation (280–320 nm) are extremely detrimental to living organisms. However, living organisms are usually protected from excessive solar UV-B radiation by feathers, fur, or pigments that absorb the radiation before it reaches sensitive physiological targets. Other means of protection include behavioral patterns and the ability to tolerate certain UV-B radiation injury because of molecular and other repair mechanisms.

Much less is known about the biological effects of UV-A radiation (320–400 nm). It can augment the biological effects of UV-B, and doses of UV-A which alone do not show any biological effect can, in the presence of certain chemical agents, result in injury to tissue (phototoxicity, photoallergy, enhancement of photocarcinogenesis).

Solar Ultraviolet Radiation

In the UV region, the sun emits like a black body of about 5200°C. This radiation is first intercepted by the ozone made by UV radiation of the sun out of oxygen molecules. The ozone layer has a maximum density at an altitude of about 25 km; above this the density is less because less and less oxygen atoms and nitrogen molecules are available for the triple collision which is needed for the formation of ozone. Below 30 km the change in the amount of ozone from normal photochemical processes becomes minute, and ozone becomes a permanent part of the stratosphere. Until about 1965, the total amount of ozone in the tropical regions was essentially constant and smaller than at high latitudes, where ozone amounts were higher and

Table 1. Albedo of total solar radiation and erythema effective weighted UV-B for different surfaces (Blumthaler and Ambach 1988)

Surface	Total solar radiation: mean albedo (%)	Erythemic solar radiation: mean albedo (%)	Remarks
Water	9.1	4.8	Clear water
Field	11.5	2.2	Varying moisture
Rock	14.4	3.7	Various sizes
Stream sand	23.8	9.8	Near stream
Grassland, corn	20.7	1.3	Varying height
New dry snow	87.0	94.4	High mountains
New wet snow	74.5	79.2	High mountains
Old dry snow	79.2	82.2	Varyingly dirty

more variable with seasons. In the past 17 years, stratospheric ozone has decreased by an average of 2%–5%, mainly because of manmade chemicals that attack ozone.

Ozone absorbs UV radiation primarily below 315 nm. In addition, air molecules scatter UV radiation more than other radiation, and therefore at least 50% of solar UV radiation reaches the ground scattered from the sky. The amount of UV radiation is also affected by other scattering and absorbing agents of the atmosphere – dust, aerosols, haze and clouds scatter, NO_x and SO_2 absorb UV radiation. The amount of UV radiation over continents as a rule is lower than over clear oceans or over tops of mountains. (For every 1000 m elevation, UV-B increases by about 15%; Schulze 1970). UV-B reaching our body will also be altered by reflection from environmental surfaces (albedo). Blumthaler and Ambach (1988) recently reported mean values for albedo of total solar radiation and erythema effective weighted UV-B for different surfaces (Table 1).

UV-B, as any other radiation, may be reflected by any surface by the combined effects of reflection, refraction, and diffraction. Over UV-B-permeable materials such as water, there is mirror-like reflectivity which follows Fresnel's law. This law says that the lower the angle of the sun is over the water, the higher the reflectivity. Consequently, the reflectivity of smooth water for UV radiation of high solar altitudes is negligibly small. It may become somewhat larger if the sea is rough. For very low angles the reflectivity may easily exceed 50%, but at these low solar altitudes, the amount of UV-B is small (less than 8% at sun angles of 30° above the horizon or less; Diffey 1987).

The amount of UV-B striking any surface varies, of course, with the direction, including the side turned away from the sun. All these exposures are markedly increased on a highly reflective surface such as snow (Buettner 1969). Diffey (1987) has estimated the annual dose of biologically effective UV radiation (to a flat surface, cloudless skies, normal ozone) for various

Table 2. Estimate of the annual dose of biologically effective UV radiation (to a flat surface, cloudless skies, normal ozone) for various latitudes in the northern hemisphere (Diffey 1987)

Geographical latitude	Annual dose (MED), total	Contribution whenever solar altitude <30°
0°	7907	307
20°	6150	228
40°	3116	240
60°	926	132

One MED (minimal erythema dose) is taken to be equivalent to an erythemally effective dose of 250 J m^2 relative to 300 nm radiation.

latitudes in the northern hemisphere (Table 2). Depending on latitude, it has been calculated that an outdoor worker may receive 25%–40% of ambient, flat surface UV exposure, while indoor workers, including a few hours on weekends, may receive 10% of that. In terms of minimal erythema doses (MED), that may represent 300–1000 MED/year for outdoor workers, and 100 MED or less for indoor workers. Furthermore, a 2-week vacation in a sunny climate may add 100+ MEDs to the dose for indoor workers (Cole et al. 1985; Diffey 1987).

Solar Exposure and Nonmelanoma Skin Cancer

Examination of the sun's role in the production of human skin cancer does not lend itself to direct experimentation. However, extensive and astute observations have strongly suggested for years the etiologic significance of light energy in the induction of these tumors (Blum 1959; Urbach 1969; Emmet 1973). Skin cancers in Caucasians are in general most prevalent in geographic areas with the greatest insolation and among people who receive the most exposure, that is among men who work outdoors. They are rare among Negroes and other deeply pigmented individuals who have the greatest protection against UV injury. Furthermore, individuals with the lightest complexion, such as those of Scottish and Irish descent, appear to be the most susceptible to skin cancer when they live in geographic areas of high exposure (Urbach et al. 1972). When skin cancers do appear in individuals from darkly pigmented races they are not distributed primarily in the sun-exposed areas as they are in light-skinned people (Oettle 1963; Davies et al. 1968). The tumors in these individuals are most commonly stimulated by other forms of trauma, such as chronic leg ulcers, irritation due to going barefoot, etc. In contrast, the distribution of skin cancers in

Bantu albinos and in patients with xeroderma pigmentosum follows sun-exposure patterns (Oettle 1963).

Together, basal cell (BCC) and squamous cell carcinomas (SCC) add up to the most frequently detected cancers in man, and have shown a significant increase in the past decades. They are also the most easily and most successfully treated human cancers. The quantitative extent to which agents other than UV exposure cause NMSC in the white population has not been established; it is, however, believed to be small. Some NMSC are caused by exposure to arsenic, pitch, or X-rays, often as occupational or industrial exposure, sometimes following treatment of skin disorders (see below). This group of tumors is found among patients of all degree of skin pigmentation who happen to be exposed to these agents. In some less developed countries, most NMSC seem to arise in neglected wounds.

NMSC is at present a serious problem because of disfigurement and the significant economic burden associated with its treatment, particularly in the United States, Europe, and Australia, and to emigrants from these regions to other parts of the world.

Anatomic Distribution of Basal Cell and Squamous Cell Cancer

Numerous studies have shown that skin cancers arise (in those susceptible, i.e., white-skinned people) primarily on sunlight-exposed sites. In the United States, about 80% of all BCC and more than half of all SCC occur on the head and neck (Urbach 1969). However, in the intensely exposed and very susceptible population of Queensland, only about 50% of BCC occur on the head and neck (Green et al. 1988). The majority of those SCC not occurring on the head and neck are found on hands and forearms; the ears of females are markedly protected.

Comparing the distribution of the sites of NMSC with studies of the pattern of insolation of the head and neck areas, it becomes clear that two-thirds of all BCC occur on skin sites receiving the highest UV doses, and that virtually all SCC occur at these sites (Urbach et al. 1972).

Race and Ethnic Extraction

It has long been known that white-skinned races have a much higher incidence of skin cancer than pigmented races. The higher incidence is attributable to the chronic effects of UV radiation. BCC in particular is very rare in pigmented races (Chuang et al. 1990).

In contrast to the anatomic distribution of SCC in whites (60% on the head and neck), Isaacson et al. (1978) found only one-third of SCC in urban blacks in South Africa to be on the head and neck. Furthermore, the male–

female ratio was 60/40, as compared to 85/15 in whites. BCC was almost absent. The age of onset was much earlier in blacks than in whites, 50% of SCC occurring before age 50.

In several carefully controlled studies, comparing white patients with NMSC to age- and sex-matched controls from the same populations, it was found that patients with skin cancer have much greater frequency of certain genetically transmitted traits than those without skin cancer (Gellin et al. 1965; O'Beirn et al. 1970; Urbach et al. 1972; Vitaliano and Urbach 1980). Skin cancer patients, as a group, have greater frequency of light eyes, complexion, and hair color than do the controls. They also sunburn more frequently and tan less easily, though the degree of tan achieved is only marginally less. Male cancer patients have experienced greater cumulative outdoor exposure than male controls. The proportions of Irish and English (including Scottish and Welsh) ancestry is higher among cancer patients, while the proportion of Slavic and other categories of national origin are smaller (Urbach et al. 1972).

Patients with NMSC differ with respect to age and sex distribution. In BCC, the two sexes are almost equally represented; almost 20% of the patients are less than 50 years of age and nearly 70% are less than 70 years old. In the SCC group, on the other hand, males outnumber females by more than 4 to 1, and almost all patients are at least 50 years of age, with more than 50% of them being over 65. Light (blue or green) eye color is also somewhat more frequent in the SCC group, but in the other coloring characteristics, complexion and hair, the two cancer groups are not significantly different. The two groups are also indistinguishable with respect to tanning and sunburning characteristics and national origins. They differ significantly in respect to total outdoor exposure, with a much larger fraction of the SCC group appearing in the maximum exposure category (Vitaliano and Urbach 1980).

These studies and the clinical impressions of many observant physicians show a distinct association of skin cancer with light-colored eyes, fair complexion, light hair color, poor tannability, ease of sunburning, and a history of repeated sunburns. Furthermore, there is an increase in Celtic stock among skin cancer patients.

But this is clearly not the whole explanation. There are many people with origins other than Celtic who match these characteristics. It is apparent that the Celts appear to inherit, but are by no means the sole possesors of a sun-sensitive, poorly adapting skin. It is clear that genetic factors are of great importance. In the three careful epidemiologic studies of Silverstone and Searle (1970), MacDonald and Bubendorf (1964), and O'Beirn et al. (1970), the prevalence of skin cancer rises with advancing age at about the same rate in Queensland and in Galway, differing primarily by age of appearance of the first lesion. In El Paso the lesions begin early, but the slope of the prevalence curve is much lower. This is probably the result of genetic differences since the population studied in Queensland and Ireland is mainly

Celtic, while the El Paso population has few Celts and probably much Mexican admixture (Urbach et al. 1972).

Geographic Distribution

Incidence data for skin cancer, other than melanoma, must be treated with considerable reserve. Many cancer registries do not register NMSC at all, and those which do are uniformly incomplete, since most of these tumors are treated in physicians' offices and are either not reported at all or reported without histologic verification.

United States. The principal sources for incidence data of skin cancer in the United States are: the National Cancer Survey performed in eight cities in 1947, a survey in Iowa in 1950 and in New York State (excluding New York City) in 1969, the extensive data of the Texas tumor registry covering the years 1944–1966, the Third National Cancer Survey in 1974 (Cutler and Young 1975), a special survey of the US. National Cancer Institute performed in 1977–1978 (Scotto et al. 1981), and a recent report from the Kaiser-Permanente Group (Glass and Hoover 1989), All these data show a marked increase in the incidence of skin cancer in the past three decades, and a pronounced north–south gradient.

Europe. The data available for incidence and prevalence of skin cancer in Europe are fragmentary and extremely difficult to interpret, since surveys, such as they are, were performed using methods of varying rigor, and over at least three decades during which the incidence of skin cancer has greatly increased. However, it is clear that just as in the United States and in Australia, a marked north–south gradient exists.

Africa. Regarding skin cancer in Africa, the reports of Oettle (1963) and Davies et al. (1968) show that native Africans have extremely low rates of NMSC as well as of melanoma. The incidence rates in the Johannesburg Bantus and in Uganda are of the order of 1–2/100 000 (almost all are SCC of the lower extremities). Isaacson et al. (1978) reported an incidence of 1/100 000 for Soweto (South Africa) blacks.

The exception are albino natives, who are extremely prone to the development of skin cancer. In South Africa, albinism is quite common among the Bantu. Oettle (1963) estimated a crude annual incidence rate of 579/100 000 for male and 408/100 000 for female Bantu for SCC of the skin. Interestingly, the rates for BCC were estimated to be only 36/100 000 for both albino sexes combined.

India. Incidence data for skin cancer in India are not available. But it is clear that the majority of skin cancers seen in hospitals occur in white-skinned nonnatives. Among native Indians, special types of SCC of the skin are found, presumably due to extreme heat, combustion, and chronic friction, such as Kangri, Dhoti, and Chutta cancer (Urbach 1963).

Japan and Taiwan. While again incidence figures are not available, it is clear that skin cancer is uncommon in Japan and Taiwan. This is also borne out by a reversal of the usual BCC to SCC ratio seen in whites. SCC are three times as common that BCC, and may arise at the site of premalignant skin changes such as burns or chronic trauma, or are secondary to arsenic ingestion (Urbach 1963).

Australia. Probably the best NMSC surveys have been carried out in Australia. Because of the predominantly European origin of the Australian population, and the fact that large segments of the population live at low latitudes and have extensive solar exposure, NMSC has always been very common. Australia has the highest skin cancer rate in the world, and it is estimated to be three times more common than all other types of cancer combined. Several recent surveys of NMSC incidence (Marks et al. 1989; Kricker et al. 1990) reflect this situation. For the Australian population as a whole, the standardized incidence rates for NMSC were 823/100 000, for BCC 659/100 000 and for SCC 166/100 000. The effect of latitude of residence was particularly striking. The rate for people living north of 29°S was 1242/100 000 and that of people living south of 37°S was 489/100 000. Similar data have been reported in two recent smaller studies (Giles et al. 1988; Marks et al. 1983).

The difference in incidence of NMSc with difference in residential latitude is one of the strongest points in favor of solar exposure causing these tumors. A recent study in south Wales, United Kingdom, calculated the incidence rate for BCC to be 83/100 000 and for SCC 19/100 000, or a combined rate of 102/100 000. The rate for a similar Welsh-extracted population in Victora, Australia, was 672/100 000 for BCC and 201/100 000 for SCC, thus a combined rate of 873/100 000 (Marks et al. 1983)

Environmental Exposure and Changing Incidence with Time

All available evidence suggests that virtually all human SCC but only two-thirds of BCC are related to total accumulated lifetime dose of biologically effective solar UV radiation (Vitaliano and Urbach 1980). It is also clear that pigmentation of the skin confers a marked protection, that there is considerable variation in the sensitivity to UV radiation among white people, and that much of this variation is genetic (Urbach et al. 1972). It is highly associated with "ease of sunburning" and ability to tan. However, given sufficient UV exposure for sufficient time, most white people can develop NMSC. The great difference in susceptibility, which is by no means regularly distributed geographically, is one of the major confounding factors for any dose–response calculation in man. Recent studies have shown that skin cancer incidence in the United States is increasing by about 2% per year, although no change in ambient UV radiation during this time period is apparent (Glass and Hoover 1989).

Potential Effect of Changes in Stratospheric Ozone

Of the total solar radiant energy that reaches earth, approximately 5% consists of UV radiation. Depending on sun angle (i.e., air mass, time of day) the biologically most effective UV radiation comprises 10% or less of the total UV radiation. Because ozone begins to absorb UV radiation significantly at about 325 nm, the segment of the solar UV spectrum that would be augmented in the event of diminution of stratospheric ozone concentration includes only the small waveband between 290 and 325 nm. Wavelengths longer than 325 nm are not appreciably influenced by changes in ozone concentration. Although the total energy that would be added to the solar (and even solar UV radiation) insolation would be small, this region has notable photochemical efficiency in biological systems.

The balance between increasing biological effectiveness of decreasing wavelengths in the UV spectrum and increasing absorption by ozone of the shorter wavelengths becomes critical when considering the biological implications of solar UV radiation changes as a function of alteration of the stratospheric ozone layer. For most biological action spectra, it is clear that changes in atmospheric ozone result in increases in biologically effective UV irradiance disproportionately greater than might be indicated by simply integrating the increasing total UV energy flux.

Extensive studies of the relative biological effectiveness of wavelengths in the UV-B (i.e., action spectra) on such diverse biological materials as purified DNA, bacteria, plant and human cells in tissue culture, and human skin and eye in vivo have shown that wavelengths of 290 nm are 1000–10 000 times as effective in producing damage (thymine dimer production, single and double strand breaks in DNA, production of mutations, cell killing, production of skin erythema and skin cancer) than wavelengths of 330 nm.

Based on the most recent action spectrum for skin erythema (McKinlay and Diffey 1987), which appears to be an acceptable surrogate for a skin carcinogenesis action spectrum (De Gruijl 1992), it has been estimated that a 1% decrease in total ozone column would increase biologically effective (action spectrum weighted) UV-B radiation by 1.6%. This could result in an increase of 2.7% for BCC and 4.6% for SCC. Should the total ozone column be reduced by 5%, the carcinogenic irradiance would increase by 8%. This could increase BCC by 14% and SCC by 25%.

A recent report of the Ozone Trends Panel (Watson and Ozone Trends Panel 1988) estimates that in the 20-year period from 1966 to 1986, total column ozone has decreased by 2%–3%, depending on latitude. Since the decreases were greater in the winter months (when very much less UV-B reaches the ground) than in the summer, the annual average increases are somewhat deceptive as far as biologically effective UV-B is concerned.

As a matter of fact, Scotto et al. (1988) have reported that in an 11-year period (1974–1985) there was no increase in ground-level, biologically effective UV-B, as measured by Robertson–Berger meters, which have a response spectrum very similar to the biological hazard spectrum of McKinlay and Diffey (1987).

It is most likely that this lack of UV radiation increase is due to metereological, climatic, and environmental factors taking place in the troposphere, which attenuate UV-B. The decreases of stratospheric ozone over the Antarctic continent and the Northern hemisphere are real, but not likely to have as yet significantly affected present incidence rates of NMSC. Other environmental changes (such as markedly increased social exposure) must play a much greater role.

Artificial Sources of Ultraviolet Radiation

Indoor Lighting. This has become a necessary part of our existence. For several decades, there has been emphasis on distributing enough luminous intensity to enhance visual acuity and provide efficient and safe illumination.

Fluorescent light sources are widely used because of superior economy. Luminaires with acrylic sheets as diffusers have been widely used to reduce glare. These sheets absorb virtually all UV radiation emitted from fluorescent lamps. More recently, fixtures with open louvres ("egg crate") have become prevalent because they increase brightness, but at the expense of letting UV radiation pass.

Measurements of a number of commonly used fluorescent lamps in various office and store configurations showed that they emit measurable amounts of UV-B, and some even small amounts of UV-C. The visual brightness of such sources is not an adequate predictor of their UV emission, and thus of their potential for biological hazard. It is possible that under some lighting conditions over a working lifetime, the risk of cumulative UV damage might be significantly increased. Utilizing acrylic louvres lowers the risk to negligible (Cole et al. 1985).

Solaria. Most commercial tanning equipment in current use exploits the divergence in the erythema and pigmentation action spectra (Gange et al. 1986). These sources include type I UV-A fluorescent lamps (UV-B content 1%–2%, lower limit 315–320 nm), type II UV-A lamps (UV-B content 0.05%, lower limit 330–340 nm) and optically filtered, metal halide-doped mercury arc lamps (Mutzhas 1986). The usual exposure to such lamps is 30 min, resulting in an exposure of about $4.5 \times 10^5\,J/m^2$, or a pigmenting dose for skin types III and IV. Very fair persons can develop mild erythema from such a dose of UV radiation. Diffey (1987) estimated that the use of solaria 10 times per year adds a negligible risk for developing skin cancer, but that use three times weekly from age 20 to 50 (30 years) could double the likelihood of skin cancer development. Clearly, the increasing use of "sun" beds and "sun" canopies for home use gives considerable cause for concern, because no controls can be executed there.

It is clear from all studies that sunbathing during a 2-week holiday in natural sunlight in sunny climates presents a much more significant carcinogenic burden for the skin than moderate use of an UV-A solarium. Although a UV-A-induced tan does not provide as much protection against acute sunburn as a UV-B-induced tan, a similar degree of tan induced by either waveband of radiation provides similar protection against DNA damage (Gange et al. 1985). However, there is no question that additional UV-A exposure from solaria is additive to the damaging effect of solar UV-B exposure.

Photosensitizers

Every person is frequently exposed to sunlight, and many people make a conscious effort to increase their exposure to the outdoor environment. For these reasons it is reasonable to state that almost everyone is some distance along a course which will lead, eventually, to the occurrence of skin cancer. That most of us do not complete this process is attributable to the competing risk of mortality. Every year, nevertheless, hundred of thousands suffer from the accumulated effects of this universal environmental exposure.

The reason for emphasizing the inevitable and chronic nature of exposure to solar carcinogenesis is to indicate the importance of agents which can modify the process. If an agent can accelerate the development of liver cancer, for example, but cannot by itself induce liver cancer, it constitutes a hazard only in the presence of an effective carcinogen. By itself it cannot be revealed to be a carcinogen, and its potential for danger is conditional upon joint exposure with a demonstrably harmful agent. It is unlikely, therefore, to be regarded as a hazard on this basis alone. With skin cancer, in contrast, it is not the possibility of carcinogenic exposure which is in question, but only the degree. Thus any agent which can significantly influence the evolution of skin cancer can correspondingly influence its incidence.

The best known examples of photosensitizers are certain natural furocoumarins (psoralens), some of which are used for medicinal or cosmetic purposes. Combinations of psoralens and UV radiation can produce severe cutaneous burns, and it is possible that these, like acute burns of UV overexposure, can produce some carcinogenic changes. Much smaller combinations, administered clinically, produce little or no such damage, but are much more carcinogenic than the UV radiation alone (Forbes and Davies

1981). Psoralens alone are not demonstrably carcinogenic. The combination, therefore, is carcinogenic (i.e., involves photochemical carcinogenesis) or is an extremely effective enhancer of photocarcinogenesis. The effectiveness of oral psoralen in enhancing cutaneous carcinogenesis has been demonstrated clinically in man (Stern et al. 1979). It is known that some highly phototoxic psoralens, such as 8-methoxypsoralen, can form interstrand cross-links in DNA under the influence of UV radiation, and it is widely assumed that such cross-links are the basis for subsequent carcinogenic changes. The nature of the association among cross-links, phototoxicity, and photocarcinogenesis has not been defined (Grube et al. 1977). Psoralens which are not phototoxic apparently do not enhance photocarcinogenesis; moreover, not all phototoxic agents enhance photocarcinogenesis. Anthracene, for example, does not enhance photocarcinogenesis (Forbes et al. 1976); the effects of other aromatic hydrocarbons are more difficult to determine, since many are chemical carcinogens and some are destroyed by light (Davies et al. 1972). There is some indication that orthoaminobenzoic acid, a phototoxic isomer of the common sunscreen paraaminobenzoic acid, may also enhance photocarcinogenesis.

For more than 15 years, the combination of 8-methoxypsoralen and UV-A has been used a medical treatment, initially for psoriasis (Parrish et al. 1974) and then for a great variety of cutaneous disorders. As therapy it is most effective, but patients have to be treated for considerable periods of time. It was to be expected that psoralen-UVA (PUVA) therapy in man would result in development af skin cancers. Indeed, as of 1988, in a carefully followed group of 1380 patients in the United States, prolonged exposure to PUVA substantially increased the risk of SCC, but not BCC. No significant increase in malignant melanoma was found (Stern 1989). In contrast, in a very large European study, skin tumors in PUVA-treated patients seemed to occur only in those previously treated with arsenic or X-rays. The difference may lie in different ways of administering the treatment (Henseler 1989).

Chemical Agents

Coal Tar and its Derivatives

Prolonged contact of the skin with tar, pitch, tar products, soot, or mineral oil products frequently causes the development of changes called "tar keratosis," which can progress to SCC. The first description of an occupational cancer was that of scrotal cancer of chimneysweeps, which Percival Pott (1775) appropriately ascribed to prolonged contact with soot. Volkman (1875) described tar cancer in brown coal and paraffin workers and identified it with Pott's scrotal cancer. He also observed the early stages of the disease consisting of frequent irritation, "tar itch," and browning of the skin, with comedones and hyperkeratotic papules and verrucous lesions. That medicinal use of tar can cause skin cancer after many years of use was first reported by Veiel (1924).

Attempts to produce cancer with tar in animal experiments were of great importance to the understanding of tar skin, tar keratosis, and tar cancer. Yamagiva and Itchikawa (1918) were the first to produce skin cancer by chronically painting rabbit skin with coal tar. By the 1930s, chemically pure hydrocarbons, mainly phenanthrenes (Benzpyrine, etc.), had been isolated from coal tar and found to be carcinogenic for skin.

Early on it had been noted that tar itch occurred mostly on exposure to sunshine, and tar cancers appeared most commonly on sites exposed to light: face, forearms, and hands (Götz 1976). Findlay (1928) reported that application of coal tar to skin followed by UV radiation increased the probability of skin carcinogenesis and shortened the development time of tumors. Lewis (1935) observed that carcinogenic hydrocarbons added to chick embryo tissue cultures photosensitized the cells to light, causing abnormalities that resembled characteristics of malignant growths.

Mottram and Doniach (1938) compared the carcinogenic and photodynamic activity of varios hydrocarbons as well as that of tar, soot, and shale oil and found a strong correlation between these two activities. When experimental studies in animals were performed, however, investigators found either potentiation or protection during simultaneous carcinogen and UV radiation exposure (Doniach and Mottram 1940; Heller 1950). It was not until decades later that the explanation for these discrepancies became apparent, namely that not only are the carcinogenic phenanthrenes photodynamically active, but that they can be photochemically decomposed to noncarcinogenic photo-products as well (Davies et al. 1972).

The most frequent non-sunlight-exposed site for human tar cancer is the scrotum (Götz 1976), probably because of the high lipid content of that skin, constant heat, and thin epidermis.

For tar cancer to develop, patients apparently must have contact for decades, and the tumors have an incubation period of typically 20 or more years. In addition to workers exposed to tar products, contact with crude mineral, slate, and spindle oil in cotton and other spinning industries may lead to similar changes (Heller 1930; Hueper and Payne 1960).

Arsenic

Arsenic is widely distributed throughout the animal and plant kingdom and in our environment, where sources can be natural or anthropogenic. In primary rocks it is present mainly in the form of sulfides, and as such has been used as pigment since prehistoric times. The arsenic sulfides are present in substantial amounts in ores bearing gold, silver, copper, lead, tin, and zinc. When ores are roasted, arsenic sublimes to arsenic trioxide, which has caused widespread arsenicism in mining communities (Geyer 1898; Birmingham et al. 1965). Other occupational exposure has been reported due to use of arsenate of lead as fungicide in wine-producing areas in France (Thiers et al. 1967) and Germany (Roth 1956), as well as in sheep dip in Australia (Sanderson 1976).

Another source of chronic arsenicism has been from contaminated drinking water. Well-studied epidemics have occurred in Cordoba, Argentina (Arguello et al. 1938), and in Taiwan, China (Yeh 1973). Finally, inorganic arsenic has been used in medical therapy for more than 200 years. Fowler (1786) suggested that arsenic was useful in treatment of remitting fevers, and by 1888, when Hutchinson wrote about arsenic cancer, it was well established as a treatment for anemia, Hodgkin's disease and such skin diseases as psoriasis, eczema, lichen planus, and lupus erythematosus. It was also widely used in cases of epilepsy and chorea and was a constituent of an official bromide mixture.

There is a dose–response relationship between the amount of arsenic ingested and the percentage of patients with keratoses (mostly palmar and plantar) and, at a higher level, with carcinomas. The average latent period is 15 years, but there is great individual variation in response (Fierz 1966). The types of tumor which develop may also vary. Although most patients show keratoses and Bowen's disease, a minority have only multiple BCC. Arsenic is a multisystem carcinogen and significant increases in cancer of the lung, bladder, and liver have been reported in groups of patients with chronic arsenicism (Yeh 1973; Hindmarsh and McCurdy 1986).

Ionizing Radiation

Within 7 years of the discovery of roentgen rays, the first case of radiation-induced skin cancer was reported by Frieben (1902). This was a SCC occurring in an area of radio-dermatitis on the back of the hand of a worker who had used his hand as a test object in a roentgen tube factory. In the earliest period, radiation cancer was an occupational hazard afflicting primarily technologists and physicians working with X-rays and radium.

All early histological studies indicated that X-ray-induced skin cancer was of the SCC type. Once superficial radiation started to be used for treatment of benign disorders such as acne and psoriasis, it was found that BCC also occurred in radiodermatitis (Anderson and Anderson 1951). However, it appears that there is some degree of site specificity, the face and back being prone to development of BCC, other areas showing mainly SCC. Occasionally, sarcomas can develop.

It is still not known which total doses, increment doses or intervals between increments produce the maximal number of tumors in human skin. However, empirical observations by experienced radiotherapists have shown that carcinomas (1) occur only on skin showing gross visible evidence of radiodermatitis; (2) occur most profusely in radiodermatitis that has been produced by the total of many small doses administered over a considerable period (years); and (3) rarely is a new carcinomas seen in the radiation sequelae produced by large doses of X-rays given for the treatment of internal cancer (Traenkle 1963).

The responses of skin to ionizing radiation and their time of onset are known in considerable detail (Potten 1985). Studies on humans have produced increasing information about the risk of skin cancer after exposure to ionizing radiation. Skin cancer has a very low mortality rate, and the most recent reports suggest 0.2% as the best estimate (Fry 1990). Experimental data confirm that exposure to UV radiation for a long period after an intial exposure to X-rays increases the carcinogenic effects of ionizing radiation (Fry 1990), as does exposure to promoters such as TPA and PUVA (Fry et al. 1986).

The development of megavoltage instruments has practically eliminated skin damage in tumor radiotherapy, and the use of "superficial" radiation for benign disease has virtually ceased. Thus, ionizing radiation-induced skin cancer is disappearing, as those of risk in the early and middle part of the twentieth century reach the end of their normal life span.

Infrared Radiation

Infrared radiation comprises about 40% of the irradiance reaching the earth's surface (Koller 1965). Although it has long been known that SCC can arise in burn scars (Lawrence 1952; Bartle et al. 1990), it is less well known that chronic heat exposure in the physiological range is also associated with NMSC. In India, Kangri cancer is frequent in the Kashmir, an average of 45 cases having been treated yearly in the Mission hospital (Mulay 1963). A kangri is an earthenware pot, covered with wickerwork, with a jute thread handle. Burning charcoal or dried leaves are put in this pot, which is tied to the abdomen under the clothes to produce warmth. The temperature to which the skin is exposed ranges from 150° to 200°F, and burns often occur. In the areas of actual contact, every stage of chronic dermatitis is seen – from redness to thickened patches of skin and later ulcerating or fungating carcinomas. Metastasis to inguinal lymph nodes is common. In China and Japan, persons in cold regions sleep on beds of hot bricks, or have underfloor braziers which result in erythema ab igne and skin carcinoma (Akasaka and Kon 1989). Similarly, turf or peat fire cancer has been frequently reported developing on the lower legs of rural Irish women who had extensive exposure to open hearths burning peat (Cross 1967). The cutaneous findings of reticulated chronic skin erythema with diffuse pigmentation and development of later keratotic lesions have been named erythema ab igne and related to chronic heat exposure. Kligman and Kligman (1984) showed experimentally that infrared radiation is capable of causing significant elastic fiber hyperplasia, and greatly enhances that due to UV irradiation of skin. Although carcinogenesis studies are few and controversial, there is evidence that moderate heating of mouse skin causes UV-induced skin tumors to develop more quickly and more frequently than in room temperature controls (Bain et al. 1943; Owen and Knox 1978). It would appear that significantly more investigative work needs to be done in this field.

References

Akasaka T, Kon S (1989) Two cases of squamous cell carcinoma arising from erythema ab igne. Nippon Hifuka Gakkai Zasshi 99:735–742

Anderson NP, Anderson HE (1951) Development of basal cell epithelioma as a consequence of radiodermatitis. Arch Dermatol Syphilol 63:586–596

Arguello RA, Ceuget DD, Tello EE (1938) Cancer y arsenicismo regional éndemico en Cordoba. Rev Argent Dermatosifilol 22:461–472

Bain JA, Rush HP, Kline BE (1943) Effect of temperature on ultraviolet carcinogenesis with wavelength of 2800–3400 Å. Cancer Res 3:610–612

Bartle EJ, Sun JH, Wang XW, Schneider BK (1990) Cancers arising from burn scars. A literature review and report of twenty-one cases. J Burn Care Rehabil 11:46–49

Birmingham DJ, Key MM, Holaday DA, Perone VB (1965) An outbreak of arsenical dermatoses in a mining community. Arch Dermatol 91:457–464

Blum HF (1959) Carcinogenesis by ultraviolet light. Princeton University Press, Princeton

Blumthaler M, Ambach W (1988) Solar UVB albedo of various surfaces. Photochem Photobiol 48:85–88

Buettner KJK (1969) The effect of natural sunlight on human skin. In: Urbach F (ed) The biologic effects of ultraviolet radiation. Pergamon, Oxford, pp 237–249

Chuang TY, Popecsh A, Su WPD, Chute CG (1990) Basal cell carcinoma. J Am Acad Dermatol 22:413–417

Cole C, Forbes PD, Davies RE, Urbach F (1985) Effect of indoor lighting on normal skin. In: Wurtman RJ, Baum MJ, Potts JP Jr (eds) The medical and biological effects of light. Ann NY Acad Sci 453:305–316

Cross F (1967) On a turf (peat) fire cancer: malignant change superimposed on erythema ab igne. Proc R Soc Med 60:1307–1308

Cutler SJ, Young JL (1975) Third National Cancer survey: incidence data. Natl Cancer Inst Monog 41:75–787

Davies JNP, Tauk R, Meyer R, Thursten P (1968) Cancer of the integumentary system in Ugandan africans. J Natl Cancer Inst 41:31–51

Davies RE, Dodge HA, Austin Wa (1972) Carcinogenicity of DMBA under various light sources. In: Proceedings of the 6th international congress for photobiology, Bochum (abstr 347)

De Gruijl F (1992) Action spectra for photocarcinogenesis. In: Urbach F (ed) The physiologic effects of UV-A radiation. Valdemar Publishing Co. Overland Park, KS, pp 91–98

Diffey BL (1987) Analysis of the risk of skin cancer from sunlight and solaria in subjects living in northern Europe. Photodermatology 4:118–126

Doniach I, Mottram JC (1940) On the effect of light upon the incidence of tumors in painted mice. Am J Cancer 39:234–240

Emmet EA (1973) Ultraviolet radiation as a cause for skin cancer. Crit Rev Toxicol 2:211–255

Fierz U (1966) Katamnestische Untersuchungen über die Nebenwirkungen der Therapie der Hautkrankheiten mit anorganischem Arsen. Arch Klin Exp Dermatol 227:286–290
Findlay GM (1928) Ultraviolet light and skin cancer. Lancet 2:1070–1073
Forbes PD, Davies RE (1981) Enhancement of photocarcinogenicity by 8-MOP. In: Cahn J, Forlot P, Grupper C, Maybeck A, Urbach F (eds) Psoralens in cosmetics and dermatology. Pergamon, Oxford, pp 365–370
Fowler I (1786) Medical reports on the effect of arsenic in the cure of agues, remitting fever and periodic headaches. Johnson, London
Frieben A (1902) Cancroid des rechten Handrückens nach lang dauerden Einwirkung von Roentgenstrahlen. Fortschr Geb Roentgenstr 6:106–108
Fry RJM (1990) Radiation protection guidelines for the skin. Int J Radiat Biol 57:829–839
Fry RJM, Storer JB, Burns FJ (1986) Radiation induction of cancer of the skin. Br J Radiol Suppl 19:58–60
Gange RW, Park YK, Kagetsu N, Blackett AD, Parrish JA (1986) Action spectra for cutaneous responses to ultraviolet radiation. In: Urbach F, Gange RW (eds) The biologic effects of UVA radiation. Praeger, New York
Gellin GA, Kopf AW, Andrade R (1965) Basal cell epitheliomas: a controlled study of associated factors. Arch Dermatol 91:38–45
Geyer L (1898) Über die chronischen Hautveränderungen beim Arsenicismus und Betrachtungen über die Massenerkrankungen in Reichenstein in Schlesien. Arch Dermatol Syphilol 43:221–280
Giles GG, Marks R, Foley P (1988) Incidence of non-melanotic skin cancer treated in Australia. BMJ 296:13–18
Glass AG, Hoover RN (1989) The emerging epidemic of melanoma and skin cancer. JAMA 262:2097–2100
Götz H (1976) Tar keratosis. In: Andrade R, Gumport SL, Popkin G, Rees TD (eds) Cancer of the skin. Saunders, Philadelphia, pp 492–523
Green A, Beardmore G, Hart V, Leslie D, Marks R, Staines D (1988) Skin canceer in a Queensland population. J Am Acad Dermatol 19:1045–1052
Grube DD, Ley RD, Fry RJM (1977) Photosensitizing effects of 8-Methoxypsoralen on the skin of hairless mice: II. Strain and spectral differences for tumorigenesis. Photochem Photobiol 25:269–276
Heller I (1930) Occupational cancers. J Ind Hyg 12:169–197
Heller W (1950) Experimentelle Untersuchungen über dem Lichtkrebs. Lichtkrebserzeugung durch Photosensibilisierung. Strahlentherapie 81:529–548
Henseler J (1989) Risk of non-melanoma skin tumors in patients treated with long-term photochemotherapy (PUVA). In: Fitzpatrick TB, Forlot P, Pathak MA, Urbach F (eds) Psoralens. Libbey, London, pp 377–386
Hindmarsh JT, McCurdy RF (1986) Clinical and environmental aspects of arsenic toxicity. Crit Rev Clin Lab Sci 23:315–347
Hueper WC, Payne WW (1960) Carcinogenic studies on petroleum asphalt, cooling oil and coal tar. AMA Arch. Pathol 65:608–614
Hutchinson J (1888) On some examples of arsenic keratosis of the skin and arsenic cancer. Trans Pathol Soc Lond 39:352–363
Isaacson C, Selser G, Kaye V et al. (1978) Cancer in urban blacks of South Africa. S African Cancer Bull 22:49–62
Kligman LH, Kligman AM (1984) Reflections on heat. Br J Dermatol 110:367–375
Koller LR (1965) Ultraviolet radiation. Wiley, New York, p 105
Kricker A, English DR, Randell PL, Heenen PJ, Clay CD, Delaney TA, Armstrong BK (1990) Skin cancer in Geralton, Western Australia: a survey of incidence and prevalence. Med J Aust 152:399–407

Lawrence EA (1952) Carcinoma arising in scars of thermal burns. Surg Gynecol Obstet 95:579–588
Lewis MR (1935) The photosensitivity of chick embryo cells growing in media containig certain carcinogenic substances. Am J Cancer 25:305–309
MacDonald EJ, Bubendorf E (1964) Some epidemiologic aspects of skin cancer. In: Tumors of the Skin. Yearbook Medical Publishers, Chicago, pp 23–46
Marks R, Ponsford MW, Selwood TS, Goodman G, Mason G (1983) Non-melanotic skin cancer in Victoria. Med J Aust 142:619–622
Marks R, Jolley D, Dorevitch AP, Selwood TS (1989) The incidence of non-melanotic skin cancers in an Australian population: results of a five-year prospective study. Med J Aust 150:475–478
McKinlay AF, Diffey BJ (1987) A reference action spectrum for ultraviolet induced erythema in human skin. In: Passchier WF, Bosnajkovic BFM (eds) Human exposure to ultraviolet radiation: risks and regulations. Exerpta Medica, Amsterdam, pp 83–88
Mottram JC, Doniach I (1938) The photodynamic action of carcinogenic agents. Lancet 1:1156–1159
Mulay DM (1963) Skin cancer in India. In: Urbach F (ed) The biology of cutaneous cancer. Natl Cancer Inst Monogr 10:215–224
O'Beirn SF, Judge P, Urbach F, MacCon CF, Martin F (1970) Skin cancer in County Galway. In: Proceedings of the 6th national cancer conference. Lippincott, Philadelphia, pp 489–500
Oettle AC (1963) Skin cancer in Africa. In: Urbach F (ed) The biology of cutaneous cancer. Natl Cancer Inst Monogr 10:197–214
Owen DW, Knox JM (1978) Influence of heat, wind and humidity on ultraviolet radiation injury. Natl Cancer Inst Monogr 50:161–167
Parrish JA, Fitzpatrick TB, Tanenbaum L et al. (1974) Photochemotherapy of psoriasis with oral methoxsalen and long-wave ultraviolet light. N Engl J Med 291:1207–1211
Pott P (1775) Chirurgical observations relative to cataract, the nose, the cancer of the scrotum, the different kinds of ruptures, and the mortification of the toes and feet. Hower, Clarke and Pollius, London, 63
Potten CS (1985) Radiation and skin. Taylor and Francis, London
Roth F (1956) Über die chronische Arsenvergiftung der Moselwinzer unter besonderer Berücksichtigung des Arsenkrebses. Z Krebsforsch 61:287–319
Sanderson KV (1976) Arsenic and skin cancer. In: Andrade R, Gumport SL, Popkin GL, Rees TD (eds) Cancer of the skin. Saunders, Philadelphia, pp 473–491
Schulze R (1970) Das Strahlenklima der Erde. Steinkoppf, Darmstadt
Scotto J, Fears RR, Fraumeni JF Jr (1981) Incidence of non-melanoma skin cancer in the United States. Publ No (NIH) 82-2433. National Cancer Institute, Bethesda
Scotto J, Cotton G, Urbach F, Berger D, Fears T (1988) Biologically effective ultraviolet radiation: Surface measurements in the United States 1974–1985. Science 239:762–764
Silverstone H, Searle JHA (1970) The epidemiology of skin cancer in Queensland. Br J Cancer 24:235–253
Stern RS (1989) PUVA: its status in the United States 1988. In: Fitzpatrick TB, Forlot P, Pathak MA, Urbach F (eds) Psoralens. Libbey, London, pp 367–376
Stern RS, Thibodeau LA, Kleinerman RA, Parrish JA, Fitzpatrick TB (1979) Risk of cutaneous carcinoma in patients treated with oral methoxsalen photochemotherapy for psoriasis. N Engl J Med 300:809–813
Thiers H, Colomb D, Moulin G, Cohn L (1967) Le cancer cutané arsénical des viticulteurs du Beaujolais. Ann Dermatol Syphilogr 94:133–158
Traenkle HL (1963) X-ray induced skin cancer in man. In: Urbach F (ed) The biology of cutaneous cancer. Natl Cancer Inst Monogr 10:423–432

Urbach F (1969) The geographic pathology of skin cancer. In: Urbach F (ed) The biologic effects of ultraviolet radiation. Pergamon, Oxford, pp 635–650
Urbach F, Rose BB, Bonnem M (1972) Genetic and environmental interactions in skin carcinogenesis. In: Environmental cancer. Williams and Wilkins, Baltimore, pp 353–371
Veiel F (1924) Teerkrebs beim Menschen. Arch Dermatol Res 148:142–145
Vitaliano PP, Urbach F (1980) The relative importance of risk factors in nonmelanoma carcinoma. Arch Dermatol 116:454–456
Volkman R (1875) Über Teer, Parraffin und Rubkrebs (Schornsteinfeger Krebs). In: Volkman R (ed) Beiträge zur Chirurgie. Breitkopf, Leipzig, p 370
Watson RT, Ozone Trends Panel (1988) Present state of knowledge of the upper atmosphere 1988. An assessment report. NASA reference publication 1208. NASA, Washington
Yamagiwa K, Itchikawa K (1918) Experimental study of the pathogenesis of carcinoma. J Cancer Res 3:1–12
Yeh S (1973) Skin cancer in chronic arsenicism. Hum Pathol 4:469–485

Ultraviolet Carcinogenesis: Environmental Effects of Ozone Depletion

J.C. van der Leun[1], F.R. de Gruijl[1], M. Tevini[2], and R.C. Worrest[3]

[1] Institute of Dermatology, University Hospital Utrecht, Heidelberglaan 100, NL-3584 CX Utrecht, The Netherlands
[2] Botanisches Institut II der Universität Karlsruhe, Kaiserstr. 12, W-7500 Karlsruhe 1, Fed. Rep. of Germany
[3] Consortium for International Earth Science Information, 1825 K Street NW, Washington, DC 20006, USA

Experimental Ultraviolet Carcinogenesis

Ultraviolet (UV) radiation is a useful agent in the study of skin carcinogenesis. The radiation administered in experiments may be selected for spectral composition and measured accurately (Forbes et al. 1982). The doses of UV radiation given to experimental animals may be in the same range as those received by people in daily life. The tumors induced appear on the skin and are accessible to observation from an early stage. In hairless mice, the tumors caused by UV radiation are predominantly squamous cell carcinomas, which are also found in human skin after prolonged sun exposure. Experimental studies make it possible to investigate the influence of wavelength, dose (de Gruijl et al. 1983), dose rate, etc. The wavelength-dependence, or "action spectrum," is becoming known to a better approximation step by step. It extends throughout the entire UV wavelength range, with wavelengths differing in effectiveness by up to 4 orders of magnitude (de Gruijl and van der Leun 1992). The dose–effect relationship found in experiments with mice is basically of the same type as found in human epidemiology.

The knowledge gained in 60 years of experimental work on UV carcinogenesis (Blum 1959) may be used in estimations of the risk of skin cancer for man. These include estimations of the risk by phototherapies, cosmetic tanning, and stratospheric ozone depletion (Slaper and van der Leun 1987).

Environmental Effects of Ozone Depletion

Of the risk factors above, that with the most difficult control and with the most far-reaching consequences is stratospheric ozone depletion (Russell Jones 1987; Graul and Forth 1990). According to the 1991 Update by the United Nations Environmental Programme (UNEP) (van der Leun

Recent Results in Cancer Research, Vol. 128

et al. 1991), the effects of ozone depletion will extend far beyond the area of skin cancer and may be summarized as follows:

Solar Interactions

- Significant global scale decreases in total ozone have occurred over the past 10 years.
- All other factors being constant, there is no scientific doubt that decreases in total ozone will increase UV-B radiation at ground level.
- Tropospheric ozone and aerosols may have masked the consequences of stratospheric ozone depletion for UV-B in some industrialized regions.
- It is likely that in areas remote from anthropogenic emissions, the UV-B changes due to stratospheric ozone depletion would be only partially compensated by tropospheric ozone and aerosol increases.
- There are no reliable estimates of the direction or magnitude of effects of any cloud cover trends on UV-B.
- Efforts to improve local and regional air quality may bring to light the increases in UV-B associated with the depletion of stratospheric ozone.

Human Health

- The induction of immunosuppression by UV-B (Kripke and Fischer 1976) has now been demonstrated in humans, not only those of light pigmentation, but also deeply pigmented individuals (Vermeer et al. 1991). This places at risk of the potential adverse impacts of UV-B on the immune system all of the world's populations, including possible increases in the incidence or severity of infectious disease.
- An increased number of adverse ocular effects have been associated with exposure to UV. These include age-related far sightedness, deformation of the lens capsule, and nuclear cataract (a form of cataract which previous information excluded from consideration). These effects appear to be independent of pigmentation. Estimates of risk would increase slightly if one were to include nuclear cataract among the forms of cataract increasing with ozone depletion. It is now predicted that, all other things being equal, a sustained 10% decrease in ozone will be associated with between 1.6 and 1.75 million additional cases of cataract per year world-wide.
- Recent information on the relationship of nonmelanoma skin cancer to UV exposures confirms previous findings and has allowed refinement of the carcinogenic action spectrum. Incorporation of this new information into the risk estimation process has led to slightly lower predictions. It is now predicted that a sustained 10% decrease in ozone will be associated with a 26% increase in nonmelanoma skin cancer. All other things

remaining constant, this would mean an increase in excess of 300 000 cases per year world-wide.

Terrestrial Plants

- Continued research on plant responses to UV-B radiation underscores the concern for agriculture, forestry, and natural ecosystems as the ozone layer is depleted (Teramura et al. 1990).
- Growth and photosynthesis of certain plants (e.g., seedlings of rye, maize, and sunflower) can be inhibited even under ambient levels of UV-B radiation.
- Certain environmental factors, both biotic (e.g., plant diseases and competition with other plants) and abiotic (e.g., carbon dioxide, temperature, heavy metals, and water availability), can interact with the effect of UV-B radiation in plants. This makes it difficult to work out quantitative predictions.
- Although most research to date has been with plants from temperate regions, data also show that certain tropical species may be adversely affected by enhanced UV-B radiation.

Aquatic Ecosystems

- Marine phytoplankton produces at least as much biomass as all terrestrial ecosystems combined. Recent results show that the aquatic ecosystem is already under UV-B stress and there is concern that an increase in UV-B radiation will cause detrimental effects.
- One consequence of losses in phytoplankton is reduced biomass production which is propagated throughout the whole food web. This may result in losses of biomass for human consumption.
- The marine phytoplankton is a major sink for atmospheric carbon dioxide. Any reduction of these populations would decrease the uptake of carbon dioxide and so augment the greenhouse effect. Also, phytoplankton production of DMS (dimethylsulfate), which acts as a precursor of cloud nucleation, would be reduced, hence potentially affecting global climate.
- A UV-B induced decrease in microorganisms fixing atmospheric nitrogen would require significant substitution by artificial fertilizers, e.g., in rice production.

Tropospheric Air Quality

- Chemical reactivity in the troposphere is expected to increase in response to increases in UV-B.

- Tropospheric ozone concentrations could rise in moderately to heavily polluted areas, but should decrease in unpolluted regions (with low oxides of nitrogen levels), as recently confirmed by measurements in the Antarctic.
- Other potentially harmful substances (hydrogen peroxide, acids, and aerosols) are expected to increase in all regions of the troposphere due to the enhanced chemical reactivity.
- These changes could exacerbate problems of human health and welfare, increase damage to the biosphere, and might make current air quality goals more difficult and expensive to attain.

Materials Damage

- UV-B radiation is particularly effective in light-induced degradation of wood and plastic products, leading to discoloration and loss of strength. Increased UV-B content in sunlight will cause more rapid degradation, resulting in increased costs of using higher levels of conventional light stabilizers, possible design of new stabilizers, and faster replacement of the affected products.
- Available research data are inadequate to reliably estimate the damage from higher UV-B levels to materials. Very limited relevant data are available for important classes of materials such as wood, plastic coatings, plastics used outdoors, and rubber. Data pertaining to performance of plastic in near-equator regions of the world, with the harshest exposure environments, are particularly needed.
- Some ongoing work relating to exposure of plastic under desert conditions is likely to contribute some of the needed data within the next few years. This may lead to improved assessment of damage to plastics resulting from partial ozone depletion, at that time.

Key Areas of Uncertainty

The key areas of uncertainty are the following:

- Quantification of the primary effects on food production and quality, on forestry, and on natural ecosystems.
- Clarification and quantification of influences on human health, especially the immune system, and occurrences of melanomas and cataracts.
- Effects on biota of the enhanced UV radiation during the Antarctic springtime ozone depletion (Smith et al. 1992).

References

Blum HF (1959) Carcinogenesis by ultraviolet light. Princeton University Press, Princeton

de Gruijl FR, van der Leun JC (1992) Action spectra for photocarcinogenesis. In: Urbach F (ed) Biological responses to ultraviolet A radiation, Valdenmar, Overland Park, pp 91–97

de Gruijl FR, van der Meer JB, van der Leun JC (1983) Dose-time dependency of tumor formation by chronic UV exposure. Photochem Photobiol 37:53–62

Forbes PD, Davies RE, Urbach F, Berger D, Cole C (1982) Simulated stratospheric ozone depletion and increased ultraviolet radiation: effects on photocarcinogenesis in hairless mice. Cancer Res 42:2796–2803

Graul EH, Forth W (1990) Das "gute" Ozon. Dtsch Ärztebl 87:2284–2291

Kripke ML, Fischer MS (1976) Immunologic parameters of ultraviolet carcinogenesis. J Natl Cancer Inst 57:211–215

Russell Jones R (1987) Ozone depletion and cancer risk. Lancet ii:443–446

Slaper H, van der Leun JC (1987) Human exposure to ultraviolet radiation: quantitative modelling of skin cancer incidence. In: Passchier WF, Bosnjakovic BFM (eds) Human exposure to ultraviolet radiation: risks and regulations. Elsevier, Amsterdam, pp 155–171

Smith RC, Prézelin BB, Baker KS, Bigidare RR, Boucher NP, Coley T, Karentz D, MacIntire S, Matlick HA, Meuzies D, Ondrusek M, Wan Z, Waters KJ (1992) Ozone depletion: ultraviolet radiation and phytoplankton biology in Antarctic Waters. Science 255:952–959

Teramura AH, Sullivan JH, Lydon J (1990) Effects of UV-B radiation on soybean yield and seed quality: a six year field study. Physiol Plant 80:5–11

van der Leun JC, Tevini M, Worrest RC (eds) (1991) Environmental effects of ozone depletion: 1991 update. Panel report pursuant to article 6 of the Montreal protocol on substances that deplete the ozone layer, under the auspices of the United Nations Environmental Programme (UNEP), P.O. Box 30552, Nairobi, Kenya

Vermeer M, Schmieder GJ, Yoshikawa T, van der Berg JW, Metzman MS, Taylor JR, Streilein JW (1991) Effects of ultraviolet B light on cutaneous immune response of humans with deeply pigmented skin. J Invest Dermatol 97:729–734

Experimental Ultraviolet Carcinogenesis

M.L. Kripke

Department of Immunology, University of Texas M.D. Anderson Cancer Center, 1515 Holcombe Boulevard, Box 178, Houston, TX 77030, USA

Introduction

Much of our information on UV carcinogenesis has come from investigations carried out in animal models. Skin cancers have been induced experimentally with UV radiation in a variety of laboratory animals, including mice, rats, guinea pigs, and opossums. The types of tumors vary depending on the species, but in mice they are usually squamous cell carcinomas and an undifferentiated type of tumor usually classified as a spindle cell tumor or fibrosarcoma. Many factors influence the induction of tumors by UV radiation; among different mouse strains, the same conditions of UV irradiation can produce tumors of different histologic types (squamous cell carcinomas versus spindle cell tumors), different body sites (ears versus dorsal skin), and different latent periods (Kripke 1977). Other factors affecting UV carcinogenesis include the age at first irradiation, skin thickness and pigmentation, UV dose and regimen, and, of course, the wavelength distribution of the UV light source (Blum 1959). Recent studies in inbred mouse strains have demonstrated, in addition, that there is an important immunological component to UV carcinogenesis (Kripke 1981).

Immunological Factors in Ultraviolet Carcinogenesis

Studies on the immunogenicity of skin cancers induced in inbred mice demonstrated that these tumors are highly antigenic. Upon transplantation into syngeneic animals, most of these tumors are rejected by the immune system of the recipient mouse. The tumors will grow progressively in immunosuppressed mice, however, demonstrating that they are tumorigenic in the absence of immunological resistance (Kripke 1974). This finding raised the question of how such highly antigenic tumors were able to grow progressively in the primary host without being rejected by the host's immune

Recent Results in Cancer Research, Vol. 128

system. A series of transplantation studies demonstrated that early in the course of chronic UV irradiation, before primary tumors were detectable, the mice lost their ability to reject UV-induced tumors (Kripke and Fisher 1976). This result demonstrated that UV irradiation had a systemic effect on the mice that interfered with tumor rejection. The importance of the systemic effect in carcinogenesis was shown by experiments in which mice were exposed to UV radiation for a short period of time to induce the systemic effect, and then they were exposed to a carcinogenic regimen of UV radiation at a distant site. Animals exposed to UV radiation at a distant site developed tumors much more rapidly than mice given only the carcinogenic regimen (De Gruijl and van der Leun 1982).

The systemic alteration brought about by UV irradiation was immunological in nature. This conclusion was based on experiments in which lymphoid cells from UV-irradiated mice were transfered to lethally X-irradiated recipients. Such mice were unable to reject UV-induced tumors, whereas mice given lymphoid cells from normal, unirradiated donors were able to resist tumor challenge (Fisher and Kripke 1977). Further studies demonstrated that suppressor T lymphocytes were responsible for the effect (Fisher and Kripke 1977, 1978; Spellman and Daynes 1977) and that the suppressor T lymphocytes inhibited the rejection of primary UV-induced skin cancers during carcinogenesis (Fisher and Kripke 1982). These studies demonstrated that exposing the skin to UV radiation caused a profound systemic change in immune function and that the immunosuppressive effects of UV radiation were an important component of UV carcinogenesis.

Mechanisms of Ultraviolet-Induced Immunosuppression

One intriguing question raised by these findings is how exposing the skin to UV radiation results in activation of suppressor T lymphocytes specific for antigens on UV-induced skin cancers. Over the past 15 years, many investigators have attempted to answer this question by studying the effects of UV radiation on immune processes (Kripke 1984). Although many facets of the question remain unanswered, we now have some working models with which to explain the phenomenon.

Clues for understanding the effects of UV radiation on tumor immunity have come largely from studies on the effects of UV radiation on other types of immune responses, particularly the delayed and contact hypersensitivity reactions. An important line of investigation relating to the mechanism of suppressor T lymphocyte induction by UV radiation arose from studies on the immunologic function of epidermal Langerhans cells. These cells are present in mammalian skin and have a dendritic morphology that forms a network throughout the epidermis. These bone-marrow-derived cells express MHC class II antigens and are now thought to be the major antigen-presenting cells of the epidermis (Stingl et al. 1978). During investigations of the function of epidermal Langerhans cells, it was noted that these cells were morphologically altered and decreased in number after exposure of murine (Toews et al. 1980) and human (Aberer et al. 1981) skin to UV radiation. Furthermore, application of a contact sensitizing chemical to the UV-irradiated skin resulted in the induction of specific immunologic tolerance, instead of the expected contact hypersensitivity (CHS) response (Toews et al. 1980), and antigen-specific suppressor T lymphocytes were present in the spleens of the animals (Elmets et al. 1983).

Based on these observations, it was postulated that damage to Langerhans cells by UV radiation alters the antigen-presentation pathway, thereby leading to activation of the suppressor pathway of the immune response instead of the effector pathway (Toews et al. 1980; Elmets et al. 1983). In an analogous manner, new UV-associated antigens present in the skin of UV-irradiated mice might also be expected to activate the suppressor pathway of the immune response, leading to the development of suppressor T lymphocytes specific for antigens present on UV-induced skin cancers. In support of this notion, we have shown recently that during the early stages of UV carcinogenesis in the mouse, epidermal Langerhans cells are morphologically altered and their antigen-presenting activity is impaired (Alcalay et al. 1989).

In addition to its direct effects on immune cells in the skin, UV radiation can alter certain immune responses initiated at distant, unexposed sites (Kripke 1984). Generally, higher doses of UV radiation than those needed to cause morphological alterations of Langerhans cells are required to suppress distant responses. The two types of immune responses impaired by acute, high doses of UV radiation are contact and delayed-type hypersensitivity (DTH); in both instances, the decreased response is associated with the presence of antigen-specific suppressor T lymphocytes in the spleen of the UV-irradiated, sensitized mice. Other immune responses, such as antibody production and allograft rejection, are not diminished by either high or low doses of UV radiation (Kripke 1984). The mechanism of distant immunosuppression by UV radiation is not well understood; however, recent studies suggest that soluble mediators released by UV-irradiated keratinocytes may be involved. Schwarz and colleagues (1986) demonstrated that intravenous injection of culture fluid from UV-irradiated murine keratinocytes suppressed the induction of contact hypersensitivity. Such supernatants also inhibit the induction of the DTH response and lead to the induction of antigen-specific suppressor T lymphocytes (Ullrich et al. 1990). The identity of these mediators has not been established, but there seem to be several such factors (Kim et al. 1990), each perhaps acting at a different step of the immune response. It remains to be determined why only some, and not all, immune responses are affected by UV radiation and how the soluble mediators cause activation of the suppressor pathway. Nonetheless, these findings provide another model to explain how UV radiation could lead to the production of tumor-specific suppressor T lymphocytes in mice exposed chronically to UV radiation.

Local Effect of Ultraviolet Radiation on Tumor Growth

In addition to the suppressor T cell-mediated systemic effect of UV radiation on the growth of UV-induced tumors, we have recently described a new, local effect of UV radiation on tumor growth in mice. This effect is manifested by the earlier appearance and higher incidence of tumors transplanted subcutaneously into UV-irradiated skin (Romerdahl et al. 1988). This effect is localized to the site of UV irradiation and is transient, disappearing within 1 week after cessation of UV irradition. Although these investigations were originally directed toward elucidating the role of UV radiation in melanoma development, we have found that this effect of UV radiation is not limited to melanomas, but extends to other immunogenic tumors as well, including UV-induced skin tumors (Donawho and Kripke 1991). Recent studies demonstrated that the local effect of UV radiation on tumor growth is absent in immunosuppressed mice, suggesting that it is immunologically mediated. This hypothesis is supported by experiments showing that the rejection of tumor cells in preimmunized mice was prevented when the challenge dose of tumor cells was given in the UV-irradiated site, but not when they were injected into an unexposed site (C. Donawho and M.L. Kripke, unpublished data). These studies suggest that UV radiation alters the local environment in a way that prevents the entry activity of immune effector cells in the UV-irradiated site. This effect appears to be unrelated to the UV-induced alteration in the number and function of epidermal Langerhans cells, but the exact nature of the alteration and the mechanism by which UV irradiation causes it are unknown at the present time.

Relevance to Humans

The majority of our information on the role of the immune system in UV carcinogenesis has come from studies on laboratory animals. However, there is increasing evidence that UV radiation causes immunological alterations in humans as well, and that the immune system is an important defense mechanism against the development of human skin cancer. UV radiation causes the same type of morphological alterations in Langerhans cells in human skin as it does in murine skin (Aberer et al. 1981), and alterations in the proportions and functions of circulating leukocytes have been noted in normal human subjects after exposure to artificial and natural sources of UV radiation (Morison et al. 1979; Hersey et al. 1983). In addition, there are changes in the antigen-presenting function of cells in human epidermis in response to suberythemal doses of UV radiation (Cooper et al. 1985; Baadsgaard et al. 1988). Recently, it was demonstrated that sensitization through UV-irradiated skin resulted in inhibition of contact sensitization in 40% of normal individuals and in more than 90% of persons who had previously had one or more skin cancers (Yoshikawa et al. 1990). This study demonstrated that local UV-induced immune suppression occurs in humans, as well as in laboratory rodents, and suggested that susceptibility to this immunosuppressive effect of UV irradiation may constitute an additional risk factor for the development of UV-associated skin cancers in humans. The finding that immunosuppressed individuals are at increased risk of developing UV-associated skin cancers also supports the notion that immunological factors are important in UV carcinogenesis in humans (Walder et al. 1971; Penn 1988).

Conclusions

The role of sunlight exposure in the development of human skin cancers was recognized around a century ago, and it has been apparent for more than two decades that UV-induced lesions in DNA are responsible for its carcinogenic activity (Cleaver 1968). Only recently, however, have we begun to realize that UV radiation also contributes to the process of skin cancer induction by means of its effects on the immune system. Studies in animal models demonstrated that exposing the skin to UV radiation could have profound, systemic, immunosuppressive effects, some of which interfered with host defenses against the development of UV-induced skin cancer. A growing body of evidence supports the notion that UV radiation can also suppress immune functions in humans, and recent studies suggest, in addition, that UV-induced immunosuppression may contribute to UV carcinogenesis in humans as well as in the mouse.

References

Aberer W, Schuler G, Stingl G, Honigsmann H, Wolff K (1981) Ultraviolet light depletes surface markers of Langerhans cells. J Invest Dermatol 76:202–210

Alcalay J, Craig JN, Kripke ML (1989) Alterations in Langerhans cells and Thy-1^+ dendritic epidermal cells in murine epidermis during the evolution of UV-induced skin cancers. Cancer Res 49:4591–4596

Baadsgaard O, Fox D, Cooper KD (1988) Human epidermal cells from ultraviolet light-exposed skin preferentially activate autoreactive $CD4^+2H4^+$ suppressor-induced lymphocytes and CD8+ suppressor/cytotoxic lymphocytes. J Immunol 140:1738–1744

Blum H (1959) Carcinogenesis by ultraviolet light. Princeton University Press, Princeton

Cleaver JE (1968) Defective repair replication of DNA in xeroderma pigmentosum. Nature 218:652–656

Cooper KD, Fox P, Neises G, Katz SI (1985) Effects of ultraviolet radiation on human epidermal cell alloantigen presentation: initial depression of Langerhans cell-dependent function is followed by the appearance of $T6^-Dr^+$ cells that enhance epidermal alloantigen presentation. J Immunol 134:129–137

DeGruijl FR, van der Leun J (1982) Systemic influence of pre-irradiation of a limited skin area on UV-tumorigenesis. Photochem Photobiol 35:379–383

Donawho C, Kripke ML (1991) Evidence that the local effect of UV radiation on the growth of murine melanomas is immunologically mediated. Cancer Res 51:4176–4181

Elmets CA, Bergstresser PR, Tigelaar RE, Wood PJ, Streilein JW (1983) Analysis of the mechanism of unresponsiveness produced by haptens painted on skin exposed to low dose ultraviolet radiation. J Exp Med 158:781–794

Fisher MS, Kripke ML (1977) Systemic alteration induced in mice by ultraviolet light irradiation and its relationship to ultraviolet carcinogenesis. Proc Natl Acad Sci USA 74:1688–1692

Fisher MS, Kripke ML (1978) Further studies on the tumor-specific suppressor cells induced by ultraviolet radiation. J Immunol 121:1139–1144

Fisher MS, Kripke ML (1982) Suppressor T lymphocytes control the development of primary skin cancers in ultraviolet-irradiated mice. Science 216:1133–1134

Hersey P, Haran G, Hasic E, Edwards A (1983) Alteration of T cell subsets and induction of suppressor T cell activity in normal subjects after exposure to sunlight. J Immunol 131:171–174

Kim TY, Kripke ML, Ullrich SE (1990) Immunosuppression by factors released from UV-irradiated epidermal cells: selective effects on the generation of contact and delayed hypersensitivity after exposure to UVA or UVB radiation. J Invest Dermatol 94:26–32

Kripke ML (1974) Antigenicity of murine skin tumors induced by ultraviolet light. J Natl Cancer Inst 53:1333–1336

Kripke ML (1977) Latency, histology, and antigenicity of tumors induced by ultraviolet light in three inbred mouse strains. Cancer Res 37:1395–1400

Kripke ML (1981) Immunologic mechanisms in UV radiation carcinogenesis. Adv Cancer Res 34:69–106

Kripke ML (1984) Immunological unresponsiveness induced by ultraviolet radiation. Immunol Rev 80:87–102

Kripke ML, Fisher MS (1976) Immunologic parameters of ultraviolet carcinogenesis. J Natl Cancer Inst 57:211–215

Morison WL, Parrish JA, Bloch KJ, Krugler JI (1979) In vivo effect of UV-B on lymphocyte function. Br J Dermatol 101:513–519

Penn I (1988) Tumors of the immunocompromised patient. Annu Rev Med 39:63–73

Romerdahl CA, Donawho C, Fidler IJ, Kripke ML (1988) Effect of UV-B radiation on the in vivo growth of murine melanoma cells. Cancer Res 48:4007–4010

Schwarz T, Urbanska A, Gschnait F, Luger TA (1986) Inhibition of the induction of contact hypersensitivity by a UV-mediated epidermal cytokine. J Invest Dermatol 87:289–291

Spellman CW, Daynes RA (1977) Modification of immunologic potential by ultraviolet radiation: II. Generation of suppressor cells in short-term UV-irradiated mice. Transplantation 24:120–126

Stingl G, Katz SI, Clement L, Green I, Shevach EM (1978) Immunologic functions of Ia-bearing epidermal Langerhans cells. J Immunol 121:2005–2013

Toews GB, Bergstresser PR, Streilein JW (1980) Epidermal Langerhans cell density determines whether contact hypersensitivity or unresponsiveness follows skin painting with DNFB. J Immunol 124:445–453

Ullrich SE, McIntyre BW, Rivas JM (1990) Suppression of the immune response to alloantigen by factors released from UV-irradiated keratinocytes. J Immunol 145:489–498

Walder BK, Robertson MR, Jeremy D (1971) Skin cancer and immunosuppression. Lancet 2:1282–1283

Yoshikawa T, Rae V, Bruins-Slot W, Van den Berg J-W, Taylor JR, Streilein JW (1990) Susceptibility to effects of UVB radiation on induction of contact hypersensitivity as a risk factor for skin cancer in humans. J Invest Dermatol 95:530–536

Xeroderma Pigmentosum Patients from Germany (the Mannheim XP Collection): Clinical and Biochemical Characteristics

H.W. Thielmann

German Cancer Research Center, W-6900 Heidelberg, Fed. Rep. of Germany

I am assuming that most readers are familiar with the human genodermatosis *xeroderma pigmentosum* (XP). It is a rare genetic disease with hypersensitivity to ultraviolet (UV) radiation and numerous malignancies on sun-exposed areas of the skin and the eye because of an inability to repair DNA damage inflicted by harmful UV radiation.

The earliest skin symptom of the disease is erythema, followed by a great number of pigmented macules, skin atrophy, and dryness (Jung 1986). Subsequently, patients develop various benign skin tumors and actinic keratoses, and by the median age of 8 years patients have developed malignant skin tumors such as squamous cell carcinomas, melanomas, and basaliomas. Some individuals suffer, in addition, from progressive neurologic degeneration.

XP is a paradigm for the idea that carcinogenesis involves DNA damage and that DNA repair plays a protective role. Since XP is one of the very few diseases in which cancer results from defective DNA repair, it has undergone intense clinical and biochemical study. Nevertheless, at present our knowledge has still not reached the point at which we could offer a clear biochemical explanation of the disorder.

Studies on XP have been conducted in the United States, Holland, Japan, and Egypt – not in Germany, at least not systematically. Therefore, in 1980, Prof. Dr. Jung from Mannheim Medical School and my group at the Cancer Research Center in Heidelberg set out to conduct a study on German XP patients using highly consistent clinical and biochemical criteria. Our aims were (1) to trace back clinical XP symptoms to the precise magnitude of the DNA repair defect and (2) to use several biochemical DNA repair parameters for identifying enzyme activities whose inadequate function is responsible for the XP defect.

Our study has meanwhile become known as the Mannheim XP Collection and comprises more than 100 patients, 66 of them have been thoroughly investigated, both clinically and biochemically (Table 1).

Recent Results in Cancer Research, Vol. 128

Table 1. Mannheim Xeroderma Pigmentosum Collection, 1991; skin tumors in XP patients

XP complementation group	Number of cases	Skin tumors			Predominant skin tumor
		Basal cell carcinoma	Squamous cell carcinoma	Lentigo maligna melanoma	
A	3	3	3	2	–
C	31	22	22	11	Basal cell carcinoma and squamous cell carcinoma
D	16	9	6	14	Lentigo maligna melanoma
E	3	3	–	–	Basal cell carcinoma
XP variant	13	13	6	4	Basal cell carcinoma
Total	66	50	37	31	

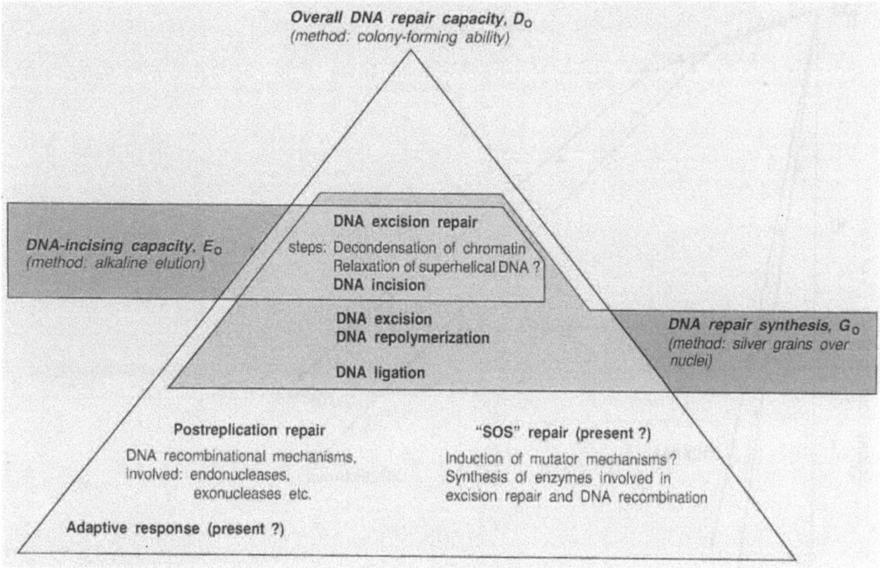

Fig. 1. Schematic representation of DNA repair mechanisms which are reflected by the analytical methods used: Colony-forming ability ("overall (or total) repair capcity"), all DNA-restoring or bypassing mechanisms; DNA repair synthesis, which includes the distinct steps DNA incision, excision, and DNA repolymerization; and DNA-incising capacity, reflecting repair-specific DNA incision only

These 66 patients could be classified according to the international complementation groups (these are genetically and biochemically distinct subforms of XP): 3 patients were assigned to group A, 31 to group C, 16 to group D, and 3 to group E, while 13 were of the XP variant type. So far, representatives of group B have not been found in the Mannheim XP Collection (Jung 1986; Thielmann et al. 1991a). Assignment of two patients to group F (or G) is preliminary.

A striking clinical aspect was that the frequency of histogenetically different skin tumors varied from one XP complementation group to another (Jung 1986): squamous cell carcinomas predominated in group C, lentigo maligna melanomas were most frequent in group D, and basal cell carcinomas occurred preferentially in group E and XP variants.

Using fibroblast strains from each patient, three key parameters of DNA repair were determined, namely colony-forming ability, DNA repair synthesis, and DNA-incising capacity (Fig. 1). *Colony-forming ability* reflects overall (or total) DNA repair capacity, including DNA excision repair, postreplication repair, and "SOS" functions – provided human fibroblasts are capable of activating such functions. *DNA repair synthesis* monitors the first three steps of the excision cascade. *DNA-incising capacity* (Thielmann et al. 1985; Popanda and Thielmann 1988) represents the ability of a cell

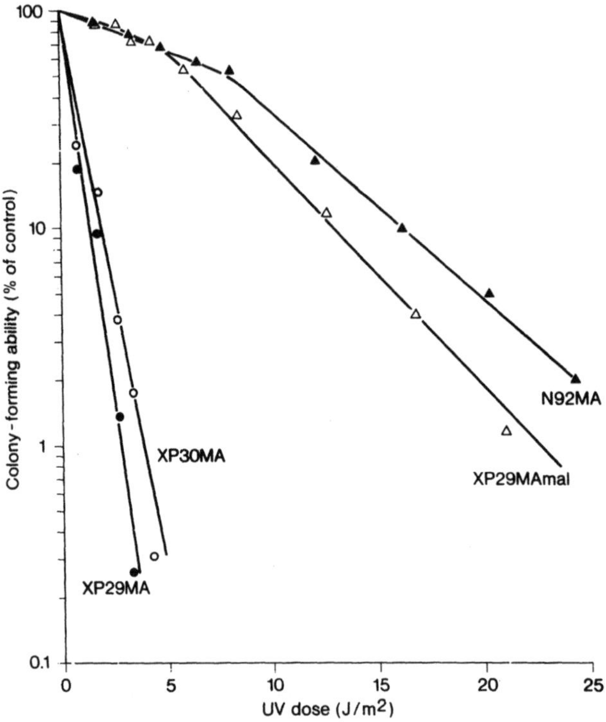

Fig. 2. Colony-forming ability of normal and XP fibroblast strains as a function of the UV dose. *XP29MA*, *XP30MA*, representatives of the Mannheim XP Collection with a strong repair defect; *N92MA*, normal control strain; *XP29MAmal*, malignant derivative of XP29MA

strain to carry out the very first step of the excision repair cascade in a dose-dependent fashion.

Dr. Edler, the biostatistician at the Cancer Research Center, strongly advised us not to restrict the analyses to single determinations but to establish dose–response relationships throughout. The reason for proceeding in this fashion was quite obvious: the more dose levels we included into an experimental series, the more accuratly the dose–response relationship could be measured. Dose–response experiments were therefore performed without exception, the resulting curves were analyzed by linear regression, and the slope of each regression line was used as the characteristic term for the whole dose–response experiment: the term D_o for overall or total DNA repair, G_o for DNA repair synthesis, and E_o for the DNA-incising capacity.

First, we determined *overall* or *total repair*. Figure 2 shows typical curves: colony-forming ability as a function of the UV dose. As a general feature, normal repair-competent fibroblasts give rise to flat curves, while repair-deficient XP fibroblasts yield steep curves because they are not able to

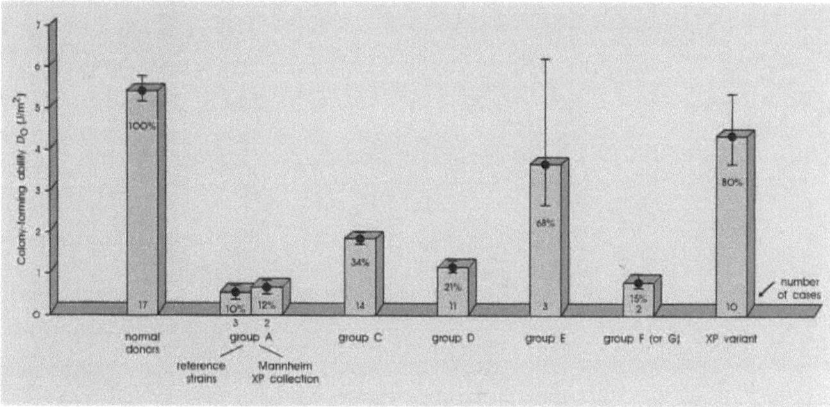

Fig. 3. Colony-forming ability, D_o, of fibroblast strains of the Mannheim XP Collection after UV irradiation. The *height of the columns* represents the weighted means of the XP complementation groups; *bars* reflect 95% confidence limits. *Numbers* at the *base* of *columns* designate the number of XP cases investigated. *Numbers* in the *middle* of *columns* express the weighted mean (as a percentage) of an XP complementation group

restore their damaged DNA to the level of integrity required for unrestrained cell proliferation.

The slope of the linear portion of the curve, called D_o, served as a measure of total repair.

Figure 3 shows a comparison of total repair capacity of all XP strains investigated. To obtain an appropriate control, post-UV D_o values of 17 normal fibroblast strains were averaged by calculating the weighted mean. This mean was set at 100%. Analogously, D_o values of all XP strains which belonged to distinct complementation groups were averaged and the resulting weighted means expressed as a percentage of the control. It can be seen from the Fig. 3 that XP group A has the strongest defect in overall repair (only 10% of that of normal controls), followed by groups F (or G; 15%), D (with 21% residual repair), C (34%), and E (68%), and the XP variant strains (80%).

From these results the question arose whether the observed reductions in overall repair were due to a defect in damage excision of the same magnitude (see Fig. 1 for repair mechanisms operating in a eukaryotic cell). To check for this possible connection, *dose-dependent DNA repair synthesis* was determined. As mentioned, this parameter monitors the first three reactions of the excision repair cascade, namely DNA incision, excision, and DNA repolymerization (Fig. 4). The analytical method chosen was the autoradiographic quantitation of thymidine which was incorporated during a 3-h repair interval after UV irradiation (see Fig. 5).

Again, for reasons of experimental accuracy, dose–response experiments were performed. However, evaluation of the results necessitated counting of

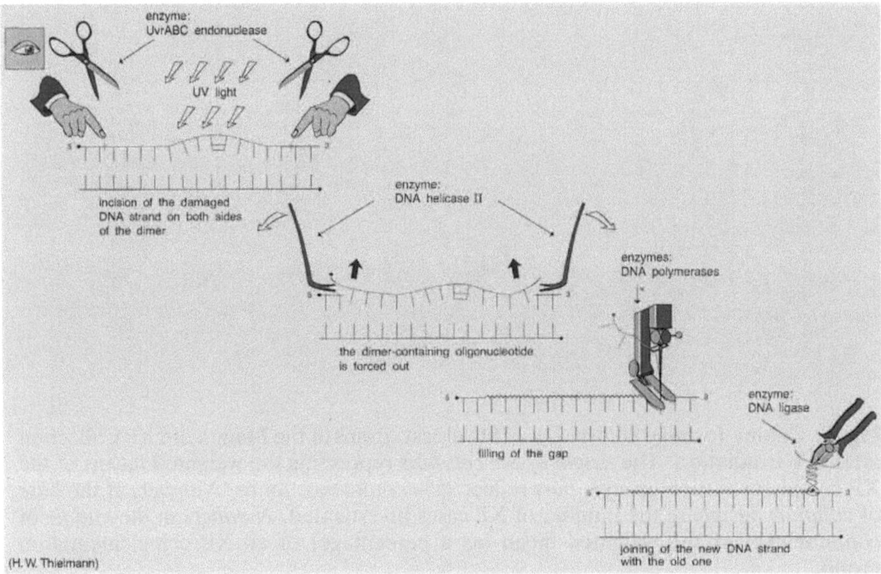

Fig. 4. Cascade of excision repair of UV-induced pyrimidine dimers in human fibroblasts, as inferred from available information on *Escherichia coli*

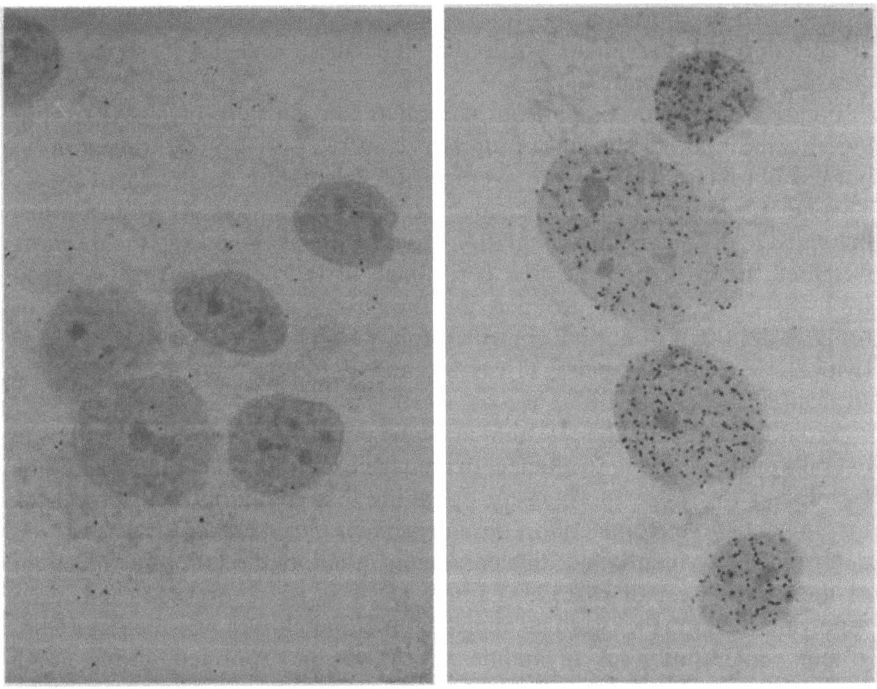

Fig. 5. Autoradiographic quantitation of thymidine (silver grains over fibroblast nuclei) incorporated during a 3-h repair interval after UV irradiation (dose 8 J/m^2). *Left*, XP12BE (complementation group A); *right*, normal control strain

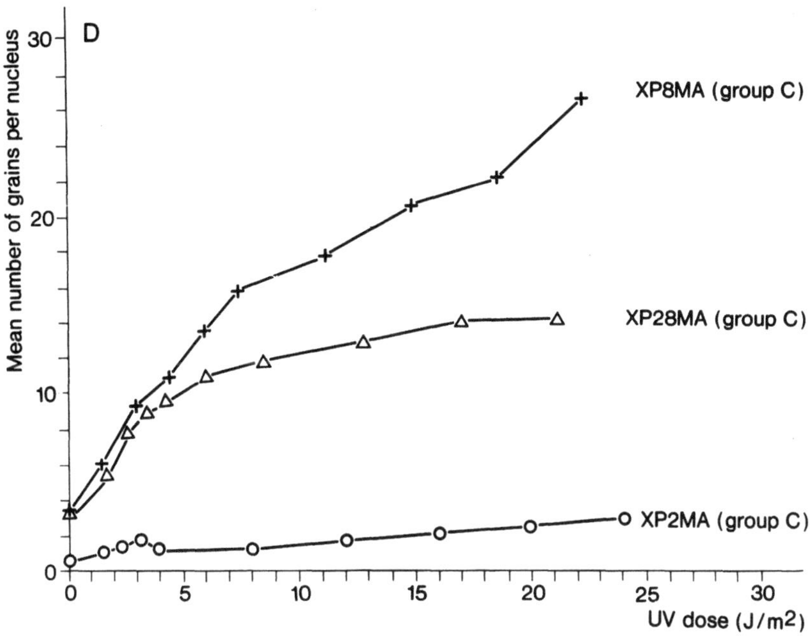

Fig. 6. DNA repair synthesis (expressed as the mean number of grains per nucleus) in XP group C fibroblast strains as a function of the UV dose

the number of grains over a 100 fibroblast nuclei for each UV dose. Since one dose–response experiment included 10 UV dose levels, 1000 fibroblast nuclei had to be evaluated to obtain one of the curves shown in Fig. 6.

Regression analysis yielded the slope of the regression line, and from this slope the comprehensive term G_o was deduced. G_o is the relative measure of DNA excision repair of a particular fibroblast strain. As in the case of colony-forming ability, the absolute G_o values of 18 normal control strains were averaged by calculating the weighted mean. This mean was set at 100% (see column "control" in the second row of Fig. 7). Compared with this control, XP groups A and F (or G) again have the strongest repair defect, followed by groups C, D, and E, and the XP variant strains. Comparison of total repair (columns in the foreground) with damage excision (columns in the background) shows that reduction of both parameters, D_o and G_o, was practically identical for all complementation groups, except for group D. Thus, the conclusion is justified that the defects observed in total repair capacity were quantitatively due to the poor functioning of the first three steps of the DNA excision repair cascade.

Again, the question may be asked: Were these reductions in both total repair and DNA repair synthesis caused by an impaired DNA-incising capacity, impaired even to the same extent? To check for this relationship,

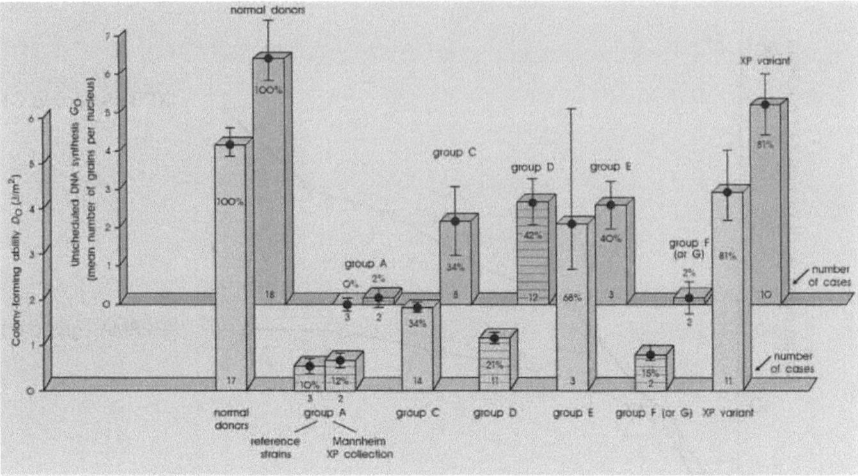

Fig. 7. Colony-forming ability, D_o (columns in the *foreground*), and DNA repair synthesis, G_o (columns in the *background*), of fibroblast strains of the Mannheim XP Collection after UV irradiation. For further details, see legend to Fig. 3

repair-specific incisions in the genome were measured for all XP fibroblast strains, applying a wide range of UV doses. The technique of alkaline elution served as analytical tool (Kohn et al. 1976).

The curves shown in Fig. 8a represent the primary elution data of a normal strain. In accordance with theoretical principles, elution velocity is inversely related to the length of the DNA fragments (Kohn et al. 1976). Repair-proficient fibroblasts exhibit a characteristic pattern: the higher the UV dose, the more enzyme-catalyzed strand breaks were introduced into genomic DNA and, consequently, the smaller in size the DNA fragments became (after denaturation in alkali). XP cells responded to UV irradiation in the fashion depicted in Fig. 8b. Since almost no DNA eluted from the filters, DNA-incising activity must have been very low.

To obtain a precise quantitation of the incision performance of a cell strain, the initial velocities of the elution curves were normalized by converting them to enzyme-catalyzed breaks per 10^6 nucleotides, by means of reference cells in which (in separate experiments) a defined number of DNA breaks had been introduced with γ-radiation (Thielmann et al. 1985; Popanda and Thielmann 1988). After this conversion, breaks were plotted against the UV dose (Fig. 9). By doing so, we obtained dose–response curves and calculated the regression lines. The slopes of these lines were called E_o, which is our measure of the DNA-incising capacity of a cell strain; it includes the information residing in 10 dose-dependent elution curves (Thielmann et al. 1985; Popanda and Thielmann 1988).

It should be mentioned that DNA incision is a very complex reaction. In the eukaryotic nucleus, genomic DNA doesn't hang around like a telephone

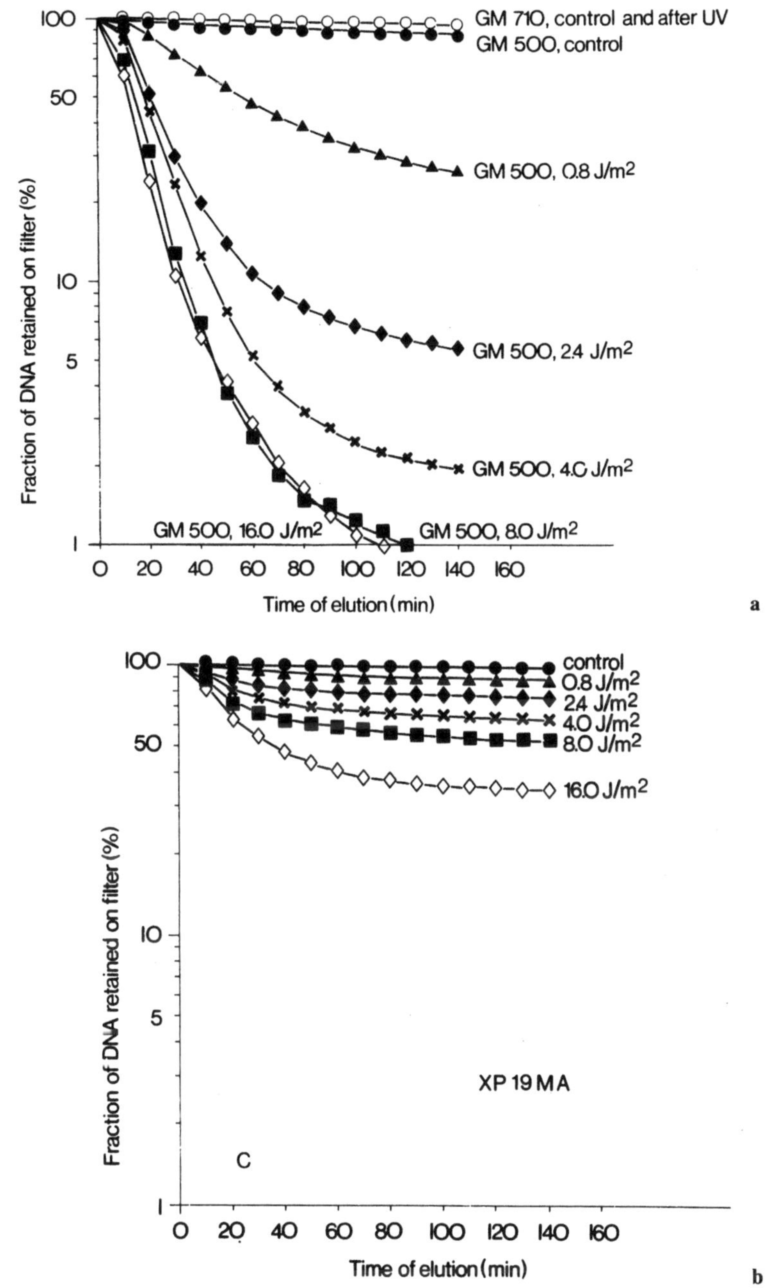

Fig. 8a,b. Alkaline elution profiles of DNA from **a** a normal fibroblast strain (strain GM500) and **b** an XP strain (XP19MA, complementation group D) after irradiation of cells with the indicated doses of UV light

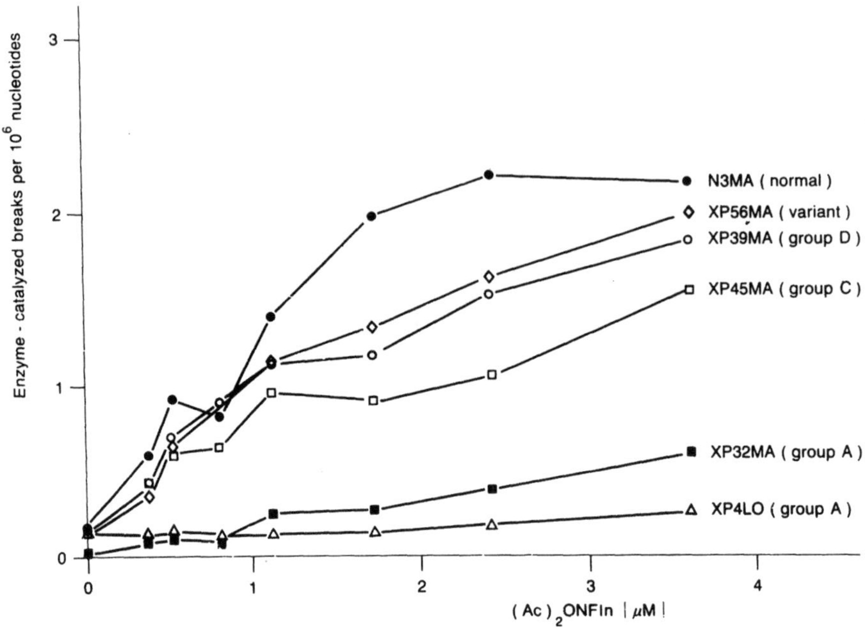

Fig. 9. Dose–response curves representing induction of enzyme-catalyzed single-strand breaks per 10^6 nucleotides in normal and XP fibroblasts as a function of the concentration of *N*-acetoxy-2-acetylaminofluorene. Very similar results were obtained when cells were exposed to UV light

wire, but is densely packed into nucleosomes and interphase chromosomes (Saenger 1984a). If DNA near damaged sites is to be incised, in order to elicit excision repair, the chromatin architecture must be loosened, nucleosomes must disintegrate, and histones must be detached from DNA, otherwise the damaged sites will not become accessible to excision repair enzymes (Lieberman 1982). In building up chromatin, DNA overwinds when coiling around the histone octamer, and this toroidal strain occurring in DNA is relaxed enzymically. Therefore, DNA freed of histones (see Fig. 10) must be negatively supercoiled with abot −1⅛ supercoil turns per nucleosome (Saenger 1984b). The coiled structure might be a bad substrate for repair enzymes.

To facilitate damage excision, topoisomerase II could have the function of relaxing superhelical DNA, rendering it a good substrate for repair enzymes. In fact, we found that DNA incision in UV-exposed fibroblasts – XP and normal alike – was inhibitable with inhibitors of topoisomerase II, such as *m*-AMSA, coumermycin, and novobiocin (Thielmann et al. 1991b). Figure 11 shows alkaline elution curves reflecting UV-irradiated normal cells in the absence (control) and presence of the topoisomerase II inhibitor

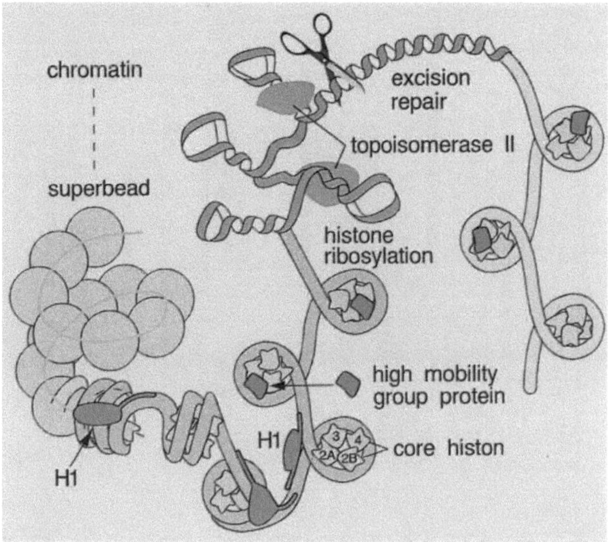

Fig. 10. Exposure of damaged DNA sites through disintegration of chromatin architecture. (Adapted from Saenger 1984b)

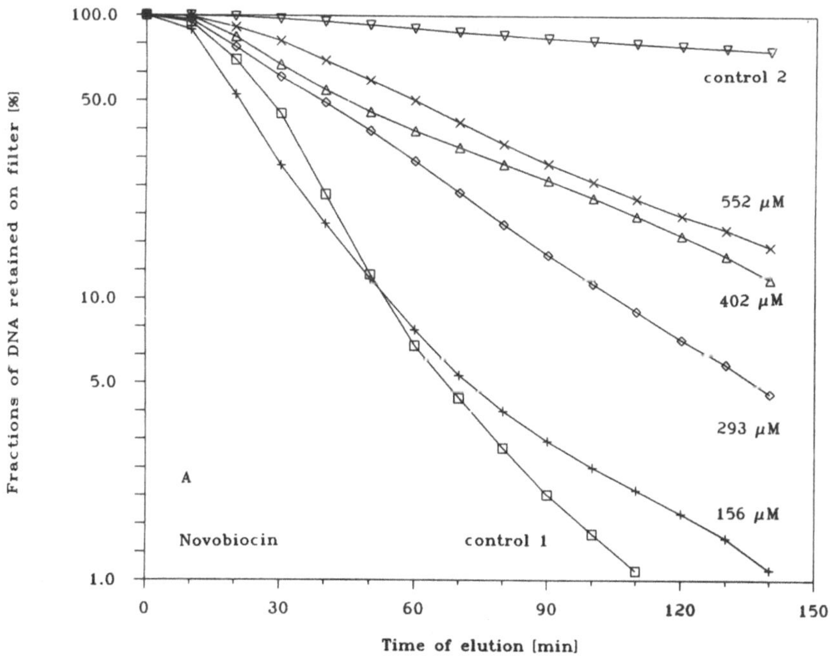

Fig. 11. Alkaline elution profiles of normal fibroblasts (strain N143MA) treated with UV light and the topoisomerase II inhibitor novobiocin. Cells of control 1 were UV-irradiated but not exposed to the inhibitor; cells of control 2 were not irradiated but treated with 552 μM novobiocin

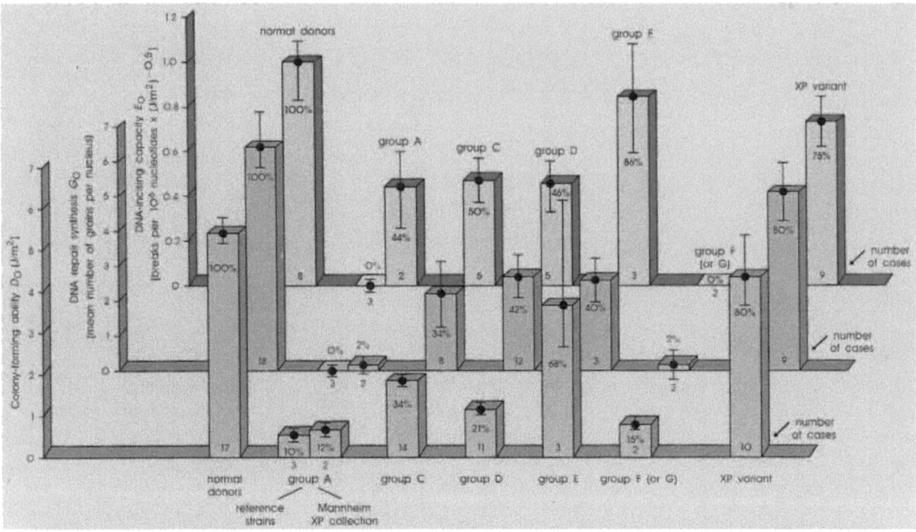

Fig. 12. Colony-forming ability, D_0 (columns in the *foreground*), DNA repair synthesis, G_0 (columns in the *middle row*), and DNA-incising capacity, E_0 (columns in the *background*) of fibroblast strains of the Mannheim XP Collection after UV irradiation. The *height of the columns* represents the weighted means of the XP complementation groups; *bars* reflect 95% confidence limits. *Numbers* at the *base* of *columns* designate the number of XP cases investigated. *Numbers* in the *middle* of *columns* express the weighted mean (as a percentage) of an XP complementation group

novobiocin. One can see that increasing novobiocin concentrations stepwise lower elution velocity. The effect may be explained by assuming that the step preceding DNA incision, namely relaxation of superhelical DNA by topoisomerase II, was inhibited. As a consequence, incision itself could not take place.

It is worth noting that the same inhibitors of topoisomerase II (including mitoxantrone and doxorubicin) decreased post-UV DNA repair synthesis in saponin-permeabilized human fibroblasts – again, in both normal ones and XP. For further data, the reader is referred to Popanda and Thielmann (1991). All data considered, it seems that topoisomerase II *does* play a role in excision repair.

Turning back to the DNA-incising capacity of XP cell strains, we can compare (Fig. 12) both total repair (columns in the first row) and excision repair (columns in the middle row) with DNA-incising capacity (columns in the last row) of representatives of various XP complementation groups. We can see that reduction of both weighted means of D_0 and G_0 values (columns in the first and second rows) is paralleled by a reduction of the weighted means of the DNA-incising capacity (columns in the last row) of similar magnitude and, therefore, must be due to a defective incision step. The only exceptions are two group A cases of the Mannheim XP Collection.

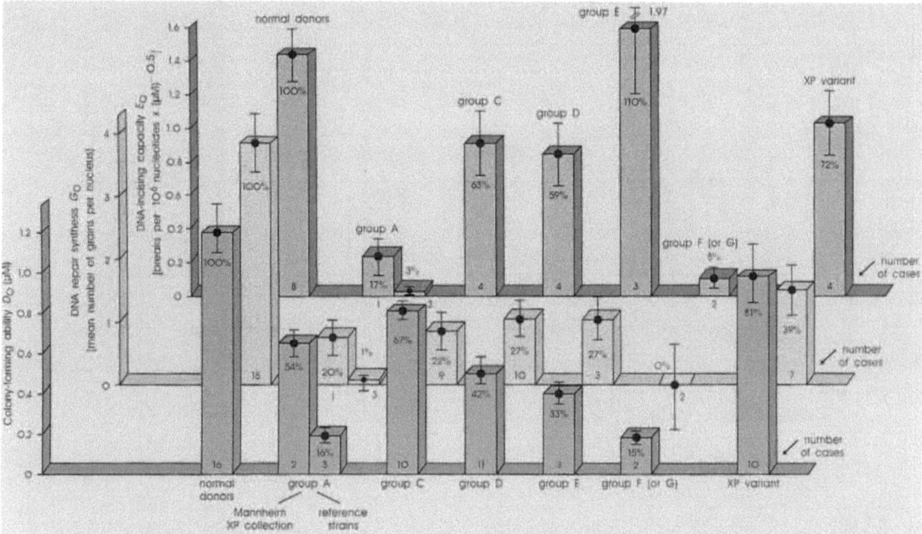

Fig. 13. Comparison of D_o (columns in the *foreground*), G_o (columns in the *middle row*), and E_o (columns in the *background*) of XP fibroblast strains of the Mannheim XP Collection after treatment with the ultimate carcinogen *N*-acetoxy-2-acetylaminofluorene. *Numbers* on columns are as in Fig. 12

Surprisingly, the 10 XP variant strains show a decrease in the weighted means of all three DNA repair parameters by 20%, and it is quite clear that reduction of the DNA-incising capacity is responsible for a similar decrease in the two other repair parameters. We are aware that this result contradicts the literature. According to the literature, XP variants are not defective in excision but in postreplication repair, i.e., in gene product(s) required for replication beyond the damaged sites (Cleaver et al. 1981).

We furthermore asked whether the mechanisms which excise UV-induced pyrimidine dimers were identical with those which remove DNA adducts formed by "UV-like" carcinogens such as *N*-acetoxy-2-acetylaminofluorene. Both DNA modifications have in common that they cause steric distortions and localized denaturation of the double helix (Thielmann and Hecht 1980) which extent over a distance of several nucleotides adjacent to the modified base residues. We repeated the series of experiments described above, but using *N*-acetoxy-2-acetylaminofluorene instead of UV light and obtained results (Fig. 13) which were similar to those shown in Fig. 12. In general, the corresponding D_o, G_o and E_o values after treatment with *N*-acetoxy-2-acetylaminofluorene were found to match those after UV irradiation.

Again, reductions in both total repair (columns in the foreground) and DNA repair synthesis (columns in the middle row) were mainly due to defective DNA-incising capacity (columns in the background). However, there were exceptions (for detailed data, see Thielmann et al. 1991a), one of which may be briefly described in order to demonstrate that from a rigorous

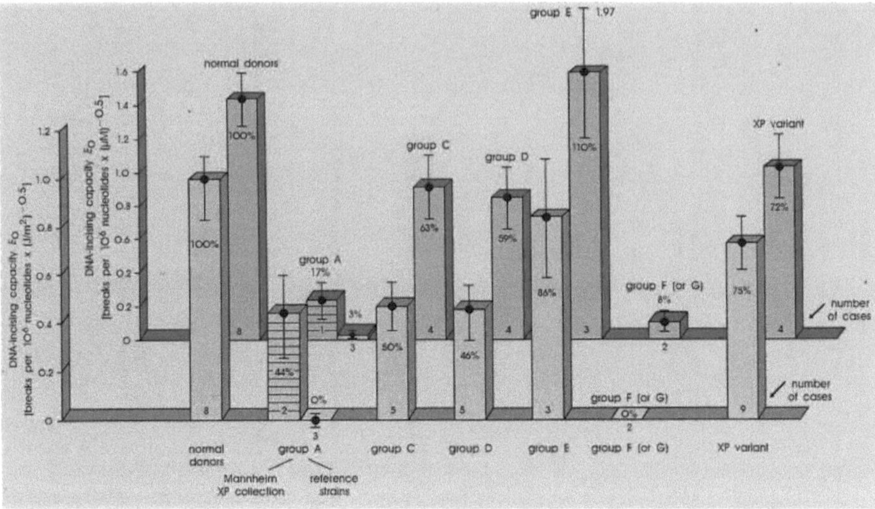

Fig. 14. DNA-incising capacities, E_o, of XP fibroblast strains of the Mannheim XP Collection after irradiation with UV light (columns in the *foreground*) or *N*-acetoxy-2-acetylaminofluorene (columns in the *background*). Designations are as in Fig. 12

comparison of the DNA repair parameters evidence can be deduced as to the enzymology of repair mechanisms. As Fig. 13 shows, XP group E was perfectly able to incise DNA damaged with *N*-acetoxy-2-acetylaminofluorene, but was very defective in DNA repair synthesis. These data strongly hint at impaired DNA excision of carcinogen-modified nucleotides (enzymes: DNA helicases or exonucleases) and/or gap filling (enzymes: DNA polymerases δ or ε) in XP group E cell strains.

Interesting is a comparison of the DNA-incising capacities of fibroblast strains from various XP complementation groups after UV irradiation (Fig. 14, columns in the background) and after treatment with *N*-acetoxy-2-acetylaminofluorene (columns in the foreground). From Fig. 14 it is obvious that reductions in the DNA-incising capacities of XP complementation groups are the same, irrespective of whether cell strains were irradiated or treated with the carcinogen (Popanda and Thielmann 1988). There is only one exception in group A. Therefore, we may conclude that the same excision repair mechanisms which remove pyrimidine dimers excise – to a large extent – DNA adducts formed by UV-like carcinogens (Fig. 15).

Regarding overall repair after treatment with methyl methanesulfonate, the weighted mean D_o values of XP complementation groups did not reveal higher sensitivity towards this alkylating carcinogen than that of controls (Fig. 16) (Thielmann et al. 1986). However, when *N*-methyl-*N*-nitrosourea was used as repair-challenging carcinogen, the weighted mean of six XP group D strains was found to be lowered by 27% (see Fig. 16) (Thielmann et al. 1986).

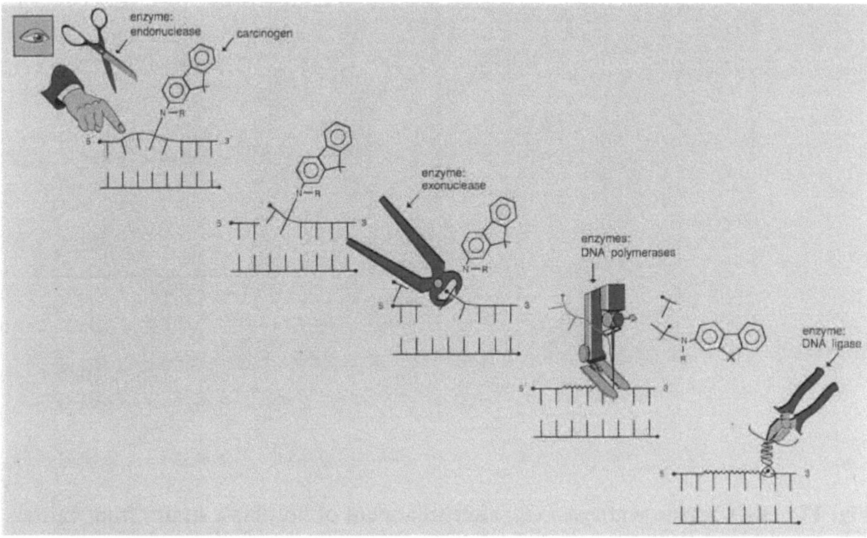

Fig. 15. Steps in a hypothetical excision repair cascade by which *N*-acetoxy-2-acetylaminofluorene/DNA adducts are removed from genomic DNA of human fibroblasts.

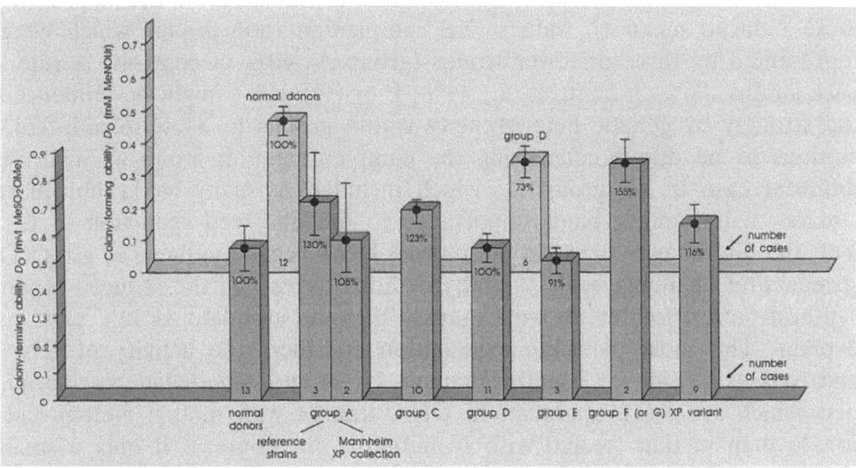

Fig. 16. Colony-forming ability, D_o, after treatment of fibroblast strains from various XP complementation groups with methyl methanesulfonate (columns in the *foreground*) or *N*-methyl-*N*-nitrosourea. For the meaning of the *numbers* on columns, see legend to Fig. 12

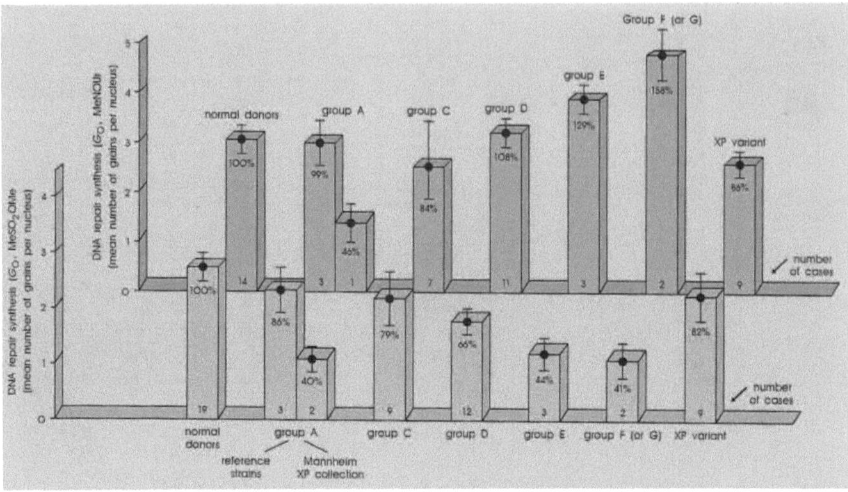

Fig. 17. DNA repair synthesis, G_o, after treatment of fibroblast strains from various XP complementation groups with methyl methanesulfonate (columns in *foreground*) or *N*-methyl-*N*-nitrosourea (columns in *background*). For further details, see legend to Fig. 12

By contrast, DNA repair synthesis was normal in all XP complementation groups after treatment with *N*-methyl-*N*-nitrosourea but exhibited considerable reductions after methyl methanesulfonate treatment. When appraising these reduced mean G_o values, XP complementation groups which were represented by three or fewer strains (group A, 40% of controls; A reference strains, 86% of controls; E, 44%; F or (G) 41%) might be influenced too strongly by genetic heterogeneity within groups to allow reliable conclusions to be drawn concerning the complementation group as such. A different case is XP group D, which included as many as 11 fibroblast strains; their number lends importance to the observed reduction in G_o. Yet, the discrepancy between the normal DNA repair synthesis in group D strains after challenge with *N*-methyl-*N*-nitrosourea and the reduced repair synthesis after treatment with methyl methanesulfonate is not easy to explain. The most plausible explanation considers the activity of DNA glycosylases specific for 7-methylguanine, 1-, 3-, and 7-methyladenine (products which are more abundant in DNA treated with methyl methanesulfonate than in that treated with *N*-methyl-*N*-nitrosourea). If only a small shortage of DNA glycosylases exists in XP cell strains it could have manifested in decreased DNA repair synthesis.

Treatment with *N*-methyl-*N*-nitrosourea revealed normal DNA excision repair synthesis but reduced overall repair. This hints at defective mechanisms other than excision repair or at impaired 6-methylguanine-DNA methyltransferase activity.

The biochemical and clinical data may be summarized as follows (see also Thielmann et al. 1991a): All three repair parameters, D_o, G_o, and

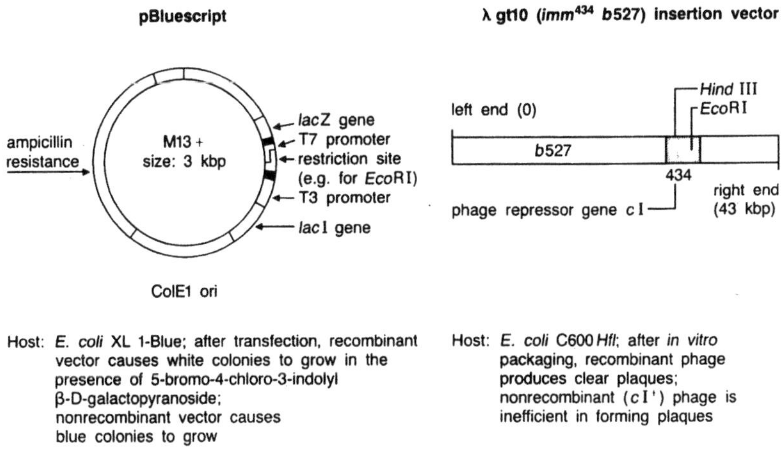

Fig. 18. Vectors λgt10 and pBluescript which were used for constructing cDNA libraries from a normal and various XP cell strains

E_o, correlated in the first approach with the clinical XP symptoms of the patients, in particular with the age at onset of the dermatological abnormalities and the age at which the first benign and malignant tumors occurred. However, the severity of the symptoms is (of course) not simply a function of the DNA-incising capacity, but is influenced by other factors as well: compensating repair mechanisms, since it was apparent that in some XP strains total repair (D_o values) exceeded DNA-incising capacity (E_o values) (see, e.g., XP group F (or G) in Fig. 12), and individual sunlight exposure.

Still, at present, the best biochemical explanation of the clinical symptoms of our XP cases is that there is a more or less defective incision of genomic DNA damaged either by UV light or "UV-like" chemical carcinogens. These findings are not entirely new. In no way is the Mannheim XP Collection the first study on XP, but we have acquired the biochemical data on DNA repair in a way that makes the underlying enzymology amenable to biostatistical analyses.

Differences in gene expression occur between normal and XP fibroblast strains. The genetic heterogeneity of the basic defect of XP was demonstrated by somatic cell hybridization (de Weerd-Kastelein et al. 1972), which resulted in the establishment of at least seven XP subforms (for literature, see Cleaver 1990). These genetically and biochemically distinct subgroups indicate that several gene products are involved in the repair of UV-damaged DNA and that mutations at different loci within repair genes can cause defective repair, which leads to the clinical state of XP. In principle, defective repair genes could be expressed in XP cells at levels different from those of

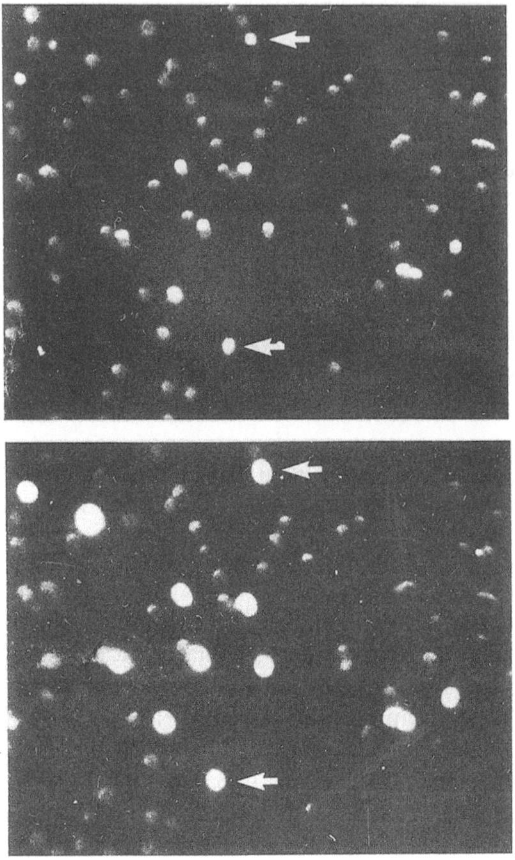

a

b

Fig. 19a,b. Detection of cDNA clones in the λgt10 library from XP89MA (complementation group D) after hybridization with radiolabelled in vitro transcripts of the pBluescript library from a normal fibroblast strain (**a**) and that of XP89MA (**b**). Second round of hybridization. Contact prints (identical exposure) of two replica filters are shown. *Arrows* point to identical sites on the autoradiographs

normal cells. Therefore, we set out to check for differences in gene expression using the technique of differential hybridization of complementary (c)DNA libraries (Lu and Werner 1988; Lu et al. 1990). These libraries were constructed from RNA of normal and XP strains in two vectors, λgt10 and pBluescript (Thielmann et al. 1991c) (Fig. 18).

XP strains included one representative of the complementation groups A, C, and D, and one XP variant strain. From each XP λgt10 cDNA library, about 16000 clones were differentially screened in that plaque lifts were hybridized with in vitro transcripts made from cDNA in the pBluescript vector from (1) the same XP strain (example: Fig. 19b) and (2) the normal control strain (Fig. 19a). With this analysis, eight different clones were

Table 2. Intensity of signals obtained by cDNA Southern hybridization with radiolabeled inserts of different clones

cDNA of λgt10 plaque	Size of insert (bp)	Signal intensities				Sequence characteristics
		XP12BE (XP group A)	XP79MA (XP group C)	XP89MA (XP group D)	XP13MA (XP variant)	
A1	1567	+	+	+	+	subunit I of cytochrome *c* oxidase
A4	192	+	+	+	+	mitochondrial 16S rRNA
A7	281	+	+	+	+	mitochondrial 16S rRNA
C13	1127	=	+	=	=	apocytochrome *b*
C14	1127	−	+	=	−	apocytochrome *b*
D1	1889	+	+	+	+	subunit I of cytochrome *c* oxidase
D5	1309	+	+	+	+	subunit I of cytochrome *c* oxidase
D8	2300	=	=	+	=	5′ end: pregnancy-specific β1-glycoprotein 3′ end: *Kpn*I element

Symbols: XP cDNA hybridization signals of higher (+), equal (=), or lower (−) strength than that of cDNA from the normal strain N17MA.

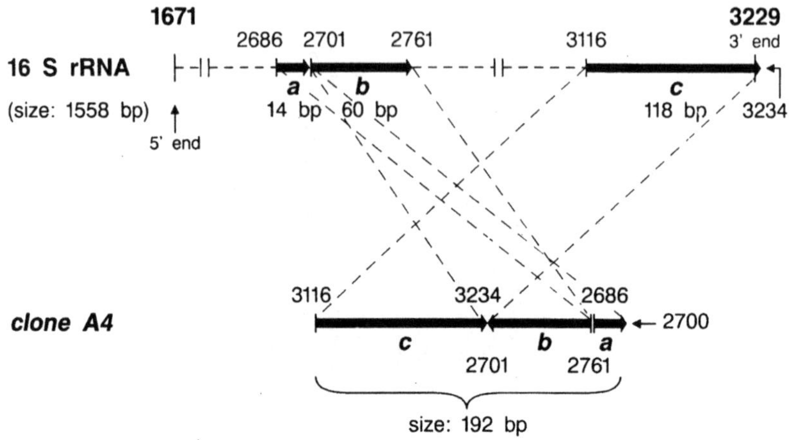

Fig. 20. Evidence that one of the isolated differential clones (clone A4, see Table 2) reflects the transcript of a rearranged mitochondrial 16 S rRNA gene. Alignment of the 192 nucleotides of clone A4 with the mitochondrial genome as present in the data base libraries resulted in 100% homology between two sections of the A4 sequence: (1) nucleotides 1–118 (*c*; see *lower part* of the figure) matched with positions 3116–3229 of the mitochondrial 16S rRNA gene (*upper part* of the figure), including, beyond its 3′ end, four bases of the tRNA^{Leu} gene; (2) nucleotides 177–192 (*a*; *lower part* of the figure) yielded perfect homolgy with the mitochondrial 16S rRNA gene at positions 2685–2700. The remaining part of A4, nucleotides 119–176 (section *b*), which could not be aligned with the human mitochondrial sequence in the above-described aligning procedure, was reversed and the complementary sequence again aligned with the sequence of the mitochondrial genome. This step revealed 100% homology with the mitochondrial 16S rRNA gene at positions 2762–2705

detected which caused stronger signals when probed with transcripts from XP strains than with those from the normal strain (Thielmann et al. 1991c).

The cDNA clones were sequenced and identified using data base libraries. Table 2 summarizes the results. Seven of the eight clones detected coded for three mitochondrial genes, for subunit I of cytochrome *c* oxidase (overexpressed in complementation groups A, C, D, and XP variant), for apocytochrome *b* (a subunit of complex III of the respiratory chain), and for mitochondrial 16S ribosomal (r)RNA. In addition, the sequences of two clones representing essentially (1) subunit I of cytochrome *c* oxidase and (2) 16S rRNA diverged from the sequence of the human mitochondrial genome present in the data base libraries (accession number: V00662). The first clone exhibited a transition mutation in that T was found to be replaced with C at position 7080, corresponding to the exchange of phenylalanine by leucine. The second clone reflected a transcript of a mitochondrial genome rearranged in the 16S rRNA gene.

The upper part of Fig. 20 shows the normal 16S rRNA gene. The cloned sequence, however, (lower part of the figure) is pieced together of small sections of the original gene, which lay either in positions distant from each other (sequences "b" and "c") or have reversed their orientation (sequence "b"). It is obvious that a complicated rearrangement must have taken place in the mitochondrial gene to yield the peculiar cDNA sequence depicted in Fig. 20.

Mutations in, and overexpression of, mitochondrial genes tell us that something must be wrong with the mitochondria in XP. The mutant genes hint at impaired functions of the respiratory chain and impaired protein synthesis due to totally altered mitochondrial 16S rRNA. Consequently, the overexpression of mitochondrial genes which we found in XP strains may indicate that the XP cell is trying hard to compensate for a functional deficit.

This situation is reminiscent of several human encephalomyopathies (for instance, hereditary optic atrophy or myoclonus epilepsy) which are known to result from mutant mitochondria (diMauro et al. 1985; Wallace 1986; Morgan-Hughes et al. 1988; Harding et al. 1990). For example, the cause of hereditary optic atrophy is a mutation in the mitochondrial dehydrogenase gene by which the arginine in position 340 is converted to histidine (Wallace et al. 1988; Singh et al. 1989). Encephalomyopathies are characterized by several neurologic symptoms which also occur in XP, including reduced intelligence, deafness, and ataxia (Rosing et al. 1985; diMauro et al. 1986; Petty et al. 1986; Harding et al. 1988), and the neurologic symptoms are progressive as in XP.

On the basis of our data we are thus tempted to conclude that defective mitochondria may be responsible for the neurologic symptoms of XP.

Acknowledgements. This work was done in collaboration with Prof. Dr. E.G. Jung, Department of Dermatology, Mannheim Medical School. Experiments on gene expression were part of the doctoral thesis of M. Rothe, University of Heidelberg, and were carried out in collaboration with Prof. Dr. D. Werner, Institute of Cell and Tumor Biology, German Cancer Research Center, Heidelberg.

References

Cleaver JE (1990) Do we know the cause of xeroderma pigmentosum? Carcinogenesis 11:875–882

Cleaver JE, Greene AE, Coriell LL, Mulivor RA (1981) Xeroderma pigmentosum variants. Cytogenet Cell Genet 31:188–192

de Weerd-Kastelein EA, Keijzer W, Bootsma D (1972) Genetic heterogeneity of xeroderma pigmentosum demonstrated by somatic cell hybridization. Nature New Biol 238:80–83

DiMauro S, Bonilla E, Zeviani M, Nakagawa M, DeVivo DC (1985) Mitochondrial myopathies. Ann Neurol 17:521–538

Harding AE, Petty RKH, Morgan-Hughes JA (1988) Mitochondrial myopathy: a genetic study of 71 cases. J Med Genet 25:528–535

Harding AE, Holt IJ, Cooper JM, Schapira AHV, Sweeney M, Clark JB, Morgan-Hughes JA (1990) Mitochondrial myopathies: genetic defects. Biochem Soc Trans 18:519–522
Jung EG (1986) Xeroderma pigmentosum. Int J Dermatol 25:629–633
Kohn KW, Erickson LC, Ewig RAG, Friedman CA (1976) Fractionation of DNA from mammalian cells by alkaline elution. Biochemistry 15:4629–4637
Lieberman MW (1982) Alterations in chromatin structure during DNA excision repair. Basic Life Sci 20:303–314
Lu X, Werner D (1988) Construction and quality of cDNA libraries prepared from cytoplasmic RNA not enriched in poly(A)$^+$ RNA. Gene 71:157–164
Lu X, Dengler J, Rothbarth K, Werner D (1990) Differential screening of murine ascites cDNA libraries by means of in vitro transcripts of cell-cycle-phase-specific cDNA and digital image processing. Gene 86:185–192
Morgan-Hughes JA, Schapira AHV, Cooper JM, Clark JB (1988) Molecular defects of NADH-ubiquinone oxidoreductase (complex I) in mitochondrial diseases. J Bioenerg Biomembr 20:365–382
Petty RKH, Harding AE, Morgan-Hughes JA (1986) The clinical features of mitochondrial myopathy. Brain 109:915–938
Popanda O, Thielmann HW (1988) Comparison of DNA-incising capacities in fibroblast strains from the Mannheim XP collection after treatment with N-acetoxy-2-acetylaminofluorene and UV light. J Cancer Res Clin Oncol 114:459–467
Popanda O, Thielmann HW (1991) Do DNA topoisomerases play a role in the repair of UV-induced DNA damage in human fibroblasts? J Cancer Res Clin Oncol [Suppl II] 117:S76
Rosing HS, Hopkins LC, Wallace DC, Epstein CM, Weidenheim K (1985) Maternally inherited mitochondrial myopathy and myoclonic epilepsy. Ann Neurol 17:228–237
Saenger W (1984a) Principles of nucleic acid structure. Springer, Berlin Heidelberg New York, p 443 (Springer advanced texts in chemistry)
Saenger W (1984b) Principles of nucleic acid structure. Springer, Berlin Heidelberg New York, p 449 (Springer advanced texts in chemistry)
Singh G, Lott MT, Wallace DC (1989) A mitochondrial DNA mutation as a cause of Leber's hereditary optic neuropathy. N Engl J Med 320:1300–1305
Thielmann HW, Hecht R (1980) Electrophoretic mobility of PM2 DNA treated with ultimate chemical carcinogens or with ultraviolet light. J Cancer Res Clin Oncol 96:243–257
Thielmann HW, Edler L, Popanda O, Friemel S (1985) Xeroderma pigmentosum patients from the Federal Republic of Germany: decrease in post-UV colony-forming ability in 30 xeroderma pigmentosum fibroblast strains is quantitatively correlated with a decrease in DNA-incising capacity. J Cancer Res Clin Oncol 109:227–240
Thielmann HW, Edler L, Friemel S (1986) Xeroderma pigmentosum patients from Germany: repair capacity of 45 XP fibroblast strains of the Mannheim XP collection as measured by colony-forming ability and unscheduled DNA synthesis following treatment with methyl methanesulfonate and N-methyl-N-nitrosourea. J Cancer Res Clin Oncol 112:245–257
Thielmann HW, Popanda O, Edler L, Jung EG (1991a) Clinical symptoms and DNA repair characteristics of xeroderma pigmentosum patients from Germany. Cancer Res 51:3456–3470
Thielmann HW, Popanda O, Edler L (1991b) The effects of inhibitors of topoisomerase II and quinacrine on ultraviolet-light-induced DNA incision in normal and xeroderma pigmentosum fibroblasts. J Cancer Res Clin Oncol 117:19–26
Thielmann HW, Rothe M, Werner D (1991c) Enhanced expression of mitochondrial genes in xeroderma pigmentosum fibroblast strains from various complementation

groups. Sixth symposium of the Section of Experimental Cancer Research (SEK) of the German Cancer Society, Heidelberg, 10–12 April 1991. J Cancer Res Clin Oncol [Suppl] 117:B27
Wallace DC (1986) Mitochondrial genes and disease. Hosp Pract 21:77–92
Wallace DC, Singh G, Lott MT, Hodge JA, Schurr TG, Lezza AMS, Elsas II LJ, Nikoskelainen EK (1988) Mitochondrial DNA mutation associated with Leber's hereditary optic neuropathy. Science 242:1427–1430

The In Vitro Analysis of Biochemical Changes Relevant to Skin Carcinogenesis

S.H. Yuspa, K. Punnonen, E. Lee, H. Hennings, J. Strickland, C. Cheng, A. Glick, and A. Dlugosz

Laboratory of Cellular Carcinogenesis and Tumor Promotion, Division of Cancer Etiology, National Cancer Institute, Bethesda, MD 20892, USA

Phenotypic Changes in Skin Carcinogenesis

The phenotypic alterations produced in mouse skin cells during the multistage development of squamous cancer have been well documented. In normal skin, all proliferating cells are confined to the basal cell compartment where less than 10% of the cells are in S phase when pulse-labeled with DNA precursors. Two keratins, K5 (M_r 60000) and K14 (M_r 55000), are transcribed largely in basal cells, although the proteins persist in the upper layers (Roop et al. 1988). The commitment to differentiate is associated with the loss of proliferative potential, the commencement of suprabasal migration, and the expression of two suprabasal keratins, K1 (M_r 67000) and K10 (M_r 59000) in the first spinous cell layer (Roop et al. 1988). Proliferating cells do not express K1 or K10 in normal epidermis. As cells migrate into the granular cell layer, K1 and K10 transcripts diminish and the genes for filaggrin, a M_r 27000 interfilamentous matrix protein, and loricrin, a major component of the cornified envelope, are activated and the proteins synthesized (Mehrel et al. 1990; Roop et al. 1989).

In benign tumors produced by chemical initiation and promotion (papillomas), the number of proliferating cells is increased ten fold, and the expression of K5 and K14 is extended into the suprabasal compartment. The abundance of K1 and K10 transcripts and proteins is reduced although the tissue distribution remains suprabasal (Roop et al. 1988). The expression of K1 and K10 is delayed, and transcripts for these genes are rare in the first few suprabasal layers of papillomas. Some papilloma cells which express K1 or K10 are capable of proceeding through S phase as indicated by the incorporation of BrdU into nuclei of K1-positive cells after pulse labeling (Huitfeldt et al. 1991). Thus papilloma cells are hyperproliferative and display an altered response to signals which in normal cells trigger the early transcription of differentiation-specific genes and inhibit proliferation.

Recent Results in Cancer Research, Vol. 128

The expression of keratinocyte-specific differentiation markers in carcinomas is highly disturbed (Roop et al. 1988). K14 protein and transcripts are diffusely expressed in carcinomas while protein and transcripts for K1 and K10 are essentially absent. Both loricrin and filaggrin are greatly diminised in carcinomas, and transcripts for these markers are in low abundance. The near absence of detectable transcripts and protein for suprabasal keratins, loricrin, and filaggrin provides a marker for malignant conversion in the mouse skin carcinogenesis model. In addition, carcinomas express keratins, such as K13 and K19, which are never expressed in normal skin but are characteristic of internal epithelia (Nischt et al. 1988). By contrast, the proliferation rate (as measured by labeling index) in carcinomas is similar to that of papillomas (Burns et al. 1976) suggesting that the changes in differentiation-related gene expression are central to the conversion phenotype.

Analysis of the Benign Neoplastic Phenotype In Vitro

Considerable insight regarding the regulation of normal skin growth and differentiation has evolved from studies of keratinocytes in cell culture (Yuspa et al. 1989b). Extracellular Ca^{2+} is a major determinant of the differentiation state of epidermal cells. In medium containing 0.05 m*M* Ca^{2+}, keratinocytes have a basal cell phenotype, whereas in medium containing 0.12 m*M* Ca^{2+}, the suprabasal markers are induced in a process regulated transcriptionally (Yuspa et al. 1989b). The expression of suprabasal markers induced by Ca^{2+} is coordinated in a temporal sequence similar to that seen in skin in vivo (Yuspa et al. 1989b). When extracellular Ca^{2+} is >0.3 m*M*, the expression of the suprabasal markers is reduced, but cultured keratinocytes stop proliferating and form cornified envelopes, the latter event being a consequence of activation of the envelope crosslinking enzyme, epidermal transglutaminase (Lichti and Yuspa 1988). Epidermal cells from initiated skin and benign or malignant skin tumors, as well as cells exposed to chemical carcinogens in vitro, are resistant to the induction of differentiation by Ca^{2+} in vitro (Yuspa et al. 1989a). This has formed the basis for a method to select for cells with the neoplastic phenotype (Yuspa and Morgan 1981) and is consistent with a defect in the response to differentiation signals as a fundamental change in neoplastic transformation of skin cells (Yuspa 1985).

Activation of the ras^{Ha} oncogene is an early event in skin carcinogenesis and highly associated with the acquisition of the benign phenotype (Balmain and Brown 1988). When the v-ras^{Ha} oncogene is introduced into normal cultured mouse basal keratinocytes (0.05 m*M* Ca^{2+}) by a defective retroviral vector, the proliferation rate of the cultured population increases five fold (Yuspa et al. 1983), consistent with the hyperproliferation seen in benign tumors. Furthermore, the infected cells are resistant to terminal differentiation in >0.1 m*M* Ca^{2+} medium, although the proliferation rate is markedly reduced at the elevated concentrations of Ca^{2+} (Yuspa et al. 1985). Transfer of v-*ras*^{Ha} keratinocytes from culture to a prepared skin graft bed produces papillomas on recipient mice (Roop et al. 1986), consistent with the complete initiating activity of this single genetic change.

Further analyses of v-*ras*^{Ha} keratinocytes have indicated that the expression of both protein and messenger (m)RNA for the suprabasal differentiation markers is inhibited in 0.12 m*M* Ca^{2+} medium. However, the switch to higher Ca^{2+} medium is associated with expression of two new keratins, K8 and K18 (Cheng et al. 1990). Previously, K8 was shown to be expressed in SV40 immortalized human keratinocytes (Morris et al. 1985) and transiently in developing human hair follicles (Dale and Holbrook 1987). These results are consistent with a Ca^{2+}-dependent change in the program of epidermal gene expression in these initiated cells.

Biochemical Pathways Involved in Differentiation of Normal Epidermis and v-*ras*^{Ha} Keratinocytes

The expression of differentiation markers in cultured keratinocytes is tightly linked to specific changes in intracellular Ca^{2+} (Ca_i), phosphatidylinositol (PI) metabolism (Jaken and Yuspa 1988; Lacal et al. 1987), and protein kinase C activation. However, the immediate Ca_i response to a change in extracellular Ca^{2+} is identical in control and v-*ras*^{Ha} keratinocytes when measured by digital image analysis of changes in fluorescence of the Ca^{2+}-sensitive dye Fura 2 (Kruszewski et al. 1991). Sustained Ca_i responses over a 24-h measurement period are also nearly identical for v-*ras*^{Ha} and control keratinocytes. A pharmacologically induced increase in Ca_i caused by exposure to 6.5 μ*M* ionomycin did not restore expression of differentiation markers in v-*ras*^{Ha} cells but did cause the cells to cornify and slough from the culture dish (Kruszewski et al. 1991). This suggests that the lack of marker expression in v-*ras*^{Ha} cells is not due to a resetting of the Ca_i requirements for gene activation to a higher level. Together, these results indicate that a direct alteration in Ca_i response does not account for the influence of v-*ras*^{Ha} on keratinocyte gene expression.

In other cell types, the *ras*^{Ha} oncogene can influence PI metabolism, probably by virtue of its G protein character (Fleischman et al. 1986; Huang et al. 1988; Lacal et al. 1987). Whether this is specific to *ras* oncogenes and germane to their transforming activity is in dispute. However, G proteins and likely to be essential in the activation of the phospholipase C, which regulates PI metabolism. The relevance of PI metabolism to the differentiation of keratinocytes (Hennings et al. 1989; Jaken and Yuspa 1988; Ziboh et al. 1984) suggests that alterations in this pathway via *ras*^{Ha} activation could be important in producing the initiated phenotype. Introduction of the v-*ras*^{Ha} gene into normal keratinocytes increases basal levels of inositol phosphates and diacylglycerols (DAG) over controls in 0.05 m*M* Ca^{2+},

Table 1. Basal levels of diacylglycerols (DAG) and inositol phosphates are elevated in neoplastic keratinocytes

	Normal	v-*ras*^{Ha}	308	SP-1
DAG	100 ± 8	233 ± 15	638 ± 100	530 ± 70
Inositol phosphates	100 ± 7	311 ± 5	210 ± 22	295 ± 14

The results have been expressed as a percentage of the control value, mean ± SEM, $n = 3$. The amount of diacylglycerols was analyzed using a diacylglycerol kinase assay (Preiss et al. 1987), and that of the inositol phosphates was measured using perchloric acid extraction together with high-pressure liquid chromatography analysis of the metabolites (Lee and Yuspa 1991a).

indicating a greater steady-state rate of PI metabolism (Table 1). PI turnover is increased even further when the cells are switched to 0.12 m*M* or 1.4 m*M* Ca^{2+} (Lee and Yuspa 1990). Similar changes in inositol phosphates and DAG levels were measured in benign neoplastic keratinocytes which have a mutated and activated c-*ras*^{Ha} gene (Table 1; Lee and Yuspa 1991b). The activity of DAG as an endogenous ligand and activator of protein kinase C (PKC) suggests that this enzyme system could be disturbed by the activation of the *ras*^{Ha} oncogene.

Significance of Protein Kinase C in the Development of the Benign Phenotype

p21^{ras}-mediated alterations in phospholipid metabolism have been associated with altered PKC function in several systems, presumably as a result of increased DAG levels. Evidence suggesting either PKC activation (Huang et al. 1988; Lacal et al. 1990; Vaidya et al. 1991) or downregulation (as a result of chronic stimulation by DAG) (Haliotis et al. 1990; Weyman et al. 1988; Wolfman and Macara 1987; Wolfman et al. 1987) has been presented for different cell types in which an activated *ras* gene was expressed. PKC is an important regulator of epidermal differentiation since the PKC activator 12-*O*-tetradecanoylphorbol-13-acetate (TPA) induces epidermal transglutaminase activity and stimulates the production of cornified envelopes, two markers of terminal differentiation (Yuspa et al. 1982). Furthermore, treatment of cultured keratinocytes with TPA prevents the expression of K1 and K10, loricrin, and filaggrin in response to Ca^{2+} (Dlugosz et al. 1990; Molloy and Laskin 1987). PKC-mediated signaling is altered in v-*ras*^{Ha} keratinocytes and neoplastic keratinocyte cell lines since the cells do not cornify in response to TPA, and marker expression in response to Ca^{2+} is constitutively inhibited (Cheng et al. 1990; Hennings et al. 1987). It is unclear whether these changes are related to chronic activation or downregulation of PKC.

Eight biochemically distinct isoforms of PKC have been described: PKC α, β_I, β_{II}, γ, δ, ε, ζ, and η (Kikkawa et al. 1989; Osada et al. 1990). Since PKC isozymes are functionally heterogeneous, the specific pattern of isozymes expressed in a cell or tissue is likely to determine responsiveness to exogenous PKC activators or endogenous diacylglycerols. To evaluate the effects of *ras* gene activation on PKC expression in cultured keratinocytes, transcripts encoding each of the isoforms were quantified by northern blot analysis. $Poly(A)^+$-enriched RNA was isolated from cultured primary mouse keratinocytes, v-ras^{Ha} keratinocytes, and the two benign neoplastic cell lines 308 and SP-1. In all keratinocytes examined, transcripts encoding PKC, α, δ, ε, ζ, and η were detected, with quantitative changes seen for several isoforms in neoplastic cells. A major difference between v-ras^{Ha} keratinocytes and normal cells is the increased abundance of PKC η mRNA in v-ras^{Ha} cells when cultured in 0.12 m*M* Ca^{2+} medium. SP-1 cells, but not 308 cells, also exhibit a Ca^{2+}-dependent enhancement of PKC η transcript levels. As reliable antibody probes become available for identifying the individual PKC isoforms, we will extend our analysis to the protein level. Our present results at the mRNA level indicate that expression of individual isozymes may be altered during neoplasia in mouse keratinocytes.

Results of studies using the protein kinase inhibitor staurosporine provide additional evidence implicating PKC in keratinocyte differentiation, and altered PKC function as an important determinant of the neoplastic phenotype. Staurosporine was reported to preferentially inhibit PKC activity (Tamaoki et al. 1986), but subsequent reports have demonstrated a lack of selectivity among several classes of kinases (Ruegg and Burgess 1989). Staurosporine failed to block TPA-mediated differentiation of cultured primary mouse keratinocytes and itself induced morphological differentiation, epidermal transglutaminase activity, and formation of cornified envelopes (Sako et al. 1988). The similar effects of staurosporine and TPA in cultured keratinocytes suggested that the same signaling pathway was mediating responses to both agents. In support of this hypothesis, staurosporine elicited several additional responses characteristic of PKC activators, such as induction of ornithine decarboxylase activity, inhibition of ^{125}I-labeled epidermal growth factor (EGF) binding, and induction of c-*fos* mRNA (Dlugosz and Yuspa 1991). In cultures where PKC was downregulated by exposure to 60 n*M* bryostatin, staurosporine-mediated effects on ^{125}I-EGF binding and cornified envelope formation were inhibited. These data suggest that staurosporine is acting, paradoxically, as a functional PKC agonist in primary keratinocytes. Although the underlying mechanism has not been determined, the narrow effective dose range for most staurosporine-mediated PKC agonist responses (5–10 n*M*) is consistent with the existence of a specific ultimate target for this agent, perhaps one of the PKC isoforms.

Because of its ability to induce differentiation in primary keratinocytes, the response to staurosporine was examined in neoplastic 308 and SP-1 cells. Staurosporine induces epidermal transglutaminase activity and causes

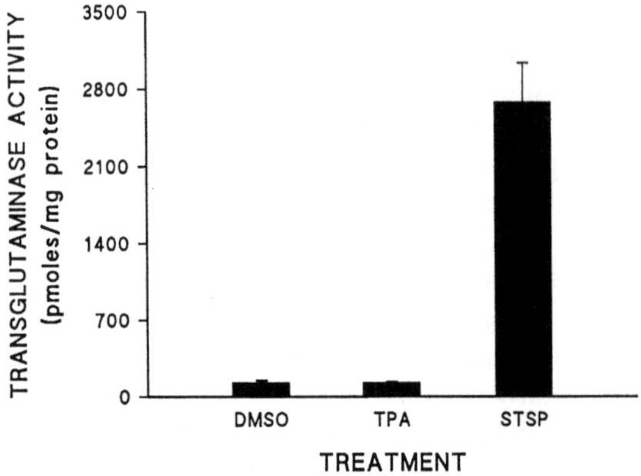

Fig. 1. Staurosporine induces epidermal transglutaminase activity in neoplastic SP-1 cells. Cells were exposed to 0.1% dimethylsulfoxide (DMSO), 160 n*M* TPA, or 10 n*M* staurosporine (*STSP*) for 24 h and keratinocyte transglutaminase activity determined by measuring covalent cross-linking of [^{3}H]putrescine to dimethylcasein (Lichti and Yuspa 1988)

cornification of neoplastic keratinocytes which are completely unresponsive to TPA (Fig. 1). Staurosporine was also effective in vivo when applied to tumors produced by grafting 308 or SP-1 cells onto the backs of nude mice (Strickland et al. 1988). Weekly application of staurosporine inhibited growth of tumors derived from both of these cell lines in a dose-dependent manner (Strickland et al. 1991), whereas TPA was ineffective. While the mechanism underlying this response has not been defined, it may be related to the unique ability of this drug to induce terminal differentiation of neoplastic keratinocytes through PKC activation.

Pharmacological Mimicry of the v-*ras*^{Ha} Phenotype

Striking changes have been described in transforming growth factor α (TGF-α) and TGF-β expression in v-*ras*^{Ha} keratinocytes (Glick et al. 1991) and these raised the possibility that an autocrine pathway was involved in the *ras*^{Ha} phenotype. Therefore, the phenotype of v-*ras*^{Ha} keratinocytes may be reproduced in normal cells by exposure to the same extrinsic factor(s). When grown in medium with 0.05 m*M* Ca^{2+}, primary keratinocytes exposed to TGF-α for 3 days were stimulated to proliferate and were morphologically similar to v-*ras*^{Ha} keratinocytes. Exposure of these cultures to higher Ca^{2+} medium indicated that TGF-α could inhibit the expression of K1 and other markers of differentiation. These results were consistent with the hypothesis that TGF-α was involved in the hyperproliferation and altered differentiation response of v-*ras*^{Ha} keratinocytes.

Despite similar changes in expression of certain phenotypic markers, TGF-α-treated primary cells were not resistant to Ca^{2+}-induced cornification and sloughing. In contrast, v-*ras*^{Ha} keratinocytes persisted in higher Ca^{2+} medium, although growth arrested, and resumed proliferation when recultured in medium with <0.10 m*M* Ca^{2+}. These observations suggested that TGF-α alone was not capable of reproducing the in vitro phenotype of v-*ras*^{Ha} keratinocytes. Since a sustained increase in inositol phosphate metabolism was an additional characteristic of neoplastic keratinocytes (Lee and Yuspa 1991b), AlF^- was used in addition to TGF-α to produce a combined effect. Cells exposed to AlF^- assume a bipolar morphology which is distinctly different from v-*ras*^{Ha} keratinocytes or normal cells treated with TGF-α. AlF^- blocked the expression of differentiation markers and terminal differentiation in response to elevated Ca^{2+} (Lee and Yuspa 1991a). However, keratinocyte growth was not stimulated by AlF^- in 0.05 m*M* Ca^{2+} medium. When combined with TGF-α, AlF^- appears to be synergistic in inducing characteristics of v-*ras*^{Ha} keratinocytes. The combination of TGF-α and AlF^- was sufficient to maintain normal keratinocytes for prolonged periods in 0.5 m*M* Ca^{2+} medium, a characteristic of v-*ras*^{Ha} keratinocytes that was not seen in response to TGF-α alone. These data suggest that cooperation between extrinsic or autocrine factors (TGFs) and intrinsic biochemical changes (increased inositol phosphate metabolism) may be involved in producing the phenotype of v-*ras*^{Ha} keratinocytes. Agents designed to counteract either of these pathways might be effective approaches to reverse benign skin neoplasms.

References

Balmain A, Brown K (1988) Oncogene activation in chemical carcinogenesis. Adv Cancer Res 51:147–182

Burns FJ, Vanderlaan M, Sivak A, Albert RA (1976) Regression kinetics of mouse skin papillomas. Cancer Res 36:1422–1427

Cheng C, Kilkenny AE, Roop D, Yuspa SH (1990) The v-ras oncogene inhibits the expression of differentiation markers and facilitates expression of cytokeratins 8 and 18 in mouse keratinocytes. Mol Carcinog 3:363–373

Dale BA, Holbrook KA (1987) Developmental expression of human epidermal keratins and filaggrin. Dev Biol 22:127–151

Dlugosz AA, Yuspa SH (1991) Staurosporine induces protein kinase C agonist effects and maturation of normal and neoplastic mouse keratinocytes in vitro. Cancer Res 51:4677–4684

Dlugosz AA, Pettit GR, Yuspa SH (1990) Involvement of Protein kinase C in Ca2+-mediated differentiation on cultured primary mouse keratinocytes. J Invest Dermatol 94:519

Fleischman LF, Chahwala SB, Cantley L (1986) ras-Transformed cells: altered levels of phosphatidylinositol-4,5-biphosphate and catabolites. Science 231:407–410

Glick AB, Sporn MB, Yuspa SH (1991) Altered regulation of TGF-beta 1 and TGF-alpha in primary keratinocytes and papillomas expressing v-Ha-ras. Mol Carcinog 4:210–219

Haliotis T, Trimble W, Chow S et al. (1990) Expression of ras oncogene leads to down-regulation of protein kinase C. Int J Cancer 45:1177–1183
Hennings H, Michael D, Lichti U, Yuspa SH (1987) Response of carcinogen-altered mouse epidermal cells to phorbol ester tumor promoters and calcium. J Invest Dermatol 88:60–65
Hennings H, Kruszewski FH, Yuspa SH, Tucker RW (1989) Intracellular calcium alterations in response to increased external calcium in normal and neoplastic keratinocytes. Carcinogenesis 10:777–780
Huang M, Chida K, Kamata N et al. (1988) Enhancement of inositol phospholipid metabolism and activation of protein kinase C in ras-transformed rat fibroblasts. J Biol Chem 263:17975–17980
Huitfeldt HS, Heyden A, Clausen OPF, Thrane EV, Roop D, Yuspa SH (1991) Altered regulation of growth and expression of differentiation-associated keratins in benign mouse skin tumors. Carcinogenesis 12:2063–2067
Jaken S, Yuspa SH (1988) Early signals for keratinocyte differentiation: role of Ca2+-mediated inositol lipid metabolism in normal and neoplastic epidermal cells. Carcinogenesis 9:1033–1038
Kikkawa U, Kishimoto A, Nishizuka Y (1989) The protein kinase C family: heterogeneity and its implications. Annu Rev Biochem 58:31–44
Kruszewski FH, Hennings H, Tucker RW, Yuspa SH (1991) Differences in the regulation of intracellular calcium in normal and neoplastic keratinocytes are not caused by *ras* gene mutations. Cancer Res 51:4206–4212
Lacal JC, de la Pena P, Moscat J, Garcia-Barreno P, Anderson PS, Aaronson SA (1987) Rapid stimulation of diacylglycerol production in Xenopus oocytes by microinjection of H-ras p21. Science 238:533–536
Lacal JC, Cuadrado A, Jones JE et al. (1990) Regulation of protein kinase C activity in neuronal differentiation induced by the N-ras oncogene in PC-12 cells. Mol Cell Biol 10:2983–2990
Lee E, Yuspa SH (1990) Keratinocytes infected with a virus containing v-ras^{Ha} have elevated inositol phosphate metabolism. Proc Am Assoc Cancer Res 31:76
Lee E, Yuspa SH (1991a) Aluminum fluoride stimulates inositol phosphate metabolism and inhibits expression of differentiation markers in mouse keratinocytes. J Cell Physiol 148:106–115
Lee E, Yuspa SH (1991b) Changes in inositol phosphate metabolism are associated with terminal differentiation and neoplasia in mouse keratinocytes. Carcinogenesis 12:1651–1658
Lichti U, Yuspa SH (1988) Modulation of tissue and epidermal transglutaminases in mouse epidermal cells after treatment with 12-O-tetradecanoylphorbol-13-acetate and/or retinoic acid in vivo and in culture. Cancer Res 48:74–81
Mehrel T, Hohl D, Rothnagel JA et al. (1990) Identification of a major keratinocyte cell envelope protein, loricrin. Cell 61:1103–1112
Molloy CJ, Laskin JD (1987) Specific alterations in keratin biosynthesis in mouse epidermis in vivo and in explant culture following a single exposure to the tumor promoter 12-O-tetradecanoylphorbol-13-acetate. Cancer Res 47:4674–4680
Morris A, Steinberg ML, Defendi V (1985) Keratin gene expression in simian virus 40-transformed human keratinocytes. Proc Natl Acad Sci USA 82:8498–8502
Nischt R, Roop DR, Mehrel T et al. (1988) Aberrant expression during two-stage mouse skin carcinogenesis of type I 47-kDa Keratin, K13, normally associated with terminal differentitation of internal stratified epithelia. Mol Carcinog 1:96–108
Osada S, Mizuno K, Saido TC et al. (1990) A phorbol ester receptor/protein kinase, $nPKC_n$, a new member of the protein kinase C family predominatly expressed in lung and skin. J Biol Chem 265:22434–22440

Preiss JE, Loomis CR, Bell RM, Neidel JE (1987) Quantitative measurement of sn-1,2-diacylglycerols. Methods Enzymol 141:294–300
Roop DR, Lowy DR, Tambourin PE et al. (1986) An activated Harvey ras oncogene produces benign tumours on mouse epidermal tissue. Nature 323:822–824
Roop DR, Krieg TM, Mehrel T, Cheng CK, Yuspa SH (1988) Transcriptional control of high molecular weight keratin gene expression in multistage mouse skin carcinogenesis. Cancer Res 48:3245–3252
Roop DR, Nakazawa H, Mehrel T et al. (1989) Sequential changes in gene expression during epidermal differentiation. In: Rogers GE, Reis PJ, Ward KA, Marshall RC (eds) The biology of wool and hair. Chapman and Hall, London, pp 311–324
Ruegg UT, Burgess GM (1989) Staurosporine, K-252 and UCN-01: potent but nonspecific inhibitors of protein kinases. Trends Pharmacol Sci 10:218–220
Sako T, Tauber AI, Jeng AY, Yuspa SH, Blumberg PM (1988) Contrasting actions of staurosporine, a protein kinase C inhibitor, on human neutrophils and primary mouse epidermal cells. Cancer Res 48:4646–4650
Strickland JE, Greenhalgh DA, Koceva-Chyla A et al. (1988) Development of murine epidermal cell lines which contain an activated rasHa oncogene and form papillomas in skin grafts on athymic nude mouse hosts. Cancer Res 48:165–169
Strickland JE, Dlugosz AA, Hennings H, Yuspa SH (1991) Staurosporine inhibits tumor formation from grafted mouse papilloma cell lines. Proc Am Assoc Cancer Res 32:127
Tamaoki T, Nomoto H, Takahashi I, Kato Y, Morimoto M, Tomita F (1986) Staurosporine, a potent inhibitor of phospholipid/Ca++ dependent protein kinase. Biochem Biophys Res Commun 135:397–402
Vaidya TB, Weyman CM, Teegarden D, Ashendel CL, Taparowsky EJ (1991) Inhibition of myogenesis by the H-ras oncogene: implication of a role for protein kinase C. J. Cell Biol 114:809–820
Weyman CM, Taparowsky EJ, Wolfson M, Ashendel CL (1988) Partial down-regulation of protein kinase C in C3H 10T1/2 mouse fibroblasts transfected with the human Ha-ras oncogene. Cancer Res 48:6535–6541
Wolfman A, Macara IG (1987) Elevated levels of diacylglycerol and decreased phorbol ester sensitivity in ras-transformed fibroblasts. Nature 325:359–361
Wolfman A, Wingrove TG, Blackshear PJ, Macara IG (1987) Down-regulation of protein kinase C and of an endogenous 80-kDa substrate in transformed fibroblasts. J Biol Chem 262:16546–16552
Yuspa SH (1985) Cellular and molecular changes during chemical carcinogenesis in mouse skin cells. In: Huberman E, Barr SH (eds) Carcinogenesis. Raven, New York, pp 201–209
Yuspa SH, Morgan DL (1981) Mouse skin cells resistant to terminal differentiation associated with initiation of carcinogenesis. Nature 293:72–74
Yuspa SH, Ben T, Hennings H, Lichti U (1982) Divergent responses in epidermal basal cells exposed to the tumor promoter 12-O-tetradecanoylphorbol-13-acetate. Cancer Res 42:2344–2349
Yuspa SH, Vass W, Scolnick E (1983) Altered growth and differentiation of cultured mouse epidermal cells infected with oncogenic retrovirus: contrasting effects of viruses and chemicals. Cancer Res 43:6021–6030
Yuspa SH, Kilkenny AE, Stanley J, Lichti U (1985) Keratinocytes blocked in phorbol ester-responsive early stage of terminal differentiation by sarcoma viruses. Nature 314:459–462
Yuspa SH, Kilkenny AE, Roop DR et al. (1989a) Consequences of exposure to initiating levels of carcinogens in vitro and in vivo: altered differentiation and growth, mutations, and transformation. In: Slaga TJ, Klein-Szanto AJP, Boutwell

RK, Stevenson DE, Spitzer HL, D'Motto B (eds) Skin carcinogenesis: mechanisms and human relevance. Liss, New York, pp 127–135
Yuspa SH, Kilkenny AE, Steinert PM, Roop DR (1989b) Expression of murine epidermal differentiation markers is tightly regulated by restricted extracellular calcium concentrations in vitro. J Cell Biol 109:1207–1217
Ziboh VA, Isseroff RR, Pandey R (1984) Phospholipid metabolism in calcium-regulated differentiation in cultured murine keratinocytes. Biochem Biophys Res Commun 122:1234–1240

Positive and Negative Growth Control in Multistage Skin Carcinogenesis

K. Brown[1], C.J. Kemp[1], P.A. Burns[1], A.B. Stoler[1], D.J. Fowlis[2], R.J. Akhurst[2], and A. Balmain[1]

[1] Beatson Institute for Cancer Research, CRC Beatson Laboratories, Bearsden, Glasgow, Scotland, UK
[2] Department of Medical Genetics, University of Glasgow Yorkhill Hospital, Glasgow, Scotland UK

Introduction

Early studies on the multistep nature of tumour formation in mouse skin were instrumental in the evolution of the present concepts of tumour initiation, promotion and progression. More recently, the application of molecular genetics to the mouse skin model has led to the identification of a number of mutational alterations in both proto-oncogenes and tumour suppressor genes which are associated with specific stages of carcinogenesis in this particular system. This article aims to review our current understanding of the genetic and biological changes implicated in mouse skin carcinogenesis.

The clonal expansion of a malignant tumour from a single normal cell is a complex process which involves the alteration and subversion of a number of different classes of gene products. The positively acting oncogenes can induce cell growth and are found to be activated constitutively in tumours, frequently as a result of mutation, gene amplification or chromosomal translocation. Tumour suppressor genes are associated with the negative regulation of growth control, and are frequently deleted or functionally inactivated in a wide variety of human and animal tumours. Genetic alterations involving both of these classes of gene products are now thought to be required before a fully malignant tumour can evolve.

Recent studies have led to the identification of a number of tumour suppressor genes (Table 1) (Stanbridge 1990). Most of the genes shown in Table 1 were identified as a consequence of the application of genetic techniques. The basis for the approaches used was the Knudson two-hit model of carcinogenesis, in which the initial recessive mutation in a tumour suppressor gene is revealed by subsequent loss of the corresponding normal allele. This loss of heterozygosity (LOH) is therefore a useful marker for the presence of a tumour suppressor gene, as illustrated in studies by Cavenee et al. (1983) who demonstrated the existence of multiple mechanisms by which loss of heterozygosity can occur in human tumours. The search for

Recent Results in Cancer Research, Vol. 128

Table 1. Tumour suppressor genes in human tumours

Gene	Locus	Neoplasm
RB1	13q	Retinoblastoma Osteosarcoma Carcinomas of breast, lung, bladder
P53	17p	Almost all tumour types
WT1	11p13	Wilms tumour
?	11p15	Wilms tumour, carcinomas, rhabdomyosarcoma
DCC	18q22	Colon carcinoma
NF1	17q11	Neurofibromatosis
FAP	5q21–22	Colon carcinoma
MEN-1	11q13	Parathyroid, pituitary, adrenal tumours
?	3p21	Lung carcinoma
?	3p12–14	Kidney carcinoma
?	1p36	Neuroblastoma

LOH in human tumours has been aided by the diverse genetic background of the human population, and consequently the rich abundance of DNA polymorphisms. The approach, however, was not applied initially to studies of multistage carcinogenesis in animal model systems. The inbred nature of most strains of rodent used in the laboratory precludes the existence of DNA polymorphisms and thus prevents the detection of LOH. We have attempted to overcome these difficulties by generating F_1 hybrid mice, either between different inbred mouse strains carrying distinct genetic polymorphisms (Bremner and Balmain 1990) or, more recently, using interspecific hybrid mice derived by crossing *Mus musculus* inbred strains with the western Mediterranean mouse *Mus spretus* (Burns et al. 1991) (Fig. 1). Since *M. musculus* and *M. spretus* diverged some 2–3 million years ago (Robert et al. 1985), F_1 hybrids display restriction fragment length polymorphisms (RFLPs) at multiple genetic loci and are consequently extremely useful for the study of tumour suppressor gene loss during chemical carcinogenesis.

The Mouse Skin Carcinogenesis Model

The main features of the classical mouse skin carcinogenesis model are depicted in Fig. 2. In this model, initiation is achieved by a single treatment of the skin with a chemical carcinogen. This is considered to result in a population of initiated cells which remain dormant until stimulated to clonally expand upon treatment with a tumour promoter such as 12-*O*-tetradecanoylphorbol-13-acetate (TPA) (Boutwell 1974). This leads to the formation of benign well-differentiated papillomas. A proportion of these papillomas then undergo further genetic changes and progress to squamous carcinomas. An additional event in this model system involves progression of squamous

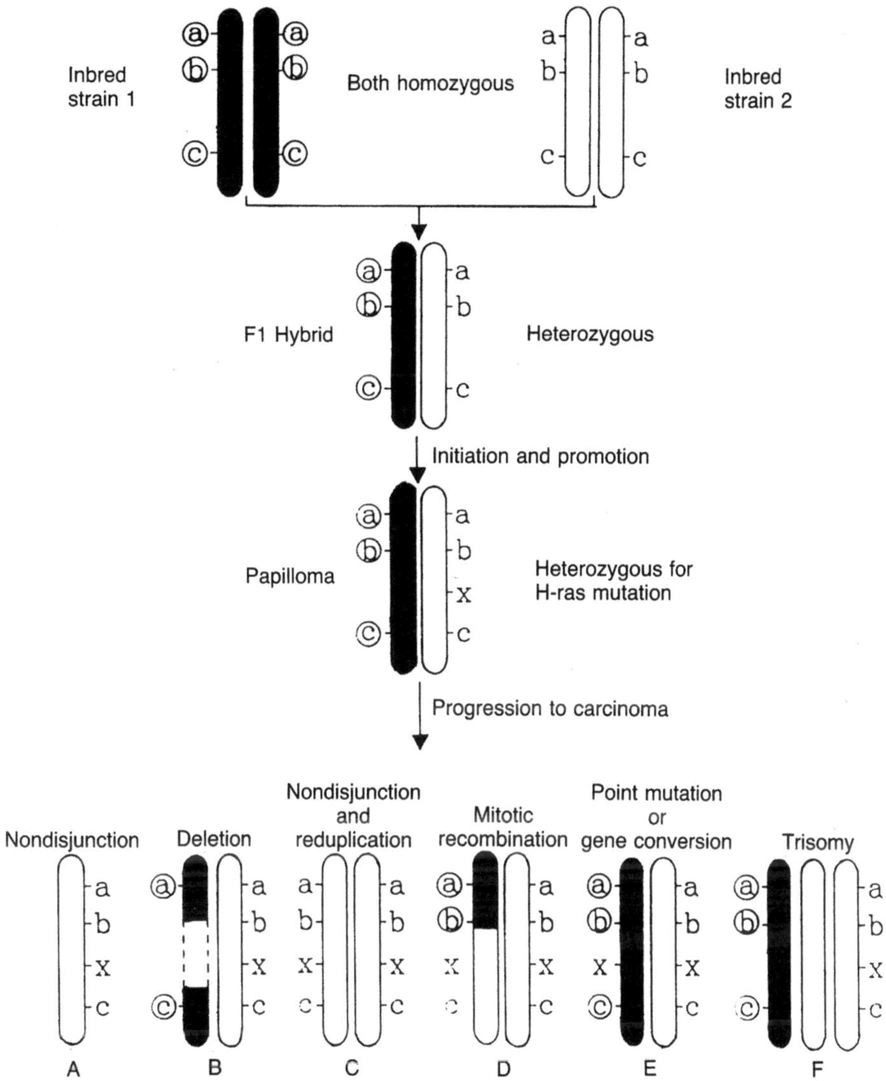

Fig. 1. The use of F_1 hybrids to characterise chromosome alterations. The example shown is for chromosome 7 from inbred strain 1 (*filled columns*) or inbred strain 2 (*open columns*). The letters *a*, *b* and *c*, denote the different alleles on chromosome 7. F_1 hybrid mice are heterozygous at each locus. *X* indicates a mutation in the Ha-*ras* gene in initiated cells, which can become hemizygous or homozygous by a variety of different mechanisms as shown

carcinomas to highly invasive undifferentiated or spindle cell carcinomas (Burns et al. 1991; Klein-Szanto et al. 1989; Buchmann et al. 1991).

The initiating event, caused by the chemical carcinogen, is in many cases the induction of a point mutation in the mouse cellular Harvey-*ras* (Ha-*ras*) proto-oncogene. The polycyclic hydrocarbon dimethylbenzanthracene

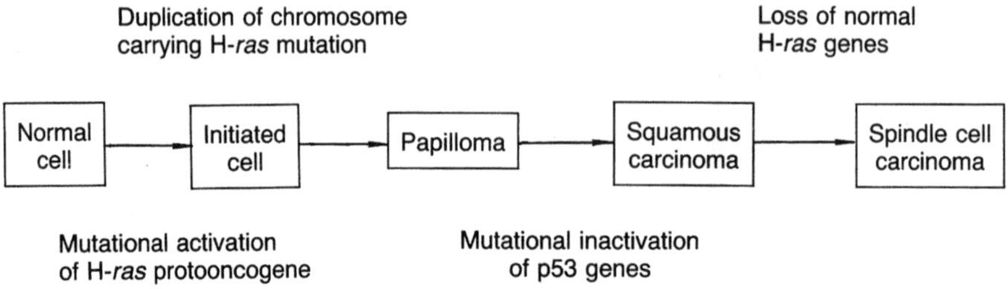

Fig. 2. Genetic alterations occurring during skin tumorigenesis. The sequence of biological events known to occur during development of skin tumours and the genetic changes detected at different stages are shown

(DMBA) gives rise to papillomas and carcinomas, a very high proportion of which show the same A→T mutation at codon 61 of the Ha-*ras* gene. Other groups have shown that DMBA extensively forms adducts with adenosine residues (S. Cheng et al. 1988), although the mechanism by which misrepair gives rise to transversion mutations of this kind is not yet known. Initiation with methylating agents such as methylnitronitrosoguanidine (MNNG) or methylnitrosourea (MNU) results in G→A mutations at codon 12 of the Ha-*ras* gene (Brown et al. 1990). A similar mutation has been observed in a number of other systems (Zarbl et al. 1985), and is thought to be the due to methylation on the O^6 position of guanosine by the carcinogen, inducing misrepair during subsequent rounds of DNA replication (Toorchen and Topal 1983). On the other hand, the carcinogen methylcholanthrene induces tumours carrying a G→T transversion mutation at codon 13 of the same target gene. The fact that the structurally different mutagenic agents give rise to tumours several months later, which nevertheless carry mutations specific for the initiating agent used, lends a great deal of support to the idea that the mutations in fact occurred at the time of treatment with the chemical initiator (for reviews, see Barbacid 1987; Balmain and Brown 1988). The equivalence of Ha-*ras* gene mutations and the initiation of skin tumorigenesis has been supported by experiments in which application of retroviruses carrying mutant Ha-*ras* genes to mouse skin or cells in culture substitutes for carcinogen treatment (Brown et al. 1986; Roop et al. 1986). More recent experiments have shown that transgenic mice harbouring mutant *ras* oncogenes which are expressed under the control of skin-specific promoters induce the formation of benign tumours (Bailleul et al. 1990). In the latter experiments the *ras* transgene was under the control of the promoter element from a keratin which is normally expressed only in terminally differentiating keratinocytes. The formation of papillomas in such transgenic mice suggests that post-commitment cells in the basal layer or suprabasal compartment can be among the target cells for chemical initiation. Indeed, it has been found that terminally differentiating human keratinocytes can be rescued from senescence by the immortalising adenovirus EIA gene product (Barrandon et al. 1989), and are potentially capable of further transformation.

Further changes either in the mutant Ha-*ras* gene copy number and/or expression are observed during tumour progression (Bremner and Balmain 1990; Quintanilla et al. 1986; B. Jandrig et al., unpublished observations). Ha-*ras* expression levels would appear to alter in a stepwise fashion, progressively in favour of the mutant allele. These changes in threshold expression levels of mutant *ras* could explain the alterations in the differentiation pattern exhibited by cells at different stages of tumorigenesis. The keratin 13 gene, normally expressed only in some internal epithelia, can be activated in papillomas expressing mutant *ras* alleles (Nischt et al. 1988; Gimenez Conti et al. 1990). The expression of mutant Ha-*ras* has been shown to induce the aberrant expression of the simple epithelial keratins K8 and K18, both in vitro (Diaz-Guerra et al. 1992; C. Cheng et al. 1990) and in vivo (M. Quintanilla et al., personal communication). Further alterations at the Ha-*ras* locus are associated with the progression of squamous cell carcinomas to spindle cell carcinomas, in which the synthesis of most of the epithelial keratins appears to be switched off, and in some cases even the simple keratins K8 and 18 are also undetectable (Diaz-Guerra et al. 1992). Spindle cells therefore represent the end of the spectrum of malignancy of epidermal keratinocytes, and are associated with over-representation of mutant *ras* alleles and/or loss of normal alleles. These are, however, not the only genes involved in this process (see below) and the identification of other important loci is an important future goal.

The Role of Tumour Suppressor Genes in Skin Tumour Progression

The interspecific *M. spretus*/*M. Musculus* hybrids are heterozygous at 70%–80% of loci examined. Consequently, their use in carcinogenesis experiments, has allowed us to apply the approach of RFLP analysis to the mouse skin model system. The recent development of polymerase chain reaction (PCR) based simple sequence length polymorphism (SSLP) has greatly increased the speed at which such analyses can be achieved (Love et al. 1990). Simple sequence repeats or microsatellites are short sequence repeats, e.g., $(AC)_n$ that are highly polymorphic in length, somatically stable and present in large numbers distributed throughout the mouse genome (Cornall et al. 1991). A large number of unique loci containing these microsatellites have now been isolated and mapped. By using a combination of these approaches (RFLP and SSLP), LOH has been examined at 25 loci covering 11 autosomes in a panel of chemically induced tumours. Markers on chromosomes 7 and 11 were frequently imbalanced or lost, whereas at least one marker on chromosomes 2, 4, 9, 12, 14, 17 and 18 retained heterozygosity in the great majority of tumours (C.J. Kemp et al., manuscript in preparation). A number of markers on chromosome 7 showed allelic imbalance in almost all papillomas and carcinomas containing mutant *ras* genes. Since the Ha-*ras* gene is on chromosome 7, these results are compatible with the trisomy of chromosome 7 seen cytogenetically (Aldaz et al. 1989). However, because of the high frequency of other changes seen on this chromosome, particularly at the *int-2* locus just distal to Ha-*ras* (Bremner and Balmain 1990), additional events involving this chromosome must also be important in tumour progression. The exact nature of these additional events is presently under study. Our previous results, showing that in some tumours, mitotic recombination had generated homozygosity at mutant Ha-*ras* alleles but retained both alleles at both *fes* and *Hbb* loci, were difficult to explain on the basis of the known map positions of these genes on chromosome 7. For this reason, we re-examined the location of Ha-*ras* in a *M. spretus*/*M. musculus* backcross and found the true location of the gene to be much closer to *int*-2 than previously thought, and in any case distal to both *fes* and *Hbb* (C.J. Kemp et al., manuscript submitted). We conclude that a gene located around the Ha-*ras*/*int-2* locus, possibly the *prad-1*/cyclin D gene which maps to this position (C.J. Kemp, unpublished results), plays an important role in tumour progression.

The tumour promoter TPA has been shown to induce a number of apparently random chromosomal changes in cells in culture and also in mouse epidermis in vivo (Furstenberger et al. 1989). The initial induction of trisomy of chromosome 7 may therefore arise as a direct consequence of TPA treatment, the trisomic cells being selected because of the increased Ha-*ras* gene dosage. In agreement with this interpretation, the non-tumour-promoting hyperplasiogenic agent retinoyl-phorbol-acetate does not induce chromosome alterations and also fails to induce papillomas after treatment of initiated mouse skin (Furstenberger et al. 1989). Thus trisomy of chromosome 7 may therefore be the equivalent of the "conversion step" postulated to be an important early event in the clonal selection of initiated cells (Furstenberger et al. 1989; Slaga 1985).

Chromosome 11 was also found to show frequent loss of heterozygosity, thought in this case the loss was observed in carcinomas but not in pre-malignant papillomas. Interestingly, the murine p53 gene is located on this chromosome. Mutational alterations of the p53 gene represent the commonest and therefore one of the most important genetic alterations yet found in human tumours. The gene codes for a nuclear phosphoprotein which appears to play a crucial role in the regulation of DNA replication. Human tumours have been found which have completely lost both p53 genes, suggesting that p53 is a tumour suppressor gene. However, other tumours appear to have mutant p53 genes which can transform cells in culture in a similar manner to classical dominant oncogenes such as Ha-*ras*.

Further studies were therefore carried out to determine whether mutational alterations of the p53 gene could be found in mouse skin tumours. Loss of alleles on chromosome 11, including the p53 allele, was found in a total of four out of 13 mouse skin carcinomas. Direct sequencing of PCR-amplified p53 alleles showed that all four carcinomas which were homozygous at the p53 locus had undergone mutational alterations (Burns et al. 1991), three of which were frameshift mutations resulting in severely truncated proteins, and the other a mis-sense mutation. Mutational alteration of p53 therefore would appear to play an important role in the development and progression of mouse skin tumours (Burns et al. 1991; A. Klein-Szanto, personal communication). The evidence to date suggests that complete loss of p53 function is associated with the transition from benign to malignant tumours, and may therefore play a role in the immortalisation of the papilloma cells, the acquisition of resistance to transforming growth factor β (TGF-β), or the loss of genetic stability which takes place at this stage of carcinogenesis.

Undifferentiated Spindle Cell Carcinomas Arise by Progression from Squamous Carcinoma Cells In Vivo

A great deal of controversy surrounds the origin of spindle cell tumours. Some pathologists consider that they arise from pre-existing squamous lesions, whereas others would categorise them as tumours of fibroblastic origin. An alteration of the ratio of mutant to normal Ha-*ras* alleles on chromosome 7 is associated with an apparent change in the morphology of tumours from the squamous to the spindle cell type (Buchmann et al. 1991). As these tumours were all initiated with DMBA, which can cause an A → T mutation at codon 61 of the Ha-*ras* gene, the mutation could conceivably have arisen independently in cells of epithelial or fibroblastic origin. We have now been able to demonstrate the squamous–spindle conversion directly using a cell line derived from a tumour which was induced in a *M. spretus*/*M. musculus* F_1 mouse by multiple treatments with DMBA. Morphologically, the line clearly showed the presence of both epithelial cells and fibroblastic cells in vitro. Single cell cloning of each cell type, followed by reinjection into nude mice, showed that the epithelial cell clone (B9) gave rise to differentiated squamous cell carcinomas whereas the fibroblastic cells formed spindle cell tumours. The clones of both cell types were shown to carry the same Ha-*ras* A → T mutation, and also the same pattern of p53 gene mutations (Burns et al. 1991). Sequence analysis showed the presence of one mutation in the *M. spretus* p53 allele, together with two independent mutations in the *M. musculus* allele, one of which was silent. Thus the pattern of four independent mutations in two genes detected in both the squamous and spindle cell types unequivocally shows that the two cell types have arisen from the same clonal origin. In addition, we conclude that the mutant p53 gene is not crucial for the progression from squamous to spindle morphology, since the mutations were present before the conversion took place. Preliminary experiments have shown that chromosome 7 alterations leading to an increase in the mutant to normal Ha-*ras* gene ratio can be detected in the spindle cell clones (Fig. 3). Experiments designed to reverse the spindle cell phenotype by expressing a transfected normal Ha-*ras* gene in a variety of spindle cells have, to date, been unsuccessful (S. Haddow et al., unpublished results). It has also not been possible to

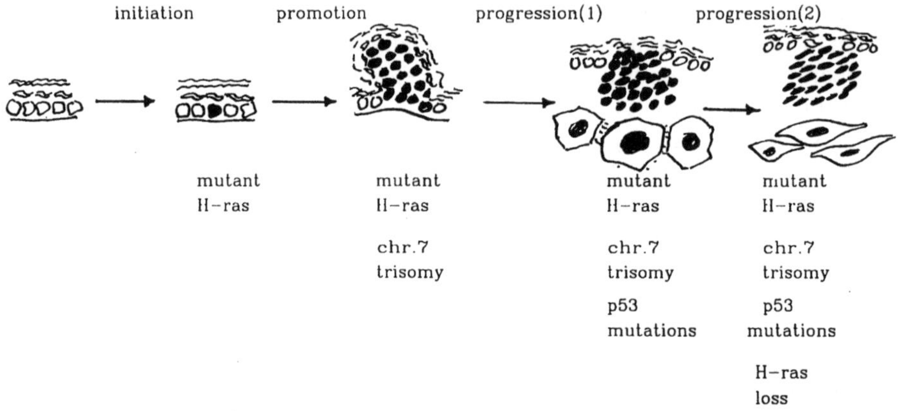

Fig. 3. Sequence of genetic events in progression and formation of the spindle cell carcinoma MSC11 the genetic events detected at each stage during

induce squamous carcinoma cells to convert to a spindle morphology by overexpression of a mutant Ha-*ras* gene, which in our hands leads to cessation of cell growth. It is therefore probable that a gene other than (or in addition to) Ha-*ras* is crucial for this particular transition.

The Spindle Cell Phenotype Is Recessive in Cell Hybrids

From the results described above, a distinct genetic alteration is associated with the progression of squamous to spindle cells. This could be a dominant event, e.g. mutation of a proto-oncogene, or a recessive change caused by loss or inactivation of a gene which controls epidermal differentiation. In an attempt to distinguish between these alternate mechanisms, we have carried out cell fusion experiments between spindle cells and a number of epidermal cell lines at different stages of carcinogenesis (A. Stoler and A. Balmain, manuscript in preparation). These include immortalised keratinocytes, papilloma cells, some of which have lost sensitivity to negative regulation by TGF-β, squamous cell carcinomas and spindle cell carcinomas. All but the spindle cell lines retain clear evidence of the expression of epithelial cell markers.

Cells from these different sources were fused to a transformed spindle-derived cell line (CarB) to form cell hybrids. The experiments showed that both immortalised cells and papillomas can suppress transformation in a spindle cell carcinoma. Tumours which did arise after a long latency were of two types, either benign epithelial cysts or well-differentiated (stage I) carcinomas. Hybrids generated with papilloma lines which had partially lost normal growth response, gave grade II carcinomas after long latency, indicating that partial reversion had occurred. The phenotype of all of these cell hybrids in vitro was that of the epithelial cell, as opposed to the spindle morphology of the tumorigenic parent. Using the squamous cell carcinoma line as the fusion parent with the spindle cells, the resulting hybrids resembled the squamous epithelial cells in both their in vivo and in vitro properties. In contrast, fusion of the spindle cell CarB with itself, or with another spindle cell carcinoma, gave rise to highly malignant hybrids with a clear spindle morphology.

Suppression of malignancy in these hybrids is therefore associated with the reestablishment of the pattern of terminal differentiation (Stanbridge 1990). A gene (or genes) which controls epidermal differentiation must be lost or functionally inactivated at this stage of skin carcinogenesis.

Negative Growth Regulation by Transforming Growth Factor β

Transforming growth factor β (TGF-β) is a potent negative growth regulator of epidermal cells (Pietenpohl et al. 1990). Previous results (Haddow et al. 1991) have shown that immortalised keratinocytes transfected with a mutant human Ha-*ras* gene and also lines derived from papillomas containing mutant Ha-*ras* genes still showed a complete inhibition of growth upon treatment with TGF-β. Some papilloma lines, however, though still non-tumorigenic had lost this response. The majority of squamous carcinomas are refractory to downregulation by TGF-β and indeed some are even slightly stimulated. It is as yet unresolved at which stage of carcinogenesis the response to TGF-β is lost, whilst the mechanistic relationships between loss of growth control and mutational alterations in proto-oncogenes or tumour suppressor genes remains completely unknown.

It appeared strange that initiated cells expressing mutant *ras* genes could still respond to TGF-β, but nevertheless underwent clonal expansion on treatment with TPA, which had previously been shown to induce high levels of TGF-β mRNA in mouse epidermis (Akhurst et al. 1988). To elucidate this apparent inconsistency, an investigation of TGF-β mRNA and protein synthesis was carried out by a combination of in situ hybridisation together with immunocytochemistry using isoform specific antibodies to TGF-β1 (Fowlis et al. 1992). TPA treatment of adult mouse skin induced TGF-β1 protein in suprabasal keratinocytes, i.e. the subpopulation of epidermal cells which had previously been shown to produce TGF-β1 mRNA (Akhurst et al. 1988). The extracellular or processed form of TGF-β1 was located mainly in the dermis, suggesting that this important regulatory protein may be involved in a paracrine mechanism of regulatory communication between epidermal and mesodermal tissues, similar to that proposed to exist in several mouse epithelia during foetal development (Lehnert and Akhurst 1988). In the context of tumour promoting activity, TGF-β could be an important mediator of the inflammatory response to TPA treatment, and/or modulate the dermal extracellular matrix to facilitate the complex series of events necessary for tissue regeneration.

The expression patterns of TGF-β in vivo in papillomas and carcinomas, induced by initiation with DMBA and promotion with TPA, were somewhat different from that seen in normal skin. Whilst both papillomas and carcinomas contained elevated levels of TGF-β_1 mRNA in the basal keratinocytes, neither the epithelial cells of the tumour nor the underlying stromal cells appeared to contain significant levels of protein. One possible explanation of this is that early tumours, though apparently still responsive to negative growth regulation by TGF-β, may evade downregulation by altered translational and/or post-translational processing of the protein. A number of other studies have indeed shown that TGF-β is subject to regulation at a number of different levels and that mRNA concentrations do not necessarily correlate with levels of protein (Glick et al. 1991; Knabbe et al. 1987). However, it should be remembered that the situation in tumours is undoubtedly extremely complex and a number of other positive and negative factors such as TGF-α or other members of the TGF-β family could also be involved.

The exact timing of the loss of growth response to TGF-β is interesting, in that it appears to precede the acquisition of fully malignant properties. Recently, the *rb* gene product has been proposed as a mediator of negative growth regulation by TGF-β in epithelial cells (Pietenpol et al. 1990; Laiho et al. 1990). However, in the mouse, as in humans, there is no evidence of *rb* being involved in the formation of skin tumours. As a significant proportion of malignant squamous carcinomas have been shown to harbour mutations in the p53 tumour suppressor gene (Burns et al. 1991; Field et al. 1991), it is possible that in epithelial tissues, negative growth regulation may be mediated by the p53 gene rather than by the *rb* gene product (Wyllie et al. 1991; H. Moses and C.C. Harris, personal communication).

Conclusions and Future Prospects

Multistage carcinogenesis in mouse skin has many similarities to tumour development in the human colon (Fearon and Vogelstein 1990). In both cases, a series of genetic events can be correlated with altered biological properties of the developing tumour cells (see Fig. 2). The advantage of the mouse model system lies in the ability to identify and isolate each stage of tumour development. Thus it has been possible to attain a greater degree of certainty as to the staging of these genetic events and to demonstrate a causal role in tumour induction. On the basis of the present evidence, we conclude that mutational activation of *ras* can be an initiating event in mouse skin carcinogenesis at least after initiation with certain chemicals. From genetic and cytogenetic studies, it is apparent that numerical chromosomal alterations take place during the promotion phase of carcinogenesis, possibly as a direct consequence of the production of DNA-damaging active oxygen species and resultant chromosomal instability induced by tumour promoters. Progression of benign tumours to squamous carcinomas involves alterations at the murine p53 locus. Possible consequences of this could be loss of responsiveness to TGF-β, or the development of the progressive aneuploidy seen in carcinomas. Interestingly, fibroblasts from Li-Fraumeni patients known to carry germline mutations in the p53 gene are genetically unstable, and accumulate alterations which appear to facilitate immortalisation in vitro (Bischoff et al. 1990).

Finally, squamous cell carcinomas can progress further to highly invasive metastatic tumours which have lost many features of epidermal differentiation. Elucidation of this step could have important consequences for our understanding of mechanisms of tumour invasion and metastasis. The recessive nature of the spindle cell phenotype suggests new approaches to the cloning of the gene(s) involved by application of reverse genetic techniques.

Acknowledgements. Our thanks to the many colleagues whose help and cooperation were invaluable in carrying out the work which is summarised in this article. The Beatson Institute is supported by generous grants from the Cancer Research Campaign of Great Britain. C.J.K. was the recipient of a Fellowship from the International Agency for Research on Cancer.

References

Akhurst RJ, Fee F, Balmain A (1988) Localized production of TGF-beta mRNA in tumour promoter-stimulated mouse epidermis. Nature 331:363–365

Aldaz CM, Trono D, Larcher F, Slaga TJ, Conti CJ (1989) Sequential trisomization of chromosomes 6 and 7 in mouse skin premalignant lesions. Mol Carcinog 2:22–26

Bailleul B, Surani MA, White S, Barton SC, Brown K, Blessing M, Jorcano J, Balmain A (1990) Skin hyperkeratosis and papilloma formation in transgenic mice expressing a ras oncogene from a suprabasal keratin promoter. Cell 62:697–708

Balmain A, Brown K (1988) Oncogene activation in chemical carcinogenesis. Adv Cancer Res 51:147–182

Barbacid M (1987) ras genes. Annu Rev Biochem 56:779–827

Barrandon Y, Morgan JR, Mulligan RC, Green H (1989) Restoration of growth potential in paraclones of human keratinocytes by a viral oncogene. Proc Natl Acad Sci USA 86:4102–4106

Bischoff FZ, Yim SO, Pathak S, Grant G, Siciliano MJ, Giovanella BC, Strong LC, Tainsky MA (1990) Spontaneous abnormalities in fibroblasts of patients with Li-Fraumeni Cancer Syndrome: aneuploidy and immortalisation. Cancer Res 50:7979–7984

Boutwell RK (1974) The function and mechanism of promoters of carcinogenesis. Crit Rev Toxicol 2:419–443

Bremner R, Balmain A (1990) Genetic changes in skin tumour progression: correlation between presence of a mutant ras gene and loss of heterozygosity on mouse chromosome 7. Cell 61:407–417

Brown K, Quintanilla M, Ramsden M, Kerr IB, Young S, Balmain A (1986) v-ras genes from Harvey and BALB murine sarcoma viruses can act as initiators of two-stage mouse skin carcinogenesis. Cell 46:447–456

Brown K, Buchmann A, Balmain A (1990) Carcinogen-induced mutations in the mouse c-Ha-ras gene provide evidence of multiple pathways for tumour progression. Proc Natl Acad Sci USA 87:538–542

Buchmann A, Ruggeri B, Klein Szanto AJ, Balmain A (1991) Progression of squamous carcinoma cells to spindle carcinomas of mouse skin is associated with an imbalance of H-ras alleles on chromosome 7. Cancer Res 51:4097–4101

Burns PA, Kemp CJ, Gannon JV, Lane DP, Bremner R, Balmain A (1991) Loss of heterozygosity and mutational alterations of the p53 gene in skin tumors of interspecific hybrid mice. Oncogene 6:2363–2370

Cavenee WK, Dryja TP, Phillips RA, Benidict WF, Godbout R, Gallie BL, Murphree AL, Strong LC, White RL (1983) Expression of recessive alleles by chromosomal mechanisms in retinoblastoma. Nature 305:779–784

Cheng C, Kilkenny AE, Roop D, Yuspa SH (1990) The v-ras oncogene inhibits the expression of differentiation markers and facilitates expression of cytokeratins 8 and 18 in mouse keratinocytes. Mol Carcinog 3:363–373

Cheng SC, Prakash AS, Pigott MA, Hilton BD, Lee H, Harvey RG, Dipple A (1988) A metabolite of the carcinogen 7,12-dimethylbenz(a)anthracene that reacts predominantly with adenine residues in DNA. Carcinogenesis 9:1721–1723

Cornall RJ, Aitman TJ, Hearne CM, Todd JA (1991) The generation of a library of PCR-analyzed microsatellite variants for genetic mapping of the mouse genome. Genomics 10:874–881

Diaz-Guerra M, Haddow S, Bauluz C, Jorcano JL, Cano A, Balmain A, Quintanilla M (1992) Expression of simple epithelial keratins in mouse epidermal keratinocytes harbouring Harvey-ras gene alterations. Cancer Res 52:680–687

Fearon ER, Vogelstein B (1990) A genetic model for colorectal tumorigenesis. Cell 61:759–767

Field JK, Spandidos DA, Malliri A, Gosney JR, Yiagnisis M, Stell PM (1991) Elevated p53 expression correlates with a history of heavy smoking in squamous cell carcinoma of the head and neck. Br J Cancer 64:573–577

Fowlis DJ, Flanders KC, Duffie E, Balmain A, Akhurst RJ (1992) Discordant TGF-b1 RNA and protein localisations during chemical carcinogenesis of the skin. Cell Growth Differ 3:81–91

Furstenberger G, Schurich B, Kaina B, Petrusevska RT, Fusenig NE, Marks F (1989) Tumor induction in initiated mouse skin by phorbol esters and methyl methanesulfonate: correlation between chromosomal damage and conversion ("stage I of tumor promotion") in vivo. Carcinogenesis 10:749–752

Gimenez Conti I, Aldaz CM, Bianchi AB, Roop DR, Slaga TJ, Conti CJ (1990) Early expression of type I K13 keratin in the progression of mouse skin papillomas. Carcinogenesis 11:1995–1999

Glick AB, Sporn MB, Yuspa SH (1991) Altered regulation of TGF-beta 1 and TGF-alpha in primary keratinocytes and papillomas expressing v-Ha-ras. Mol Carcinog 4:210–219

Haddow S, Fowlis DJ, Parkinson EK, Akhurst RJ, Balmain A (1991) Loss of growth control by TGF-β occurs at a late stage of mouse skin carcinogenesis and is independent of ras gene activation. Oncogene 6:1465–1470

Klein-Szanto AJP, Larcher F, Bonfil RD, Conti CJ (1989) Multistage chemical carcinogenesis protocols produce spindle cell carcinomas of the mouse skin. Carcinogenesis 10:2169–2172

Knabbe C, Lippman ME, Wakefield LM, Flanders KC, Kasid A, Dickson RB (1987) Evidence that transforming growth factor-beta is a hormonally regulated negative growth factor in human breast cancer cells. Cell 48:417–428

Knudson AG (1989) Epidemiology of genetically determined cancer. In: Bock G, Marsh J (eds) Genetic analysis of tumour suppression. Wiley, Chichester, pp 3–11

Laiho M, DeCaprio JA, Ludlow JW, Livingston DM, Massague J (1990) Growth inhibition by TGF-β linked to suppression of retinoblastoma protein phosphorylation. Cell 62:175–185

Lehnert SA, Akhurst RJ (1988) Embryonic expression pattern of TGF-beta 1 mRNA suggests both paracrine and autocrine mechanisms of action. Development 104:263–273
Love JM, Knight AM, McAleer MA, Todd JA (1990) Towards construction of a high resolution map of the mouse genome using PCR-analysed microsatellites. Nucleic Acids Res 18:4123–4130
Nischt R, Roop DR, Mehrel T, Yuspa SH, Rentrop M, Winter H, Scheizer J (1988) Aberrant expression during two-stage mouse skin carcinogenesis of a type I 47-kDa keratin, K13, normally associated with terminal differentiation of internal stratified epithelia. Mol Carcinog 1:96–108
Pietenpol JA, Stein RW, Moran E, Yacuik P, Schlegel R, Lyons RM, Pittelkow MR, Munger K, Howley PM, Moses HL (1990) TGF-beta 1 inhibition of c-myc transcription and growth in keratinocytes is abrogated by viral transforming proteins with pRB binding domains. Cell 61:777–785
Quintanilla M, Brown K, Ramsden M, Balmain A (1986) Carcinogen-specific mutation and amplification of Ha-ras during mouse skin carcinogenesis. Nature 322:78–80
Robert B, Barton P, Minty A, Daubas P, Weydert A, Bonhomme F, Catalan J, Chazottes D, Guenet JL, Buckingham M (1985) Investigation of genetic linkage between myosin and actin genes using an interspecific mouse back-cross. Nature 314:181–183
Roop DR, Lowy DR, Tambourin PE, Strickland J, Harper JR, Balaschak M, Spangler EF, Yuspa SH (1986) An activated Harvey ras oncogene produces benign tumours on mouse epidermal tissue. Nature 323:822–824
Slaga TJ (1985) Mechanisms involved in multistage skin tumorigenesis. Carcinog Compr Surv 10:189–199
Stanbridge EJ (1990) Human tumor suppressor genes. Annu Rev Genet 24:615–657
Toorchen D, Topal MD (1983) Mechanisms of chemical mutagenesis and carcinogenesis: effects on DNA replication of methylation at the O6-guanine position of dGTP. Carcinogenesis 4:1591–1597
Wyllie FS, Dawson T, Bond JA, Goretsky P, Game S, Prime S, Wynford-Thomas D (1991) Correlated abnormalities of transforming growth factor-β1 response and p53 expression in thyroid epithelial cell transformation. Mol Cell Endocrinol 76:13–21
Zarbl H, Sukumar S, Arthur AV, Martin-Zanca D, Barbacid M (1985) Direct mutagenesis of Ha-ras-1 oncogenes by N-nitroso- N-methylurea during initiation of mammary carcinogenesis in rats. Nature 315:382–385

The Role of Endogenous Factors in Skin Carcinogenesis

G. Fürstenberger, P. Krieg, R. Schnapke, S. Feil, and F. Marks

Research Program Tumor Cell Regulation, German Cancer Research Center, W-6900 Heidelberg, Fed. Rep. of Germany

Introduction

Based upon clinical experience Virchow introduced the concept of irritation-induced carcinogenesis in 1862 (Virchow 1863). Since then a significant body of information has been accumulated providing evidence for an intimate relationship between wounding, wound healing, and tumor development. It includes medical case reports suggesting an influence of injury or chronic irritation on human carcinogenesis (Mueller and Thornbury 1973; Sanderson and Mackie 1979) and results from several experimental models indicating that wounding, although not of itself a carcinogenic stimulus (Hasegawa et al. 1987), can act as a tumor promoter in animals exposed to initiating chemical or viral carcinogens. Thus, sarcomas develop at the site of experimental wounds in chickens infected with Rous sarcoma virus (Dolberg et al. 1985) and in v-*jun* transgenic mice (Schuh et al. 1990). Moreover, epidermal tumors arise at sites of increased mechanical stress in v-*ras* transgenic mice (Bailleul et al. 1990; Leder et al. 1990). Upon initiation with chemical carcinogens wounding induces tumor development in mouse and rat liver (Fisher and Fisher 1959: Pound and McGuirre 1978), in rat intestine (Pozharizski 1975; Chester et al. 1989), in mouse oral mucosa (Konstantinides and Smulov 1982), in rabbit ear (McKenzie and Rous 1941), and in mouse skin (Hennings and Boutwell 1970; Clark-Lewis and Murray 1978; Argyris 1980). More recently, a variety of growth factors which are produced and released in a temporarily and locally restricted manner during the wound response have been found to be constitutively expressed in tumor cells and to support tumor growth via an autocrine activation pathway (for review see Sporn and Roberts 1986; Heldin and Westermark 1989).

Recent Results in Cancer Research, Vol. 128

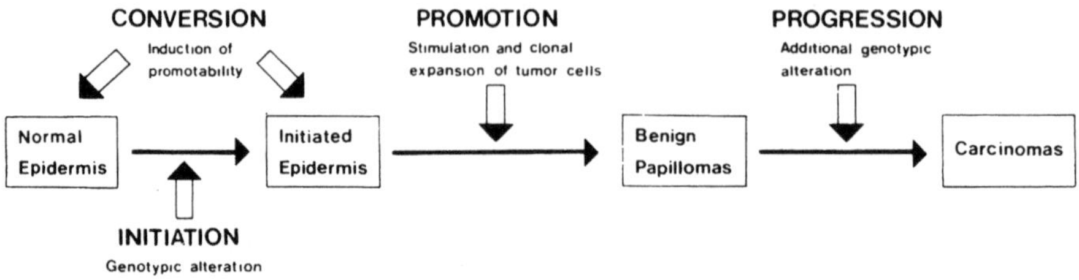

Fig. 1. Experimental multistage carcinogenesis in mouse skin. Initiation, i.e., the primary mutagenic event of carcinogenesis, does not result in tumor development unless additional processes called conversion and promotion occur. Promotion results from the chronic treatment with an incomplete tumor promoter such as 12-*O*-retinoylphorbol-13-acetate (RPA) or mezerein inducing the clonal expansion of tumor cells. Incomplete promoters are unable to promote tumor growth in initiated skin unless the tissue has been "converted" into a state of "promotability" by a short-term treatment with a complete promoter such as 12-*O*-tetradecanoylphorbol-13-acetate (TPA), wounding, or injection of TGF-α/TGF-β either prior to or after initiation. The initiation–conversion–promotion approach to mouse skin carcinogenesis results primarily in papillomas, which finally develop into carcinomas. This malignant progression can be enhanced by treatment of the papillomas with mutagenic carcinogens

Wounding Is a Converting Stimulus in the Initiation–Conversion–Promotion Protocol of Mouse Skin Carcinogenesis

Mouse skin was the first tissue where, upon preceding initiation with a chemical carcinogen, a tumor-inducing effect of repeated mechanical wounding could be unequivocally demonstrated (Hennings and Boutwell 1970; Clark-Lewis and Murray 1978; Argyris 1980), thereby mimicking the activities of the potent chemical tumor promoters of the phorbol ester type (initiation–promotion protocol of mouse skin carcinogenesis; Marks and Fürstenberger 1987; Schmidt and Hecker 1989). In fact, a hallmark of both wounding and phorbol ester application is the development of a strong inflammatory reaction, followed by a pronounced epidermal hyperplasia at the wound edges or within the treated area. This local hyperplastic transformation of the tissue is a prerequisite for the development of epidermal tumors (Marks 1990). However, the observation that phorbol esters exhibiting equipotent inflammatory and hyperplasiogenic activities evoked dramatically varying tumor-inducing potencies indicated that a permanent stimulation of epidermal cell proliferation is only a necessary but not a sufficient condition for the development of tumors in initiated mouse skin. This result led to the distinction of two classes of phorbol ester tumor promoters, converting (or complete) promoters such as the phorbol ester 12-*O*-tetradecanoylphorbol-13-acetate (TPA) and nonconverting (or incomplete) promoters such as the TPA-derivative 12-*O*-retinoylphorbol-13-acetate (RPA) or the plant poison mezerein (Slaga et al. 1980; Fürstenberger et al. 1981). Thus, in initiated mouse skin, tumors develop along a two-step protocol upon repeated treatment with a complete promoter such as TPA (initiation–promotion protocol) or along a three-step protocol upon subsequent treatment with a single application of the complete promoter TPA followed by repeated administrations of the incomplete promoter RPA (initiation–conversion–promotion protocol; Fig. 1). The TPA-induced conversion has been shown to depend on the induction of epidermal DNA synthesis, to correlate with chromosomal damage, and to be effective either before or after initiation leading to a rather long-lasting alteration of the tissue (Marks and Fürstenberger 1990).

Using this protocol incisional wounds can be shown to mimic the activity of TPA as a complete tumor promoter, pointing to critical functions of endogenous factors produced during the wound reaction (Fürstenberger and Marks 1983). These factors include cytokines, cell adhesion molecules, and peptide- and lipid-derived proinflammatory mediators generated by thrombocytes, leukocytes, fibroblasts, endothelial cells, and keratinocytes (Cunningham 1990; Barker et al. 1991; Blitstein-Willinger 1991; McKay and Leigh 1991). In this scenario, the keratinocyte occupies a central position in that it translates exogenous harmful stimuli into endogenous signals which initiate, propagate, and terminate the wound reaction, including an initial inflammatory response (attraction and activation of leukocytes and lymphocytes), proliferation of connective tissue cells, production of extracellular matrix, angiogenesis, and epithelial cell migration and proliferation, finally leading to a reepithelialization and other processes of wound healing in skin.

Wound-Related Epidermal Cytokines

Upon transient activation by exogenous stimuli or permanent activation in benign or malignant hyperproliferative skin diseases in vivo or in cell culture keratinocytes produce and release a complex cocktail of mediators and cytokines (for reviews see Cunningham 1990; Kupper 1990; Barker et al. 1991; McKay and Leigh 1991). In contrast to this "activated keratinocyte phenotype" (Kupper 1990) unstimulated epidermis produces such factors only at very low doses or in an inactive form (Fig. 2).

Epidermal cytokines include growth factors such as transforming growth factor α (TGF-α) (Coffey et al. 1987; Gottlieb et al. 1988; see below), basic fibroblast growth factor (bFGF) (Halaban et al. 1988; O'Keffe et al. 1988) and platelet-derived growth factor (PDGF) (Antoniades et al. 1991), which have been shown to stimulate the proliferation of activated keratinocytes along receptor-mediated processes in an autocrine manner. Factors produced by keratinocytes which inhibit their own growth include transforming growth factor β (TGF-β; Shipley et al. 1986; Lyons and Moses 1990; see below) and tumor necrosis factor α (TNF-α) (Pillai et al. 1989). Growth-modulatory cytokines with specificity for epithelial cells are also produced by fibroblasts,

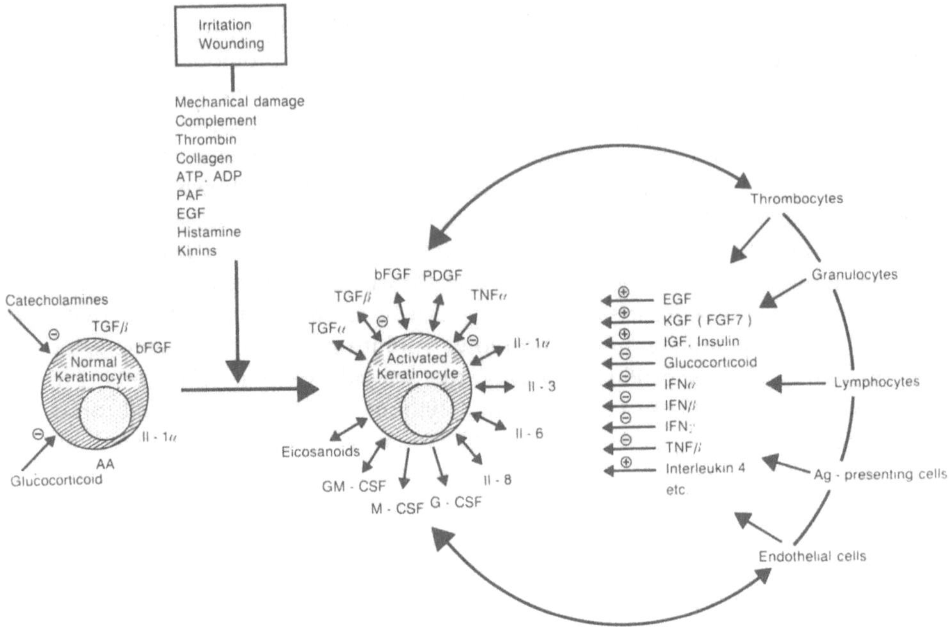

Fig. 2. Cytokine production by "activated keratinocytes." Upon irritation or injury of skin, the keratinocytes are activated to produce and secrete a complex cocktail of cytokines and lipid mediators. These factors recruit other cell types involved in repair and defense processes and activate the generation and release of additional chemical signals to the wound milieu. Many of these and the keratinocyte-derived factors control keratinocyte proliferation along para- and autocrine pathways (+, stimulation; −, inhibition). The normal (nonactivated) keratinocytes produce some factors such as IL-1α, TGF-β, bFGF and the eicosanoids as inactive precursors, in an otherwise seqestered form, or at low levels. These factors may be activated and released upon cell damage and/or stimulation of keratinocytes by so-called primary wound factors such as thrombin, ATP, platelet-activating factor (*PAF*), kinins, and others, which then may trigger the subsequent stages of keratinocyte activation (Marks 1990)

leukocytes, lymphocytes and thrombocytes, including epidermal growth factor (EGF) and keratinocyte growth factor (KGF) (Rubin et al. 1989; Bottaro et al. 1990) and the growth-inhibitory interferons α, β_1 and γ (Fig. 2) (for review see McKay and Leigh 1991). Other effects of TGF-α, TGF-β, bFGF, and PDGF are their interactions with endothelial cells and dermal fibroblast to induce angiogenesis, fibrosis, and deposition of extracellular matrix (Goustin et al. 1986; Folkman and Klagsbrun 1987; Roberts et al. 1988).

Activated keratinocytes have been shown to produce and to respond to several members of the interleukin family including interleukin-1α (IL-1α), interleukin-6 (IL-6) and interleukin-8 (IL-8), which have all been shown to stimulate keratinocyte proliferation (Fig. 2) (Grossman et al. 1989; Kupper

1990; McKenzie and Sauder 1990; Nickoloff et al. 1990). In addition, IL-8 is a potent leukocyte attractant and may thus contribute to the major pathologic alterations observed in psoriasis, i.e., leukocyte infiltration and epidermal hyperproliferation (Reusch et al. 1990; Gillitzer et al. 1991).

The cocktail of cytokines that is released from activated keratinocytes is further supplemented by the presence of colony stimulating factors (CSFs), including multi-CSF (or interleukin-3), granulocyte CSF (G-CSF), macrophage CSF (M-CSF) and granulocyte/macrophage CSF (GM-CSF) (Fig. 2; for a review see McKay and Leigh 1991).

Thus a major characteristic of the "activated keratinocyte" is its ability to produce and release cytokines and to express their corresponding receptors. Many of these cytokines, such as TGF-α, TGF-β_1, IL-1, and others, induce their own induction in an autocrine loop or stimulate the production of other cytokines, e.g., IL-1 stimulates the release of IL-6, IL-8, GM-CSF, or TGF-α from neighboring keratinocytes (Larsen et al. 1989; McKenzie and Sauder 1990; Lee et al. 1991). This complex network of cytokines is responsible for the induction of an inflammatory infiltrate and the effects on the dermis and blood vessels that give rise to the formation of the granulation tissue, this being a prerequisite for the repithelialization of wounds or to the generation of stroma, a critical condition of tumor growth (Folkman 1985; Dvorak 1986).

TGF-α and TGF-β Stimulate Wound Healing and Mimic the Converting Effect of Full Skin Wounding

Among the numerous wound-related cytokines, TGF-α and TGF-β have been shown to improve the healing of split thickness incisional wounds. Similar to in culture (Barrandon and Green 1987), TGF-α or EGF have been shown to stimulate keratinocyte proliferation and migration in vivo, thereby stimulating reepithelialization of the wound (Schultz et al. 1987). The epidermal growth inhibitor TGF-β is known to stimulate the dermal aspects of wound healing by inducing enhanced generation of connective tissue, promoting angiogenesis, and increasing the tensile strength of wounds (Mustoe et al. 1987; Quaglino et al. 1991). Moreover, TGF-β was found to stimulate the TGF-α-induced outgrowth of epidermal cells from porcine partial-thickness skin explants by accelerating the initiation and the rate of outgrowth during the migratory phase of the cultures (Hebda 1988). In experimental wounds TGF-β-induced keratinocyte migration may result in an impoverishment of keratinocytes in the immediate vicinity of the wound edges, resulting in a compensatory hyperproliferation of adjacent keratinocytes (Schnapke 1992), which may be facilitated by a decreasing gradient of TGF-β concentration in combination with stimulatory effects of "positive" growth factors such as TGF-α or others. The physiological significance of TGF-β in the wound response is further supported by the immunological demonstration of TGF-β_1 protein in the direct vicinity of a wound (Kane et al. 1991). These results point to an important role of TGF-β in both the dermal and epidermal aspects of the wound response (Wahl et al. 1989).

When injected simultaneously into carcinogen-initiated skin, TGF-α and TGF-β proved to be converting agents, i.e., to induce epidermal tumor development pending subsequent promotion with a nonconverting promoter such as the phorbol ester RPA. Alone neither TGF-α nor TGF-β exhibited such a converting effect (Fürstenberger et al. 1989). TGF-α is assumed to contribute the mitogenic component to the conversion process since it can replaced by an exogenous skin mitogen such as RPA (Fürstenberger et al. 1989) and since TGF-α has been shown to be a major autocrine growth factor for keratinocytes in vivo and in vitro (Coffey et al. 1987; Finzi et al. 1991; Vassar and Fuchs 1991). Moreover, increased expression of TGF-α messenger (m)RNA and protein is common in benign and malignant hyperproliferative skin diseases such as psoriasis and epidermal neoplasias (Finzi et al. 1988; Gottlieb et al. 1988; Elder et al. 1989; Ho et al. 1991). Interestingly, the converting tumor promoter TPA has been shown to increase TGF-α mRNA and protein in mouse epidermis in vivo (Imamoto et al. 1991). This may indicate that phorbol esters bring about their mitogenic effects by the induction of endogenous growth factors such as TGF-α or, more directly, by interacting with pathways of the intracellular transduction of mitogenic signals, for instance by activating protein kinase C (Nishizuka 1988).

As far as the role of TGF-β in conversion is concerned, it is intriguing that this cytokine has been also shown to mediate the effect of wounding on Rous sarcoma virus-induced tumorigenesis in chickens whereas EGF, TGF-α or PDGF were inactive (Sieweke et al. 1990). Moreover, the converting promoter TPA was shown to stimulate the expression of TGF-β mRNA (Akhurst et al. 1988a; Krieg et al. 1991) and protein (Akhurst et al. 1988b) in mouse epidermis in vivo, whereas the nonconverting phorbol ester RPA was significantly less potent in this respect (Krieg et al. 1991). These data provide some experimental evidence for a critical function of TGF-β in tumor development in carcinogen- or virus-initiated epithelia as suggested previously (Parkinson 1985).

The Role of TGF-β in Epidermal Carcinogenesis

The common basis of both wound healing and carcinogenesis is thought to be cellular hyperproliferation combined with the formation of supplementary structures such as the granulation tissue of a healing wound or the tumor stroma (see above; Haddow 1972; Dvorak 1986). The major difference between the two processes appears to be the transient nature of the healing process as compared to the infinite growth of tumors. According to the data discussed above, TGF-β may play an important role in the generation of both granulation tissue and tumor stroma (Roberts et al. 1988) as well as – probably in combination with TGF-α – on epithelial hyperproliferation (see above). This conclusion is supported by the observation that a single subcutaneous injection of TGF-β_1 into the neck of newborn mice could evoke a fibrous nodule exhibiting all of the characteristics of granulation tissue (Roberts et al. 1986). On the other hand, the continous generation of tumor stroma would require a permanent release of TGF-β by the overlying epithelial tumor cells.

The above-mentioned initiation – promotion protocol of mouse skin carcinogenesis provides an appropriate system to study the expression of TGF-β_1 or its isoforms β_2 and -β_3 in different stages of tumor development in vivo. Northern blot analysis of RNA from individual papillomas revealed weak TGF-β_1 expression that was only slightly elevated compared to normal epidermis. In contrast, strong overexpression of TGF-β_1 mRNA was seen in squamous cell carcinomas. TGF-β_2 mRNA levels were found to be very low in normal epidermis and in benign and malignant tumors, whereas a strong overexpression of TGF-β_3 mRNA was detected in RNA samples obtained from papillomas and carcinomas (summarized in Fig. 4). Using in situ hybridization, active synthesis of TGF-β_1 mRNA could be localized to the epithelial cells in carcinomas, whereas the level of TGF-β_1 mRNA in papillomas appeared to be beyond the level of detection (Fig. 3). Only very low levels of TGF-β_2 expression could be detected in normal and neoplastic epidermis but very high levels of TGF-β_3 transcripts were identified in the epithelial parts of papillomas and carcinomas (Schnapke 1992). Taken together, the epithelial parts of papillomas and carcinomas represent the main site of synthesis of the TGF-β isoforms. Moreover, TGF-β_1 and TGF-β_3 appear to be differentially regulated at the transcriptional level in benign and malignant tumors as compared to normal epidermis. Differential expression of TGF-β isoforms has been also observed in mouse epidermis in vivo. While treatment with the phorbol ester TPA led to a transient expression of TGF-β_1 mRNA (Akhurst et al. 1988a), retinoic acid application resulted in an enhanced expression of TGF-β_2 mRNA (Glick et al. 1989).

The immunohistochemical staining pattern using isoform-specific antibodies was found to be consistent with the results of the in situ hybridization experiments (Figs. 3, 4), demonstrating a strong expression of TGF-β_1 and TGF-β_3 protein in epithelial domains of papillomas and carcinomas. Most of the staining appeared to be localized in the extracellular matrix surrounding the cells. In contrast to Glick et al. (1991), we were unable to observe a strict compartimentalization of the expression of the TGF-β isoforms in papillomas. Using another set of antibodies these authors investigated papillomas arising from v-Ha-*ras*-transfected keratinocytes grafted onto nude mice. While TGF-β_1 was found to be abundant in the basal and spinous layers, TGF-β_2 and TGF-β_3 were expressed predominantly in the granular layers. In summary, in situ hybridization and immunohistochemical analysis provide evidence for constitutive overexpression of TGF-β_1 and TGF-β_3

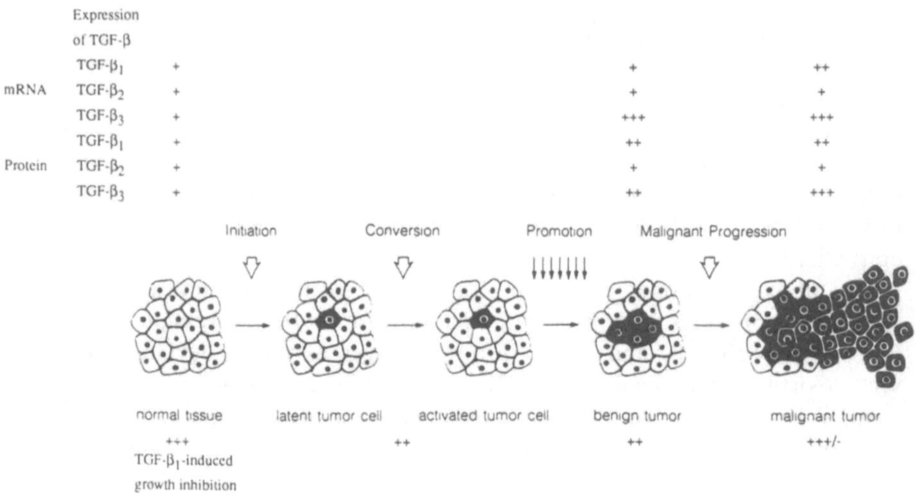

Fig. 3a–d. Expression of TGF-β_1 mRNA and protein in papillomas and carcinomas obtained by the initiation–promotion protocol. **a, b** Autoradiographs of in situ hybridizations of a papilloma and a carcinoma using a TGF-β_1 cRNA probe. Note the very weak – if at all – specific TGF-β_1 mRNA expression in the epithelial part (*E*) of the papilloma (**a**) and the strong epithelial localization (*E*) of TGF-β_1 mRNA in the carcinoma (**b**) predominantly in the stratum basale (*Sb*) and stratum spinosum (*Ss*) (*Sg*, stratum grannlosum; *Sc*, stratum corneum; D, dermis). **c, d** The imunohistochemical localization of TGF-β_1 protein in a papilloma (**c**) and a carcinoma (**d**) using a TGF-β_1-specific antibody coupled to anti-rabbit-AMCA secondary antibody. Note the predominant'y extracellur localization in the epithelial part (*E*) of the papilloma (**c**) and the carcinoma (**d**)

mRNA and protein in papillomas and carcinomas. The continuous release of TGF-β from the tumors cells could well lead to permanent induction of supporting tumor stroma which is critically required for permanent tumor growth (Dvorak 1986). During the very early phase of experimental tumor induction, e.g., in the conversion stage, TGF-β may be provided either experimentally by local injection or by the release of TGF-β into the wound area, or by de novo synthesis induced more actively by the converting tumor promoter TPA than by the nonconverting promoter RPA (see above).

In addition to this paracrine action of TGF-β, autocrine effects of the factor on the keratinocyte have to be considered. This would certainly lead

Fig. 4. Expression pattern of TGF-β isoforms in vivo and effects in vitro during multistage carcinogenesis in mouse skin. Summary of the expression of TGF-β isoforms at the mRNA and protein level in normal mouse epidermis, papilloma, and carcinoma produced along the initiation–promotion protocol and the sensitivity of normal keratinocytes and papilloma- and carcinoma-derived epidermal cells towards TGF-β_1-induced growth inhibition. For further details see text

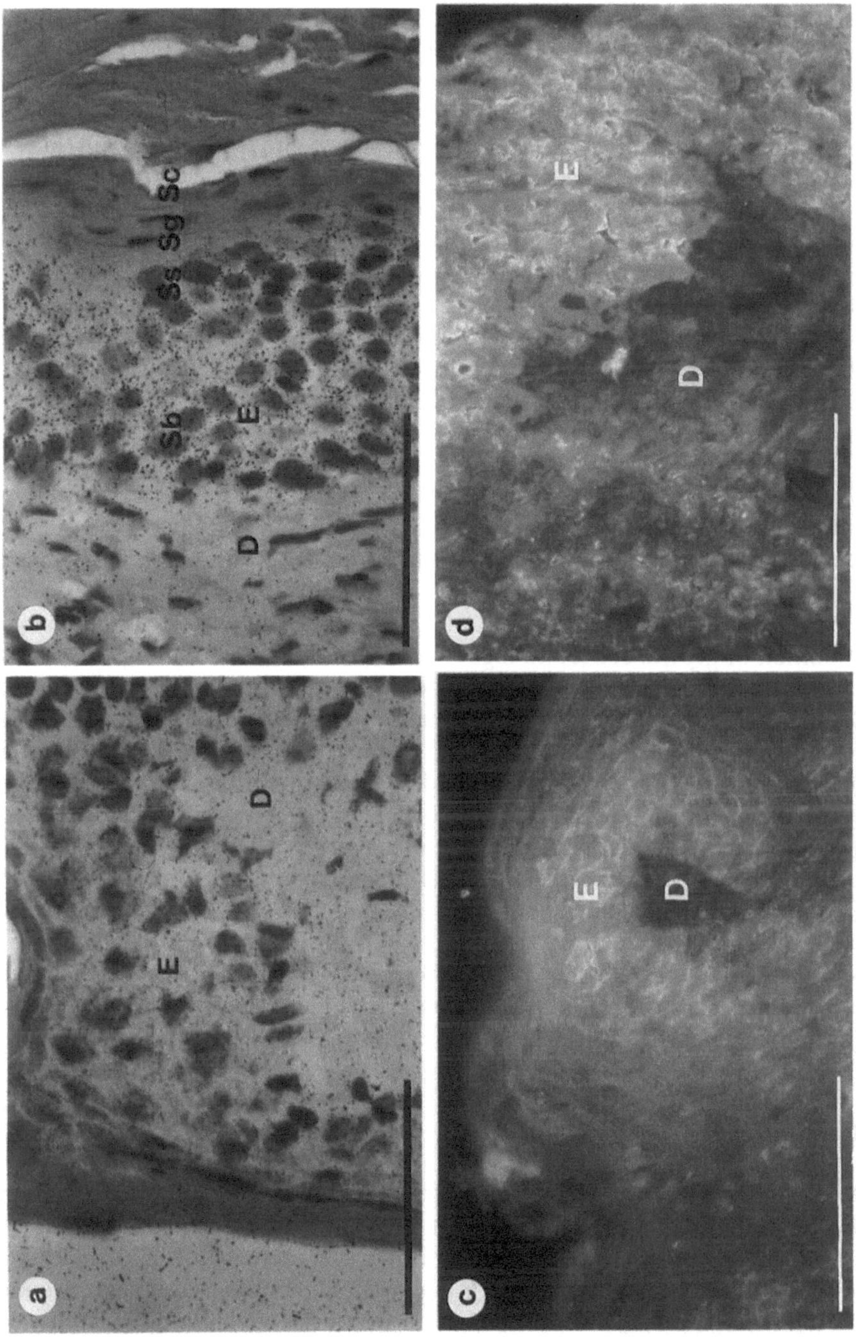
a
E
D
b
Sb
E
D
Ss
Sg
Sc
c
E
D
d
E
D

to downregulation of tumor growth provided that tumor cells respond to growth inhibition by TGF-β with comparable sensitivity to that of normal keratinocytes in vitro and in vivo (Lyons and Moses 1990). In the mouse this appears to be the case for nontumorigenic immortalized epidermal cell lines, for papilloma-derived cells, and at least for some carcinoma cell lines. However, in some malignant carcinoma cell lines the growth inhibitory response was found to be dramatically reduced or completely lost (summarized in Fig. 4; Haddow et al. 1991; Krieg et al. 1991). The conclusion that can be drawn from such studies is that growth control by TGF-β is lost – if at all – at a late stage of mouse skin carcinogenesis. A comparable late change in TGF-β sensitivity has been reported for cell lines derived from human colon adenomas and carcinomas (Manning et al. 1991). Thus, it is evident that acquisition of resistance to TGF-β may contribute to the uncontrolled growth characteristics of at least some malignant carcinomas. However, such a conclusion cannot be drawn for papillomas which rapidly grow in spite of permanent treatment with the TGF-β-inducing agent TPA (Akhurst et al. 1988a,b) or a constitutive overexpression of TGF-β (see above; Glick et al. 1991). It may be assumed that more subtle changes hardly detectable in the proliferation assays may have occurred in papilloma cells. In fact, one of the papilloma cell lines in our study (Krieg et al. 1991) showed a dose-response for TGF-β-induced inhibition of growth shifted to higher concentrations. In addition, it remains to be established that the immunoreactive protein produced by the tumor cells is indeed biologically active, mature TGF-β. Thus, the inability of tumor cells to activate latent TGF-β complexes could be a contributing mechanism to escape TGF-β-mediated negative growth regulation (Bascom et al. 1989). On the other hand, the balance between positive and negative growth factors rather than the effect of any one factor may play a critical role in the clonal selection and expansion of papilloma cells (see above; Parkinson and Balmain 1990). Two lines of evidence support this idea, namely the combined action of TGF-α and TGF-β in conversion (see above) and the strong induction by TPA of both TGF-β isoforms and TGF-α. The latter induces its own production, thus providing a strong autocrine amplification mechanism (Coffey et al. 1987; Pittelkow et al. 1989).

Conclusions

Wounding has been shown to act as a complete (converting) tumor promoter in the initiation–conversion–promotion or initiation–promotion protocol of mouse skin carcinogenesis. The converting activity of incisional skin wounding can be mimicked by the activity of the two cooperative wound factors TGF-α and TGF-β_1. Both factors are transiently induced and released upon wounding or upon treatment with the converting tumor promoter TPA; moreover, they are constitutively expressed in epidermal tumors, supporting tumor growth via both autocrine and paracrine activation pathways. Continous TGF-α production may be responsible for the increased growth rates of tumors, and overexpression and activation of the latent TGF-β isoforms may indirectly propagate tumor growth by paracrine action of the secreted factors on supporting stromal elements and – at least at late stages of tumor development – by loss of the autocrine growth inhibitory effects of TGF-β. Thus, the unbalanced coexpression of a negative growth factor such as TGF-β and a positive growth factor such as TGF-α is critical for the development of epidermal tumors in initiated mouse skin in vivo.

References

Akhurst RJ, Fee F, Balmain A (1988a) Localized production of TGF-β mRNA in tumour promoter-stimulated mouse epidermis. Nature 331:363–365

Akhurst RJ, Lehnert SS, Fee F, Balmain A (1988b) The role of transforming growth factor-β in mouse development and carcinogenesis. Biochem Soc Trans 17:595–597

Antoniades HN, Galanopoulos T, Neville-Golden J, Kiritsy CP, Lynch SE (1991) Injury induces in vivo expression of platelet-derived growth factor (PDGF) and PDGF receptor mRNAs in skin epithelial cells and PDGF mRNA in connective tissue fibroblasts. Proc Natl Acad Sci USA 88:565–569

Argyris TS (1980) Tumor Promotion by abrasion-induced hyperplasia in skin of mice. J Invest Dermatol 75:360–362

Bailleul B, Surani MA, White S, Barton SC, Brown K, Blessing M, Jorcano J, Balm in A (1990) Skin hyperkeratosis and papilloma formation in transgenic mice expressing a ras oncogene from a suprabasal Keratin promoter. Cell 62:697–708

Barker JNWN, Mitra RS, Griffiths CEM, Dixit VM, Nickoloff BJ (1991) Keratinocytes as initiators of inflammation. Lancet 337:211–214

Barrandon Y, Green H (1987) Cell migration is essential for sustained growth of keratinocyte colonies: the roles of transforming growth factor α and epidermal growth factor. Cell 50:1131–1137

Bascom CC, Sipes NJ, Coffey RJ, Moses HL (1989) Regulation of epithelial cell proliferation by transforming growth factors. J Cell Biochem 39:25–32

Blitstein-Willinger E (1991) The role of growth factors in wound healing. Skin Pharmacol 4:175–182

Bottaro DP, Rubin JS, Ron D, Finch PW, Florio C, Aaronson SA (1990) Characterization of the receptor for keratinocyte growth factor. Evidence for multiple fibroblast growth factor receptors. J Biol Chem 265:12767–12770

Chester JF, Gaissert HA, Ross JS, Malt RA, Weitzman SA (1989) Colonic cancer induced by 1,2-dimethylhydrazine: promotion by experimental colitis. Br J Cancer 59:704–705

Clark-Lewis J, Murray AW (1978) Tumor promotion and the induction of epidermal ornithine decarboxylase activity in mechanically stimulated mouse skin. Cancer Res 38:494–497

Coffey RJ, Derynck R, Wilcox JN, Bringman TS, Goustin AS, Moses HL, Pittelkow MR (1987) Production and autoinduction of transforming growth factor-alpha in human keratinocytes. Nature 328:817–820

Cunningham F (1990) Lipid mediators in inflammatory skin disorders. J Lipid Mediator 2:61–74

Dolberg DS, Hollingworth R, Hertle M, Bissel MJ (1985) Wounding and its role in RSV-mediated carcinogenesis. Science 230:676–678

Dvorak HF (1986) Tumors: wounds that do not heal. N Engl J Med 315:1650–1659
Elder JT, Fisher GJ, Lindquist PB, Bennett GL, Pittelkow MR, Coffey RJ, Ellingsworth L, Derynck R, Voorhees JJ (1989) Overexpression of transforming growth factor alpha in psoriatic epidermis. Science 243:811–814
Finzi A, Kilkenny A, Stricklan JE, Balaschak M, Bringman T, Derynck R, Aaronson S, Yuspa SH (1988) TGF-alpha stimulates growth of skin papillomas by autocrine and paracrine mechanisms but does not cause neoplastic progression. Mol Carcinog 1:7–12
Finzi E, Harkins R, Horn T (1991) TGF-α is widely expressed in differentiated as well as hyperproliferative skin epithelium. J Invest Dermatol 96:328–332
Fisher B, Fisher ER (1959) Experimental evidence in support of the dormant tumor cell. Science 130:918–919
Folkman J (1985) Tumor angiogenesis. Adv Cancer Res 43:175–203
Folkman J, Klagsbrun M (1987) Angiogenic factors. Science 235:442–447
Fürstenberger G, Marks F (1983) Growth stimulation and tumor promotion in skin. J Invest Dermatol 81:157s–161s
Fürstenberger G, Berry DL, Sorg B, Marks F (1981) Skin tumor promotion is a two-stage process. Proc Natl Acad Sci USA 78:7722–7726
Fürstenberger G, Rogers M, Schnapke R, Bauer G, Höfler P, Marks F (1989) Stimulatory role of transforming growth factors in multistage carcinogenesis: possible explanation for the tumor-inducing effect of wounding in initiated NMRI mouse skin. Int J Cancer 43:915–921
Gillitzer R, Berger R, Mielke V, Müller C, Wolff K, Stingl G (1991) Upper keratinocytes of psoriatic skin lesions express high levels of NAP-1/IL-8 mRNA in situ. J Invest Dermatol 97:73–79
Glick AB, Flanders KC, Danielpour D, Yuspa SH, Sporn MB (1989) Retinoic acid induces transforming growth factor-β_2 in cultured keratinocytes and in mouse epidermis. Cell Regul 1:87–97
Glick AB, Sporn MB, Yuspa SH (1991) Altered regulation of TGF-β_1 and TGF-α in primary keratinocytes and papillomas expressing v-Ha-ras. Mol Carcinog 4: 210–219
Gottlieb AB, Chang CK, Posnett DN, Fanelli B, Tam JP (1988) Detection of transforming growth factor alpha in normal, malignant, and hyperproliferative human keratinocytes. J Exp Med 167:670–675
Grossman RM, Krueger J, Yourish D, Granelli-Piperno A, Murphy DP, May LT, Kupper TS, Sehgal PB, Gottlieb A (1989) Interleukin 6 is expressed in high levels in psoriatic skin and stimulates proliferation of cultured human keratinocytes. Proc Natl Acad Sci USA 86:6367–6371
Goustin AS, Leof EB, Shipley GD, Moses HL (1986) Growth factors and cancer. Cancer Res 46:1015–1029
Haddow A (1972) Molecular repair, wound healing and carcinogenesis: tumor production a possible overhealing? Adv Cancer Res 16:181–234
Haddow S, Fowlis DJ, Parkinson K, Akhurst RJ, Balmain A (1991) Loss of growth control by TGF-β occurs at a late stage of mouse skin carcinogenesis and is independent of ras gene activation. Oncogene 6:1465–1470
Halaban R, Langdon R, Birchall N, Cuaono C, Baird A, Scott G, Moellmann G, McGuire J (1988) Basic fibroblast growth factor from human keratinocytes is a mitogen for melanocytes. J Cell Biol 107:1611–1619
Hasegawa R, St John M, Tibbels TS, Cohen SM (1987) Evaluation of epidermal cell kinetics following freezing or wounding of mouse skin and their potential as initiators of carcinogenesis. J Invest Dermatol 88:652–656
Hebda PA (1988) Stimulatory effects of transforming growth factor-beta and epidermal growth factor on epidermal cell outgrowth from porcine skin explant cultures. J Invest Dermatol 91:440–445

Heldin CH, Westermark B (1989) Growth factors as transforming proteins. Eur J Biochem 184:487–496

Hennings H, Boutwell RK (1970) Studies on the mechanism of skin tumor promotion. Cancer Res 30:312–320

Ho T, Horn T, Finzi E (1991) Transforming growth factor α expression helps to distinguish keratoacanthomas from squamous cell carcinomas. Arch Dermatol 127:1167–1171

Imamoto A, Beltran LM, DiGiovanni J (1991) Evidence for autocrine/paracrine growth stimulation by transforming growth factor α during the process of skin tumor promotion. Mol Carcinog 4:52–60

Kane CJM, Hebda PA, Mansbridge JN, Hanawalt PC (1991) Direct evidence for spatial and temporal regulation of transforming growth factor β_1 expression during cutaneous wound healing. J Cell Physiol 148:157–173

Konstantinides A, Smulow J (1982) Tumorigenesis at a predetermined oral site after one intraperitoneal injection of N-nitroso-N-methylurea. Science 216:1235–1237

Krieg P, Schnapké R, Fürstenberger G, Vogt I, Marks F (1991) TGF-β_1 and skin carcinogenesis: antiproliferative effect in vitro and TGF-β_1 mRNA expression during epidermal hyperproliferation and multistage tumorigenesis. Mol Carcinog 4:129–137

Kupper TS (1990) The activated keratinocyte: a model for inducible cytokine production by non-bone marrow-derived cells in cutaneous inflammatory and immune responses. J Invest Dermatol 95:146S–150S

Larsen CG, Anderson AO, Oppenheim JJ, Matsushima K (1989) Production of interleukin 8 by human dermal fibroblasts and keratinocytes in response to interleukin 1 or tumor necrosis factor. Immunology 68:31–36

Leder A, Kuo RD, Cardiff RD, Sinn E, Leder P (1990) v-Ha-ras transgene abrogates the initiation step in mouse skin tumorigenesis: effects of phorbol esters and retinoic acid. Proc Natl Acad Sci USA 87:9178–9182

Lee SW, Morhenn VB, Ilnicka M, Eugui EM, Allison AC (1991) Autocrine stimulation of interleukin-1α and transforming growth factor α production in human keratinocytes and its antagonism by glucocorticoids. J Invest Dermatol 97:106–110

Lyons RM, Moses HL (1990) Transforming growth factors and the regulation of cell proliferation. Eur J Biochem 187:467–473

Manning A, Williams AC, Game SM, Paraskeva C (1991) Differential sensitivity of human colonic adenoma and carcinoma cells to transforming growth factor β (TGF-β): conversion of an adenoma cell line to a tumorigenic phenotype is accompanied by a reduced to the inhibitory effects of TGF-β. Oncogene 6:1471–1476

Marks F (1990) Hyperplastic transformation, the response of the skin to irritation and injury. In: Galli CL, Marinovich DM, Hensby TN (eds) Skin pharmacology and toxicology. Plenum, New York, pp 121–145

Marks F, Fürstenberger G (1987) Multistage carcinogenesis- the mouse skin model. In: zurHausen H, Schlehofer JE (eds) Accomplishments in oncology, vol 2. Lippincott, Philadelphia, pp 18–30

Marks F, Fürstenberger G (1990) The conversion stage of skin carcinogenesis. Carcinogenesis 11:2085–2092

McKay IA, Leigh IM (1991) Epidermal cytokines and their roles in cutaneous wound healing. Br J Dermatol 124:513–518

McKenzie I, Rous P (1941) The experimental disclosure of latent neoplastic changes in tarred skin. J Exp Med 73:391–416

McKenzie RC, Sauder DN (1990) The role of keratinocyte cytokines in inflammation and immunity. J Invest Dermatol 95:105S–107S

Mueller CE, Thornbury JR (1973) Adenocarcinoma of the colon complicating ureterosidmoistomy: a case report and review of the literature. J Urol 109:225–227

Mustoe TA, Pierce GF, Thamason A, Gramates P, Sporn MB, Deuel TF (1987) Accelerated healing of incisional wounds in rats induced by transforming growth factor-beta. Science 237:1333–1336
Nickoloff GJ, Griffiths CEM, Barker JNWN (1990) The role of cell adhesion molecules, chemotactic factors, and cytokines in inflammatory and neoplastic skin diseases – 1990 update. J Invest Dermatol 97:106–110
Nishizuka Y (1988) The molecular heterogeneity of protein kinase C and its implication for cellular regulation. Nature 334:662–665
O'Keffe EJ, Chiu ML, Payne RE (1988) Stimulation of growth of keratinocytes by bFGF. J Invest Dermatol 90:767–769
Parkinson EK (1985) Defective responses of transformed keratinocytes to terminal differentiation stimuli. Their role in epidermal tumor promotion by phorbol esters and by deep skin wounding. Br J Cancer 52:479–493
Parkinson EK, Balmain A (1990) Chalones revisited: a possible role of transforming growth factor-β in tumor promotion. Carcinogenesis 11:195–198
Pillai S, Bikle DD, Eessalu TE (1989) Binding and biological effects of tumor necrosis factor alpha on cultured human neonatal foreskin keratinocytes. J Clin Invest 83:816–821
Pittelkow MR, Lindqusit PB, Abraham RT, Graves DR, Derynck R, Coffey RJ (1989) Induction of transforming-α expression in human keratinocytes by phorbol esters. J Biol Chem 264:5164–5171
Pound AW, McGuirre LJ (1978) Repeated partial hepatectomy as a promoting stimulus for the carcinogenic response of liver to nitroseamines in rats. Br J Cancer 37:585–594
Pozharizski KM (1975) The significance of nonspecific injury for colon carcinogenesis in rats. Cancer Res 35:3824–3830
Quaglino D Jr, Nanny LB, Ditesheim JA, Davidson JM (1991) Transforming growth factor-beta stimulates wound healing and modulates extracellular matrix gene expression in pig skin: Incisional wound model. J Invest Dermatol 97:34–42
Reusch M, Studtmann K, Schröder MJ, Sticherling M, Christophers E (1990) NAP-1/IL-8 is a potent mitogen for human keratinocytes in vitro. J Invest Dermatol 95:485 (abstr)
Roberts AB, Sporn MB, Assoian RK, Smith JM, Roche NS, Wakefield LM, Heine U, Liotta LA, Falanger V, Kelert JH, Fanci AS (1986) Transforming growth factor type β: rapid induction of fibrosis and angiogenesis in vivo and stimulation of collagen formation in vitro. Proc Natl Acad Sci USA 83:4167–4171
Roberts AB, Thompson NL, Heine U, Flanders KC, Sporn MB (1988) Transforming growth factor-β: possible roles in carcinogenesis. Br J Cancer 57:594–600
Rubin JS, Osada H, Finch PW, Taylor WG, Rudikoff S, Aaronson SA (1989) Purification and characterization of a newly identified factor specific for epithelial cells. Proc Natl Acad Sci USA 86:802–806
Sanderson KV, Mackie R (1979) Tumors of the skin. In: Rook A, Wilkinson DS, Ebling FJG (eds) Textbook of dermatology, vol 2. Blackwell, Oxford, pp 2186–2192
Schmidt R, Hecker E (1989) Biological assays for irritant, tumor-initiating and tumor-promoting activities: II. Standardized initation/promotion protocol and semiquantitative estimation or promoting (or iniatiating) potencies in the skin of NMRI mice. J Cancer Res Clin Oncol 115:516–524
Schnapke R (1992) Transformierender Wadistumsfaktor β – Expression und Effekte in Keratinocyten und während der Mehrstufen Karzinogenese in Mäusehant. Ph D thesis, University of Heidelberg
Schuh AC, Keating SJ, Monteclaro FS, Vogt PK, Breitman ML (1990) Obligatory wounding requirement for tumorigenesis in v-jun transgenic mice. Nature 346:756–760

Schultz GS, White M, Mitchell R, Brown G, Lynch J, Twardzik DR, Todaro G (1987) Epithelial wound healing enhanced by transforming growth factor α or vaccinia growth factor. Science 235:350–357
Shipley GD, Pittelkow MR, Wille JJ, Scott RE, Moses HL (1986) Reversible inhibition of normal human prokeratinocyte proliferation by type-β transforming growth factor-growth inhibitor in serum free medium. Cancer Res 46:2068–2071
Sieweke MH, Thompson NL, Sporn MB, Bissel MJ (1990) Mediation of wound-related Rous Sarcom Virus tumorigenesis by TGF-β. Science 248:1656–1660
Slaga TJ, Fischer SM, Nelson K, Gleason GL (1980) Studies on the mechanisms of skin tumor promotion: evidence for several stages of promotion. Proc Natl Acad Sci USA 77:3659–3663
Sporn MB, Roberts AB (1986) Peptide growth factors and inflammation, tissue repair and cancer. J Clin Invest 78:329–332
Vassar R, Fuchs E (1991) Transgenic mice provide new insights into the role of TGF-α during epidermal development and differentiation. Genes Dev 5:714–727
Virchow R (1863) Die krankhaften Geschwülste. 30 Vorlesungen gehalten während des Wintersemesters 1862–1863 an der Universität Berlin. Hirschwald, Berlin
Wahl SM, Wong H, McCartney-Francis (1989) Role of growth factors in inflammation and repair. J Cell Biochem 40:193–199

In Vitro Transformation and Tumor Progression

P. Boukamp, D. Breitkreutz, A. Hülsen, S. Altmeyer, P. Tomakidi, and N.E. Fusenig

Division of Carcinogenesis and Differentiation, German Cancer Research Center (DKFZ), W-6900 Heidelberg, Fed. Rep. of Germany

Introduction

In recent years, our understanding of the genetic basis of cancer has been greatly enhanced by the discovery of molecular elements involved in cell transformation such as the oncogenes, capable of neoplastically transforming certain rodent cells via DNA transfection (Land et al. 1983), and tumor suppressor genes. The latter were originally discovered by somatic cell-hybridization experiments via whole cell fusion revealing that the cancerous phenotype could be suppressed by the introduction of normal genetic information (Harris et al. 1969; Stanbridge 1976). Meanwhile, more than 50 types of oncogenes are known and an increasing number of "tumor suppressor genes" are being detected and cloned (for reviews see Stanbridge 1990; Bishop 1991).

Much of our present knowledge about the role of these genes in neoplastic transformation originated from experimental model systems using cultured rodent cells. For skin carcinogenesis, in particular, most experiments were performed with mouse cells (for review see Boyd and Barrett 1990) or the mouse skin model in vivo (Bremner and Balmain 1990). In all systems the multistage nature of carcinogenesis could be clearly demonstrated. Human cells, on the other hand, have only rarely been used, partly due to their remarkable resistance to transformation by oncogenes or other transforming agents (Sager 1984). Moreover, human cells often behave differently to rodent cells and so extrapolation from the rodent system to the human situation in the absence of experimental data might be misleading.

One of the still rare human tumor models studied in detail and clearly underlining the multistep nature of tumorigenesis was recently proposed by Fearon and Vogelstein (1990) for colorectal cancer. Here, tumors of various developmental stages can be obtained, allowing the study of both inherited and somatic genetic alterations. The authors presented a model for the genetic basis of colorectal tumors including mutational activation of oncogenes, mutational inactivation of "tumor suppressor genes" (both representing a general phenomenon), and mutations in genes probably specifically involved in distinct cancer types (e.g., DCC gene). Unlike colorectal tumorigenesis, for most other human tumors, the different stages in tumor development are often either not known or not available, and thus experimental systems might help to fill this gap.

Our recent studies have been focused on establishing cell systems as well as in vitro and in vivo models to functionally characterize normal human keratinocytes and human tumor-derived carcinoma cells (Boukamp et al. 1982, 1985, 1990a; Tilgen et al. 1983; Watt et al. 1987) as a basis for studying the causal mechanisms for tumor progression. Furthermore, we have been successful in inducing intermediate stages between these two endpoints – the normal keratinocyte and the carcinoma cell – by establishing the immortalized HaCaT keratinocyte line and its transfection with the c-Ha-*ras* oncogene (Boukamp et al. 1990b). We would like to introduce this model and discuss our current hypothesis of the multistage carcinogenic process in this system.

Cell Immortalization

Hypothetical Mechanisms of Immortalization

Normal human keratinocytes can reproducibly be immortalized by infection or transfection the DNA tumor viruses (simian virus 40 or the human papillomaviruses type 16 or 18; for reviews see Rhim and Dritschilo 1991; Fusenig et al. 1989). In contrast to the results with normal rodent cells, transfection with the *ras* oncogene did not result in permanently growing keratinocyte lines (Henrad et al. 1990; own unpublished results). In addition, we have used a different approach to achieve immortalization (as developed with mouse keratinocytes, Fusenig et al. 1985) by avoiding known oncogenic agents and, fortunately, obtained a cell line (HaCaT) which arose spontaneously from a long-term primary culture of trunk skin keratinocytes (Boukamp et al. 1988). This HaCaT cell line and another one derived from foreskin keratinocytes (Baden et al. 1987) are presently the only spontaneously immortalized keratinocyte lines that we know of.

One putative mechanism involved in escaping from senescence of the HaCaT cells might have been mutational activation of p53, which is thought to act as an oncogene in its mutated form (for review see Lane and Benchimol 1990). Moreover, it was shown that normal rodent cells can be immortalized by transfection with the mutated p53 (Jenkins et al. 1984). Thus, mutation of this gene could be a putative mechanism for immortalization of the HaCaT cells. On immunohistochemistry the HaCaT cells react strongly with antibodies against p53 which detect the wild type and the mutated form of the protein (Banks et al. 1986; Gannon et al. 1990). Similarly, on Western blot analyses the protein was clearly expressed by HaCaT cells of different passage levels, but not detectable in normal fibroblasts or the human bladder carcinoma cell line EJ. Already these data strongly argue for the presence of the long-living mutated form of the p53. By sequencing of the p53 gene in the HaCaT cells two mutations were found typical for skin cancer in sun-exposed areas (Lehmann et al. 1993). Thus, UV-induced mutations in the p53 gene might be causally related to the immortalization of HaCaT cells, although this alteration per se should not be sufficient to induce this early stage of cell transformation. Additional, culture-associated genetic changes might be required. The precursor keratinocytes of HaCaT cells were cultured at elevated temperatures and it cannot be excluded that this growth condition might have induced or facilitated genetic defects. It was recently shown that elevated temperatures increase the risk for chromosome breaks and thus for chromosomal rearrangements, one of the earliest indications for cell transformation. As early as in the second passage, the HaCaT cells showed four consistent cytogenetic changes: (a) loss of the Y chromosome and (b) three distinct chromosomal translocations leading to monosomy of 3p, 4p, and 9p and trisomy of 9q (Boukamp et al. 1988). These markers were extremely stable throughout the whole culture period, strongly suggesting their important role for the immortalized phenotype.

The hypothetical mechanism inducing immortalization here might be (1) mutation of p53 gene and (2) partial loss of senescence genes, described to be present on chromosome 1 (Sugawara et al. 1990), but also assumed for chromosomes 4 and 9 (Barrett 1991). The causal relationship of these changes to escape from senescence of the HaCaT cells is a matter of ongoing studies.

Differentiation Potential In Vitro and In Vivo

In the past, immortalization of human keratinocytes has been generally considered to have a massive impact on their differentiation properties, and this is certainly true for virally transformed cells which often express only an irregular differentiation programm (for review see Rhim 1989; Fusenig et al. 1991a). However, comparable to our spontaneously immortalized murine cell lines (Fusenig et al. 1985; Breitkreutz et al. 1986), the HaCaT cells, too, had maintained a high degree of differentiation, indicating that loss of differentiation was not an obligatory step for immortalization. HaCaT cells still largely resemble normal keratinocytes. This was particularly obvious in early passages due to the pronounced stratification including formation of large horn squames. Although stratification decreased with passages, the expression of epidermal keratins and their modulation remained stable in later passages of HaCaT cells as well (Ryle et al. 1989; Breitkreutz et al. 1989).

Another marker for epidermal differentiation is the formation of a well-structured epithelium in surface transplants, best demonstrated in our in vivo transplantation model, established for mouse skin keratinocytes (Fusenig et al. 1983; Boukamp et al. 1990a), which could successfully be modified and adapted to the requirements of nude mice. Briefly, the cells are seeded on collagen gel (type I) and then transplanted (as a monolayer attached to the collagen) onto the muscle fascia of the back of nude mice. The collagen gel thus separates the epidermal cells from the mouse mesenchyme. Within 1–2 weeks, early passage HaCaT cells developed an epidermis-like epithelium which typically exhibited the known strata of the epidermis in situ and strongly resembled transplants of normal human skin keratinocytes (Boukamp et al. 1988, 1990a). Moreover, the typical differentiation markers such as the differentiation-specific keratins K1 and K10, involucrin and filaggrin were expressed and properly distributed within the epithelium. This highly preserved differentiation was not only restricted to early passage HaCaT cells, but also maintained in those cells which had lost the ability to stratify in vitro (Breitkreutz et al. 1991).

Thus, starting with normal keratinocytes from trunk skin, we had obtained, as a first step in the transformation process, the spontaneously immortalized HaCaT cell line. These cells had maintained two important characteristics of normal cells, rendering them an excellent model to study tumor progression, namely (1) a high capacity for epidermal differentiation and (2) the non-tumorigenic phenotype throughout the whole culture period of more than 300 passages (>6 years).

These contrast to other human keratinocyte lines, which mostly show drastically reduced or almost complete loss of differentiation and tend to become tumorigenic with higher passage levels.

Tumorigenic Conversion

ras *Oncogene Transfection*

One mechanism thought to be involved in malignant conversion is the activation of proto-oncogenes, giving rise to dominantly acting oncogenes (for review see Bishop 1991), and it has recently been shown that there was a high frequency of mutations in the c-Ha-*ras* oncogene in basal and squamous cell carcinomas of the skin, while in only one case was the Kirsten *ras* gene activated (Pierceall et al. 1991). By transfection with the cellular Ha-*ras* oncogene, we could establish a significant number of tumorigenic clones. However, due to their growth behaviour in vivo as well as their tumor histology, two classes of clones could be distinguished: (1) those which grew slowly and eventually persisted, forming large epidermal cysts which on histology were classified as benign tumors; (2) a second group of clones which grew progressively and were highly differentiated squamous cell carcinomas, i.e., malignant tumors. Thus, by transfection with a c-Ha-*ras* oncogene, we obtained 12 out of 18 *ras*-expressing clones which were tumorigenic, whereby six clones formed benign and six clones malignant tumors (Boukamp et al. 1990b).

Growth Behaviour In Vivo

Benign and malignant tumor cells could additionally be distinguished by their invasive capacity, which was restricted to the malignant clones. This difference could best be demonstrated in surface transplants. Here, the benign tumor cells formed a well-differentiated superficial epithelium with no indication of invasive growth, even when the collagen was degraded. The malignant cells also formed a superficial epithelium initially, but within 1–2 weeks infiltrated the collagen and the mouse mesenchyme (Boukamp et al. 1990b). The collagen gel, primarily acting as a barrier for direct cell–cell contact between epidermal and mesenchymal cells, obviously only delays but does not prevent the onset of invasion. This situation offers the advantage of allowing the early stages preceding the actual invasion, such as angiogenesis and stroma activation, to be studied in detail. In the course of a study, preliminary experiments have shown that during the first 4–5 days the tumor cells proliferated quickly, generating 10–12 cell layers. Proliferation then drastically decreased and at day 5–7 focal infiltration of mesenchymal cells and capillaries into the collagen started, followed by migration of tumor cells into the collagen gel. Thus, before actual invasion, mesenchyme and epithelium obviously interacted via diffusible factors and thereby induced, for instance, downregulation of proliferation in the epithelial cells as well as attraction of fibroblasts and induction of angiogenesis in the mesenchyme.

Differentiation Properties In Vivo

While the capacity for invasion was restricted to malignant HaCaT-*ras* clones and clearly distinguished them from the benign tumorigenic cell clones, the two types of tumorigenic cells could not be identified by their differentiation capacity. The HaCaT-*ras* clones had maintained the capacity to synthesize differentiation-specific keratins (K1 and K10) in culture, particularly at high cell densities. In contrast to the parental HaCaT cell line, which had gradually lost the ability to stratify in culture, most of the HaCaT-*ras* clones retained this ability and could form multilayered sheets on plastic and in organotypic cultures on collagen gels (Ryle et al. 1989). Similarly, also in transplants the malignant cells were still perfectly able to form a well-differentiated epidermis-like epithelium with all the characteristic strata comparable to those of the parental HaCaT cells. In these transplants all epidermal differentiation markers (K1, K10, involucrin, filaggrin) were expressed, although for the differentiation-specific keratins K1 and K10 the onset of expression was somewhat delayed, particularly for K10, so that coexpression of the two keratins was dissociated. Moreover, even in areas where the cells invaded the host tissue, differentiation seemed quite normal, as shown by the strictly suprabasal staining for K1 (Breitkreutz et al. 1991). Thus, notwithstanding some minor variations, differentiation potential was not significantly reduced in the tumorigenic HaCaT-*ras* clones, nor was their response to differentiation inducers (Breitkreutz et al. 1989), irrespective of the level of *ras* oncogene expression and the tumorigenic growth behaviour in vivo.

Furthermore, both HaCaT cells and tumorigenic HaCaT-*ras* clones had maintained quite normal expression of adhesion molecules. There is accumulating evidence that changes in cell–cell adhesion molecules might play an important role in the invasion process. Particularly E-cadherin, also called uvomorulin or L-CAM (for review see Edelman 1986), is being discussed as a "suppressor of invasion" for epithelial cells (Vlemincks et al. 1991). We have studied the expression of uvomorulin in HaCaT-*ras* clones in northern blots and could not find any difference between the nontumorigenic, benign or malignant tumorigenic HaCaT-*ras* cells. Only in a mesenchymal-like variant of the HaCaT cells obtained after MyoD1 transfection, subsequent treatment with 5-aza-2′-deoxycytidine, and selection for reduced adhesive properties (Boukamp et al. 1992) was uvomurulin expression lost. We also determined uvomorulin expression in transplants by immunofluorescence to exclude that the gene might be specifically downregulated in vivo. However, even invading areas showed a positive staining for uvomorulin (Boukamp and Fusenig 1992).

Thus, the tumorigenic cells – both the benign and malignant ones – exhibited altered growth control in vivo as compared to the nontumorigenic cells, leading to tumor growth. In addition, the malignant cells could clearly be distinguished by their invasive capacity.

Growth Potential In Vitro

In vitro, both the benign and malignant clones exhibited altered growth regulation in culture, since they had largely lost their dependence on serum as supplier for growth factors. In medium with 10% fetal calf serum, all clones had a similar population doubling time (PDT) of about 20 h. Under serum-free conditions, the PDT drastically increased in the nontumorigenic cells, while all tumorigenic cells proliferated further at a rate of approximately 30 h PDT. This increase in growth autonomy was even more pronounced when the cells were plated at clonal density. In medium with 10% fetal calf serum all cells exhibited a colony-forming efficiency of approximately 40%–60%. Under serum-free conditions, this drastically decreased towards zero for the non-tumorigenic cells, while the tumorigenic ones still showed a colony-forming efficiency of approximately 20% (Fusenig et al. 1990). Thus, independence of serum, i.e., externally supplied growth factors, was obviously one of the characteristics gained by the tumorigenic cells, but this did not discriminate benign from malignant tumorigenic cells.

This discrimination was, however, feasible due to the different responsiveness to transforming growth factor β (TGF-β_1). In general, keratinocytes are very sensitive to TGF-β_1-induced growth inhibition, and the HaCaT cells, the nontumorigenic variants, and the benign tumorigenic HaCaT-*ras* clones had maintained this sensitivity. All malignant HaCaT-*ras* clones, on the other hand, were no longer growth-suppressed when treated with up to 5 ng/ml TGF-β_1 and some were even growth-stimulated (A. Hülsen and N.E. Fusenig, in preparation). While independence from stimulatory growth factors was obviously characteristic for all tumorigenic clones, decreased sensitivity to growth inhibition by TGF-β_1 seemed to be a marker only for the malignant HaCaT-*ras* clones.

Malignant Progression

Thus, following *ras* oncogene transfection, we obtained two distinct stable phenotypes – the benign and the malignant tumor cells. These could be distinguished by in vitro and in vivo parameters and therefore it is very likely that these two phenotypes have a genetically fixed basis. This raised the question: Were both phenotypes induced by *ras* or did they require additional processes?

ras *Expression*

First, we examined *ras* expression in these cells. Western blot analysis showed that all tumorigenic HaCaT-*ras* clones expressed the p21 oncogene product, while it was absent in nontumorigenic HaCaT-*ras* clones and in the parental HaCaT cells when using an antibody specific for the mutated p21. However, all cells clearly expressed the normal (wild-type) p21 when a panreactive antibody was used (Boukamp et al. 1990b). The oncogene expression of p21 in the tumorigenic clones, by contrast, varied from very low to high levels, so no positive correlation between level of expression and tumorigenic potential in the two groups was obvious. This strongly suggests that the amount of mutated p21 was not critical, but that a minimal level was sufficient to provide the cells with a growth advantage in vivo. This may have been induced by enhanced autocrine growth regulation and by rendering them insensitive to growth inhibition signals of the in vivo environment. So the *ras* oncogene seemed to be responsible for tumorigenic conversion, but giving rise only to benign tumors, since we have no evidence so far that it is also responsible for malignant progression (Fusenig et al. 1991b). Thus, other mechanisms have to be postulated for this step.

ras *Integration Site*

One possible mechanism involved in malignant progression might be related to the integration site of the *ras* oncogene into the HaCaT genome. For studying this question, we isolated the chromosomes carrying the *ras* oncogene from different HaCaT-*ras* clones by the technique of microcell transfer (Fournier and Ruddle 1977; Saxon et al. 1985). The cells are initially blocked in metaphase (by colcemide), but with time a significant proportion escapes the block and enters G_1. Since there is no spindle formation, the chromosomes remain unsorted and nuclear membranes are formed around single or groups of chromosomes, leading to micronuclei each containing one to a few chromosomes. The cells are then enucleated by treatment with cytochalasin B, followed by high-speed centrifugation, and the resulting microcells are fused with mouse recipient cells (A9 cell line). In these mouse cells, the human chromosomes can be identified (by G-11 staining, leading to differential staining of human and mouse chromosomes) and expanded. Clones with a single human chromosome were selected and the presence of the *ras* oncogene verified by Southern blot analysis. Finally, the respective chromosomes were identified by G-banding and the integration site of the *ras* oncogene determined by in situ hybridization. Seven individual clones were analyzed this way and revealed that the *ras* oncogene was always integrated in a different chromosome, or at least in different arms of the chromosome, strongly suggesting that integration had occurred randomly (Boukamp et al., in preparation). This largely contradicts the observation of a rather specific integration as proposed for *ras*-transfected rat fibroblasts (McKenna et al. 1988).

Cooperation with the Cytogenetic "Background" of the Recipient Cell

Due to our experimental approach, the isolatated *ras* oncogene containing chromosomes were available (in the A9 cells) for further studies. Thus, we transferred them into the parental HaCaT cells and so introduced the ras oncogene integrated in an intact chromosome. Transfection of cells is generally accompanied by additional cytogenetic rearrangements which are difficult to interpret in their functional significance. This is largely excluded by the procedure of microcell transfer, since the chromosome in question is maintained as an entity. This technique should therefore allow us to determine whether and how far the undisturbed cytogenetic background of the recipient cells may influence the action of the *ras* oncogene.

Thus, the *ras* oncogene carrying chromosomes were reisolated from the mouse cells as microcells and this time transferred into HaCaT cells of different passages. Previous detailed cytogenetic analyses of consecutive HaCaT passages had shown that a number of new marker chromosomes developed between passages 30 and 50 (S. Altmeyer and N.E. Fusenig, in preparation). *ras*-oncogene-carrying chromosomes of different HaCaT-*ras* clones were transferred into HaCaT cells of the passages >35, 19–26, and a subclone of HaCaT passage 10. The resulting individual clones were analyzed by G-11 staining and mouse chromosome contamination excluded. The clones derived from the highest HaCaT passage grew progressively as tumors in nude mice and, on histology, were locally invasive squamous cell carcinomas. With HaCaT cells of passage 19–26, the majority of clones either grew slowly and formed encapsulated benign cysts or the nodules formed after injection completely regressed, comparable to the results with the nontumorigenic HaCaT cells. When the same *ras*-containing chromosome was transferred into cells from HaCaT passage 10, they remained nontumorigenic in vivo. Thus, differences in tumor growth in vivo was not due to loss of *ras* in the nontumorigenic clones, as verified by Southern blot analysis. All clones which were further studied exhibited the same oncogene restriction pattern as the original HaCaT-*ras* clones (Southern blot analysis). Also, using in situ hybridization we could demonstrate that the chromosomes carrying the *ras* oncogene were present and unchanged in the different HaCaT clones, and *ras* RNA was also expressed in these clones as shown by northern blot analysis.

These results clearly indicated that the *ras* oncogene, integrated in the same chromosome, exerted different effects in the recipient cells, depending on their genetic background. It now remains to determine whether the actual karyotypic differences between early and later passage HaCaT cells were due to the loss of certain chromosomes (during passaging) carrying putative tumor suppressor genes, and whether this might account for the altered cooperation with the *ras* oncogene, i.e., resulting in malignant transformation. At present, we are assaying chromosomes 15 and 13, whereby chromosome 15 is of particular importance due to the presence of the thrombospondin gene, a putative suppressor gene for angiogenesis (Good et al. 1990). This could be of particular importance, since one of the major differences between the benign and malignant tumorigenic HaCaT-*ras* cells is the ability of the latter to induce massive angiogenesis in surface transplants in the early phase of invasion, while the benign and nontumorigenic clones do not possess this ability.

Conclusions

In analogy to the model developed by Vogelstein for colorectal tumorigenesis (Fearon and Vogelstein 1990), we could distinguish at least three different stages of transformation in our model of the multistep process of keratinocyte carcinogenesis:

1. Immortality, which in addition to the action of simian virus 40 or human papilloma virus genes, can possibly be induced by mechanisms such as loss of senescence genes and mutation of the p53 gene.
2. Tumorigenic conversion could be induced by the c-Ha-*ras* oncogene. According to our hypothesis, this will only lead to the benign tumorigenic phenotype, comparable with results obtained after transfection and infection studies in mouse keratinocytes in vitro and in vivo (Roop et al.

1986, Bremner and Balmain 1990). Moreover, this stage was associated with the underrepresentation of chromosome 1p and, functionally, with altered growth regulation in culture and in vivo.

3. Malignant conversion obviously required additional genetic changes probably leading to loss of "tumor suppressor genes." We are testing at present whether chromosomes 15 and 13 are particularly involved. In addition, these clones showed altered response to TGF-β_1, which might indicate a modified interaction with host stroma.

Spontaneous metastatic potential has so far not been detected in our cells. However, intravenous injection did lead to the formation of (highly differentiated) lung colonies, demonstrating that the cells are able to attach and grow at distant sites. Whether additional, at present still unknown, genetic alterations are required for metastasis, as proposed by Vogelstein (Fearon and Vogelstein 1990), or whether this propensity is already present in a minor tumor cell population requiring further selection and altered interaction with the environment, as proposed by Kerbel (1990), remains to be analyzed.

References

Baden HP, Kubilius J, Kredar JC, Steinberg ML, Wolman SR (1987) Isolation and characterization of a spontaneously arising long-lived line of human keratinocytes (NM1). In Vitro Cell Dev Biol 23:205–213

Banks L, Matlashewski G, Crawford L (1986) Isolation of human-p53-specific monoclonal antibodies and their use in the studies of human p53 expression. Eur J Biochem 159:529–534

Barrett JC (1991) Comparison of human versus rodent cell transformation: importance of cell aging. In: Rhim J, Dritschilo A (eds) Neoplastic transformation in human cell systems in vitro. Humana, Totowa

Bishop M (1991) Molecular themes in oncogenesis. Cell 64:235–248

Boukamp P, Fusenig NE (1992) Trans-differentiation from epidermal to mesenchymal/myogenic phenotype is associated with a drastic change in cell-cell and cell-matrix adhesion molecules. J Cell Biol

Boukamp P, Tilgen W, Dzarliewa RT, Breitkreutz D, Haag D, Riehl RK, Bohnert A, Fusenig NE (1982) Phenotypic and genotypic characteristics of a cell line from a squamous cell carcinoma of human skin. J Natl Cancer Inst 68:415–427

Boukamp P, Rupniak THR, Fusenig NE (1985) Environmental modulation of the expression of differentiation and malignancy in six human squamous cell carcinoma cell lines. Cancer Res 45:5582–5592

Boukamp P, Dzarliewa-Petrusevska RT, Breitkreutz D, Hornung J, Markham A, Fusenig NE (1988) Normal keratinization in a spontaneously immortalized aneuploid human keratinocyte cell line. J Cell Biol 106:761–771

Boukamp P, Breitkreutz D, Stark H-J, Fusenig NE (1990a) Mesenchyme-mediated and endogenous regulation of growth and differentiation of human skin keratinocytes derived from different body sites. Differentiation 44:150–161

Boukamp P, Stanbridge EJ, Foo DY, Cerutti PA, Fusenig NE (1990b) C-Ha-ras oncogene expression in immortalized human keratinocytes (HaCaT) alters growth potential in vivo but lacks correlation with malignancy. Cancer Res 50:2840–2847

Boukamp P, Chen J, Gonzales F, Jones PA, Fusenig NE (1992) Progressive stage of "trans-differentiation" from epidermal to mesenchymal phenotype induced by MyoD1 transfection, 5-aza-2' deoxyctidine treatment, and selection for reduced cell attachment in the human keratinocyte line HaCaT. J Cell Biol 116:1257–1271

Boyd JA, Barrett JC (1990) Genetic and cellular basis of multistep carcinogenesis. Pharmacol Ther 46:469–486

Breitkreutz D, Hornung J, Pöhlmann J, Brown-Biermann L, Bohnert A, Bowden PE, Fusenig NE (1986) Environmental induction of differentiation-specific keratins in malignant mouse keratinocyte lines. Europ J Cell Biol 42:255–267

Breitkreutz D, Boukamp P, Stark H-J, Ryle C, Fusenig NE (1989) Response of established keratinocyte lines to modulators of epidermal differentiation. In: Pharmacology and the Skin, vol 3. Karger, Basel, pp 8–14

Breitkreutz D, Boukamp P, Ryle CM, Stark H-J, Roop DR, Fusenig NE (1991) Epidermal morphogenesis and keratin expression in c-Ha-ras-transfected tumorigenic clones of the human HaCaT cell line. Cancer Res 51:4402–44409

Bremner R, Balmain A (1990) Genetic changes in skin tumor progression: correlation between presence of a mutant ras gene and loss of heterozygosity on mouse chromosome 7. Cell 61:407–417

Edelman GM (1986) Cell adhesion molecules in the regulation of animal form and tissue pattern. Annu Rev Cell Biol 2:81–116

Fearon ER, Vogelstein B (1990) A genetic model for colorectal tumorigenesis. Cell 61:759–767

Fournier REK, Ruddle FH (1977) Microcell-mediated transfer of murine chromosomes into mouse, chinese hamster, and human somatic cells. Proc Natl Sci USA 74:319–323

Fusenig NE, Breitkreutz D, Dzarliewa RT, Boukamp P, Bohnert A, Tilgen W (1983) Growth and differentiation characteristics of transformed keratinocytes from mouse and human skin in vitro and in vivo. J Invest Dermatol 81:168s–175s

Fusenig NE, Dzarliewa-Petrusevska RT, Breitkreutz D (1985) Phenotypic and cytogenetic characteristics of different stages during spontaneous transformation of mouse keratinocytes in vitro. In: Barrett JC, Tennant RW (eds) Carcinogenesis, vol 9. Raven, New York, pp 293–326

Fusenig NE, Boukamp P, Breitkreutz D, Hülsen A, Karjetta S, Stanbridge E (1989) Transformation of human skin epithelial cells in vitro: concepts and stages of transformation. In: Chadwick KH, Seymour C, Barnhard B (eds) Cell transformation and radiation-induced cancer. Hilger, Bristol, pp 45–56

Fusenig NE, Boukamp P, Breitkreutz D, Hülsen A, Petrusevska RT, Cerutti P, Stanbridge E (1990) In vitro transformation of human skin epithelial cells: role of ras oncogene in malignant progression. Toxicol In Vitro 4:627–634

Fusenig NE, Breitkeutz D, Boukamp P (1991a) Differentiation potential of cancer cells. In: Masters J (ed) Human cancer in primary culture. A handbook. Kluwer Dordrecht, pp 55–80

Fusenig NE, Boukamp P, Breitkreutz D, Hülsen A (1991b) Altered regulation of growth and differentiation at different stages of transformation of human skin keratinocytes. In: Rhim J, Dritschilo A (eds) Neoplastic transformation in human cell systems in vitro. Humana, New Jersey

Gannon JV, Greaves R, Iggo R, Lane DP (1990) Activating mutations in p53 produce a common conformational effect. A monoclonal antibody specific for the mutant form. EMBO J 9:1595–1602

Good DJ, Polverini PJ, Rastinead F, Le Beau MM, Lemons RS, Frazier WA, Bouck NP (1990) A tumor suppressor-dependent inhibitor of angiogenesis is immunologically and functionally indistinguishable from a fragment of thrombospondin. Proc Natl Acad Sci USA 87:6624–6628

Harris H, Miller UJ, Klein G, Worst P, Tachibana T (1969) Suppression of malignancy by cell fusion. Nature 223:363–368
Henrad DR, Thornley AT, Brown LM, Rheinwald JG (1990) Specific effects of ras oncogene expression on the growth and histogenesis of human epidermal keratinocytes. Oncogene 5:475–481
Jenkins JR, Rudge K, Currie GA (1984) Cellular immortalization by a cDNA clone encoding the transformation-associated phospho-protein p53. Nature 312:651–654
Kerbel RS (1990) Growth dominance of the metastatic cancer cell: cellular and molecular aspects. Adv Cancer Res 55:87–132
Land H, Parada LF, Weinberg K (1983) Tumorigenic conversion of primary embryo fibroblasts requires at least two cooperating oncogenes. Nature 304:596–602
Lane DP, Benchimol S (1990) p53: oncogene or anti-oncogene? Genes Dev 4:1–8
Lehmann TA, Modah R, Stanek J, Welsh J, Bennett WP, Stampfer M, Boukamp P, Fusenig NE, Harris CC (1993) P53 mutations in human immortalized epithelial cell lines. Carcinogenesis (in press)
McKenna WG, Nkahara K, Muschel RJ (1988) Site specific integration of Ha-ras in transformed rat embryo cells. Science 241:1325–1327
Pierceall WE, Goldberg LH, Tainsky MA, Mukhopadhyay T, Ananthaswamy HN (1991) Ras gene mutation and amplification in human nonmelanoma skin cancers. Mol Carcinog 4:196–202
Rhim JS (1989) Neoplastic transformation of human epithelial cells in vitro. Anticancer Res 9:1345–1366
Rhim JS, Dritschilo A (eds) (1991) Neoplastic transformation in human cell systems in vitro. Humana, Totowa
Roop DR, Lowy DR, Tambourin PE, Strickland J, Harper JR, Balaschak M, Spangler EF, Yuspa SH (1986) An activated Harvey ras oncogene produces benign tumours on mouse epidermal tissue. Nature 323:822–824
Ryle CM, Breitkreutz D, Stark H-J, Leigh IM, Steinert PM, Roop D, Fusenig NE (1989) Density-dependent modulation of synthesis of keratins 1 and 10 in the human keratinocyte line HaCaT and in ras-transfected tumorigenic clones. Differentiation 40:42–54
Sager R (1984) Resistance of human cells to oncogenic transformation. Cancer Cells 2:487–493
Saxon PJ, Srivatsan ES, Leipzig GV, Sameshima JH, Stanbridge EJ (1985) Selective transfer of individual human chromosomes to recipient cells. Mol Cell Biol 5:140–146
Stanbridge EJ (1976) Suppression of malignancy in human cells. Nature 260:17–20
Stanbridge EJ (1990) Human tumor suppressor genes. Annu Rev Genet 24:615–657
Sugawara S, Oshimura M, Koi M, Annab LA, Barrett JC (1990) Induction of cellular senescence in immortalized cells by human chromosome 1. Science 247:707–710
Tilgen W, Boukamp P, Breitkreutz D, Dzarliewa RT, Engstner M, Haag D, Fusenig NE (1983) Preservation of morphological, functional and karyotypic traits during long-term culture and in vivo passage of two human skin squamous cell carcinomas. Cancer Res 43:5995–6011
Vlemincks K, Vakaet Jr L, Mareel M, Fiers W, Van Roy F (1991) Genetic manipulation of E-cadherin expression by epithelial tumor cells reveals an invasion suppressor role. Cell 66:107–119
Watt F, Boukamp P, Hornung J, Fusenig NE (1987) Effect of growth environment on spatial expression of involucrin by human epidermal keratinocytes. Arch Dermatol Res 279:335–340

*Human Papillomaviruses and Cancer**

D.R. Lowy, S.A. Sedman, B.D. Cohen, and J.T. Schiller

National Institutes of Health, Bethesda, MD 20892, USA

Human papillomavirus (HPV) infection has been associated with specific human cancers, including cancer of the cervix and other genital cancers and skin cancers in patients with epidermodysplasia verruciformis. HPV does not thus far appear to be commonly associated with nongenital Bowen's disease or nongenital skin cancers, although it is found routinely in genital forms of these conditions. Other factors in addition to HPV infection appear to contribute to tumor associated with HPV, which suggests that cellular changes in addition to HPV infection may be required for frank malignancy. Only a subset of the more than 60 HPV types have been found regularly in malignancies. Among the HPVs that infect the genital tract, some, such as HPV6 and HPV11, are only rarely detected in association with genital cancers, while others, including HPV16 and HPV18, are regularly found in malignancies. The former HPV types are therefore designated "low-risk" and the latter "high-risk."

Multiple differences account for the greater biological activity of the high-risk HPV types. One striking correlation is that the high-risk HPV types can induce immortalization of cultured human keratinocytes, while low-risk HPV types lack this activity. Immortalization by the high-risk HPV types has been found to require cooperation between the viral *E6* and *E7* genes, which are the two viral genes that are preferentially retained and expressed in cervical cancers. The *E6* and *E7* genes of low-risk HPV types were each inactive when tested with a potentially cooperating gene from a high-risk HPV, although a combination of the two genes from two different high-risk HPV types could cooperate efficiently with each other. These results correlate with quantitative differences in the ability of the E7 proteins from the high-risk HPV types to bind the tumor suppressor RB protein and to be

* Since it was impossible for the authors to meet the deadline for manuscript submission, they agreed to the abstract submitted being published. The Editors.

Recent Results in Cancer Research, Vol. 128

phosphorylated by casein kinase II and with the reported ability of E6 from high-risk HPV types to bind tumor suppressor protein p53. The apparent significance of p53 binding is suggested by its ability to substitute for high-risk E6 in the keratinocyte immortalization assay.

Skin Carcinogenesis: A Health Problem Meets with a Scientific Challenge Concluding Remarks and Future Prospects

F. Marks

German Cancer Research Center, W-6900 Heidelberg, Fed. Rep. of Germany

The symposium on which this book was based was intended to bring together clinicians and experimental scientists engaged in research in skin carcinogenesis. The field of skin carcinogenesis seems to be particularly well suited for such an approach, for two reasons:

1. Among the white population skin cancer is by far the most frequent form of malignant neoplasia and, as far as malignant melanoma is concerned, also a serious threat. Skin cancer was the first neoplastic disease shown to be caused by environmental factors. More than 200 years ago, Sir Percival Pott made the revolutionary suggestion of a causal relationship between skin cancer in chimney sweeps and chronic contact with soat and tar. About a century later, Unna discussed the possibility of skin cancer being related to sun exposure and in 1902 Frieben demonstrated the skin-carcinogenic potential of X-rays. Finally, the reader may be reminded of Guiffo's results showing a transplantable or infectious agent to be involved in the generation of skin warts, which is considered to be a landmark in tumor virology. So, the three major types of exogenous factors accused of being involved in carcinogenesis were deteced using skin as a target organ (reviewed in Marks 1989).

2. After the famous coal tar experiment of Yamagiwa and Ichikawa (1914), animal skin became the classic and most widely used model for the detection of environmental carcinogens as well as for experimental purposes, and important concepts such as multistage carcinogenesis were developed for the first time by employing this model. These also include the biological characterization of key compounds of carcinogenesis such as the polycyclic aromatic hydrocarbons and the phorbol ester tumor promoters. Thus, experimental skin carcinogenesis quickly overcame the limits of dermatology, developing into an approach thought to provide general information on the induction and development of benign and malignant epithelial tumors.

Today it is generally accepted that cancer results from an accumulation of genetic defects. Recently, there has been much excitement over the so called Vogelstein model which suggests that fully malignant colorectal cancer of man is due to both mutation of protooncogenes and inactivation of suppressor genes (Fearon and Vogelstein 1990). At first glance it appears as if this model has now made the classical animal model of skin carcinogenesis outdated. It must not be overlooked, however, that the Vogelstein model, like any model of human carcinogenesis, is more or less a *descriptive* one dealing with already existing pathological states, whereas the skin model offers all kinds of experimental interactions and gradual procedures, thus permitting a much deeper insight into the basic *mechanisms* of tumor generation and tumor development.

This is true for both chemically and UV-induced epithelial skin cancer and is best exemplified by the process of tumor promotion, which is precisely defined both in operational and mechanistic terms in the animal model, whereas in human carcinogenesis it remains a matter of much speculation and debate. Moreover, the animal skin model offers rather unique possibilities of freely alternating between in vivo and in vitro conditions. The in vitro cultivation of skin cells has reached a high standard by now and allows a detailed analysis of those biochemical and cellular alterations which are the result of the critical gene mutations.

On the first day of the symposium its objectives were layed down, not only by setting up the two pillars (i.e., laboratory experiment and epidemiology) that cancer research rests on, but in particular by introducing main topics of current interest: the role of cell proliferation and cell aging in tumor development; and the heterogeneity of the target tissue, i.e., skin, and the complex interaction of this target tissue with the rest of the body. The subsequent contributions provided many variations of these basic themes, demonstrating in particular the tremendous impact of modern concepts and methods like those of molecular biology, biochemistry, immunology, etc. As one example, the successful demonstration of mutated Ha-*ras* proto-oncogenes in chemically initiated mouse skin may be mentioned. Before now everybody was convinced that initiated skin is biochemically and morphologically indistinguishable from normal skin. Now, one is forced to realize that this was a premature statement. Moreover, it has now become possible to dissect the biochemical consequences of this *ras* mutation under controlled experimental conditions using keratinocyte cell cultures. Another example is provided by the rapid progress made in the characterization of skin cell differentiation markers using monoclonal antibody techniques. It appears as if experimental dermatologists will soon compete with the immunologists in playing this sort of game. Finally, together with modern techniques of gene analysis, the breeding of hybrid and transgenic animals offers a wide field of exciting investigations into the genetic mechanisms of carcinogenesis.

Like every living organism, a cell not only proliferates but is also prone to die sooner or later. Normal cells seem to have an inborn lifespan which restricts the number of division cycles in a very strict and specific manner.

Upon neoplastic transformation this brake is released, resulting in some kind of "immortality." The molecular mechanism of this phenomenon has now become the subject of genetic analysis, which will hopefully be followed in due course by a better understanding of the biochemical events involved in the termination of the cellular lifespan. Perhaps this will help to explain the well-known but still mysterious observation that only the latency period but not the overall incidence of spontaneous neoplasia is a function of normal life expectancy in different species and that rodent cells can be transformed much more easily than human cells. Thus, cancer appears to be related to senility and may also be considered as a normal cause of death. In approaching the molecular mechanisms, one gets the impression of a very close relationship between molecular oncology and molecular gerontology.

There are, of course, many unresolved problems, such as the relationship between senescence, terminal differentiation, and apoptosis. Do epidermal cells undergo senescence and, if so, is this process restricted to the proliferative compartment or is it related to terminal differentiation? Is apoptosis an additional homeostatic control device in skin, for example in the regression of papillomas and hair follicles, and can the demonstration of a growth arrest and DNA damage gene (GADD) induced upon distress be taken as an indication for apoptotic processes to occur in skin? Or may everything be explained by terminal differentiation, at least as far as the keratinocyte is concerned?

A problem closely related to these questions and also waiting for a final solution is the control of epidermal tissue homeostasis. Is it due to the action of intercellular signals controlling both cell proliferation and perhaps apoptosis, or is it again merely an automatic consequence of terminal differentiation? A steadily increasing number of growth factors and cytokines has been found to either induce or inhibit epidermal cell proliferation (McKay and Leigh 1991; Kupper 1990; Fuchs 1990; Marks 1991), and the idea easily comes up that, while normal homeostasis is due to an equilibrium, neoplastic growth results from an disequilibrium between positive and negative signals. But what is the proper physiological role of factors such as the TGF-α/TGF-β pair? Are they really homeostatic regulators or merely wound hormones becoming active only upon skin damage? Considering the rapidly increasing knowledge of the molecular mechanisms of such factors, in particular in cell cycle control, the lack of information on their proper physiological function is especially disappointing. So, we are urgently waiting for progress in the field of skin endocrinology and skin pharmacology!

In this context, it must not be forgotten that growth control is not only a problem of molecular biology and biochemistry, but in particular of cell sociology. Several speakers have emphasized the fact that living skin is a complex organ rather than a homogeneous cell population, and that its function and proliferative behavior depend critically on precisely controlled interactions between its different components, be it the dermal and epithelial compartment, different cell types in the epidermis, or – most important for an understanding of growth control – stem cells and mature cells within the same tissue type. The precise location of putative stem cells, for example in the hair root, and the control of their function by the underlying dermal compartment and by systemic signals indicates that in skin, like in other organs, homeostasis critically depends on tissue architecture and intercellular interactions and gives an impression of the long way research still has to go to finally arrive at an understanding of tissue growth control.

Just to mention a few related questions which are still to be answered:

- Do stem cells exist in interfollicular epidermis? And if so, where precisely are they located?
- Does initiation of carcinogenesis occur in the stem cell compartment, as has been proposed to explain the persistence of the initiated state?
- What is the cell of origin of epidermal tumors?
- What kind of signals controlling epidermal functions are emitted by the dermal compartment and vice versa?
- What is the proper function of Merkel cells?

And when comparing in vivo with in vitro data we should be aware of the fact that in vivo a tumor does grow only on a stroma bed providing the proper device for energy supply and waste disposal, whereas under in vitro conditions these important prerequisites for survival are provided by the experimenter. So, many in vivo effects such as, for example, the conversion of initiated skin into a state of promotability (Marks and Fürstenberger 1990), may be related to stroma induction rather than to effects on the keratinocyte.

One of the most exciting developments of modern dermatology has led to a complete change of our view of epidermal cell functions. For a long time the keratinocyte was thought to provide only a resistant horny layer protecting the body from external injury and water loss. Now we have learned that this cell type additionally has the function of an interface in that it is a very active transmitter and receiver of intercellular signals which attract and influence many other cell types, especially those involved in wound healing and defense reactions (Milestone and Edelson 1988). Skin has been found to be an outpost of the immune system. The role of the Langerhans cell as an antigen-presenting cell provides an impressive example, and it is obvious that carcinogenesis is influenced by such interactions, as shown for immune-suppressed patients or UV carcinogenesis. There are much more fascinating aspects of skin physiology which were touched upon during this symposium. We heard of several promising attempts to apply modern experimental techniques to clinical problems. This includes the identification of differentiation markers, signal transduction pathways, regulatory genes, etc. The results are impressive enough, but – in my opinion – they are still in the stage of description rather than of elucidation of causal relationships. We hope that this situation will change rapidly in the near future as a better understanding emerges of the physiological functions of protooncogene-

and suppressor gene-encoded proteins as well as growth factors and other homeostatic regulators.

Malignant melanoma is a major clinical problem and most efforts are presently concentrating on the identification of endogenous and exogenous risk factors. So, the melanoma story provides first of all an example for the second basis of cancer research, i.e., epidemiology with all its advantages and limitations. Everybody is frightened by the steady increase of this very aggressive cancer among the white population, which has created an urgent need for better measures of prevention and treatment. We have heard of a series of studies trying to scrutinize inheritable or otherwise constitutive conditions of an increased melanoma risk, but we are still in search of the environmental risk factors which seem to be critically involved. There is evidence that sunlight might provide such a risk factor, but this evidence is not as unequivocal as in the case of squamous and basal cell carcinoma. One has gained the impression that the concept of sun exposure in childhood still may not be the final answer. As far as basic research is concerned, melanoma research lagged behind other areas of cancer research for a long time. This situation seems to be rapidly changing now to the same extent as modern experimental methods are being applied to this problem. The investigations presented during this symposium and dealing with the role of cellular adhesion molecules and growth factors in melanoma progression provided impressive examples and exciting future prospects; especially for new therapeutic approaches and diagnostic measures. As far as basal and squamous cell carcinoma is concerned the epidemiological data are absolutely clear in showing that most of these cancers result from life-long sun exposure. Actually, these diseases presently provide the most impressive if not classic examples of environmentally induced neoplasia. Such conclusions are, of course, of great interest for the general public, as shown by the ongoing debate on the hazards resulting from a destruction of the atmospheric ozone layer, from artificial tanning devices, and from an outdoor lifestyle. Moreover, diseases such as xeroderma and others may be considered as the best documented examples of the interaction between inborn defects and exogenous factors in carcinogenesis. Whether papillomaviruses belong to these exogenous factors has still to be shown.

In summary, the contributions to this symposium and to this volume have provided an exemplary insight into the present status of cancer research, which is characterized by a rapid increase in basic knowledge in contrast to the generally much slower progress in the prevention and treatment of the disease. Moreover, they demonstrate that a rather disturbing discrepancy exists between the clear-cut identification of an environmental hazard such as UV light and the acceptance of such a fact by the general public. The dramatic impact of new methods and concepts certainly justifies the hope that the molecular mechanisms of carcinogenesis will be fully revealed in the not too far distant future. An intensification of both the collaboration between scientists and clinicians and the instruction of the public is, therefore, urgently required to bridge the still widening gap between theory and practice. This symposium and this book have pursued just this aim, and it is hoped that they have fulfilled their purpose.

References

Fearon ER, Vogelstein B (1990) A genetic model for colorectal tumorigenesis. Cell 61:759–767

Fuchs E (1990) Epidermal differentiation: the bare essentials. J Cell Biol 111:2807–2814

Kupper TS (1990) The activated keratinocyte: a model for inducible cytokine production by non-bone marrow-derived cells in cutaneous inflammation and immune responses. J Invest Dermatol 94:146S–150S

Marks F (1989) Skin cancer (excluding melanomas). In: Greaves MW, Schuster S (eds) Handbook of experimental pharmacology, vol 87/II: Pharmacology of the skin II. Springer, Berlin Heidelberg New York, pp 167–194

Marks F (1991) Neoplasia and the wound response: the lesson learned from the multistage approach of skin carcinogenesis. In: Paukovits WR (ed) Growth regulation and carcinogenesis, vol I. CRC Press, Boca Raton, pp 53–82

Marks F, Fürstenberger G (1990) The conversion stage of skin carcinogenesis. Carcinogenesis 11:2085–2092

McKay IA, Leigh IM (1991) Epidermal cytokines and their roles in cutaneous wound healing. Br J Dermatol 124:513–518

Milestone LM, Edelson RL (eds) (1988) Endocrine, metabolic and immunologic functions of keratinocytes. Ann NY Acad Sci 548

Yamagiwa K, Ichikawa K (1914) Über die künstliche Epithelwucherung. Gann 8:11–142

Subject Index

Springer-Verlag and the Environment

We at Springer-Verlag firmly believe that an international science publisher has a special obligation to the environment, and our corporate policies consistently reflect this conviction.

We also expect our business partners – paper mills, printers, packaging manufacturers, etc. – to commit themselves to using environmentally friendly materials and production processes.

The paper in this book is made from low- or no-chlorine pulp and is acid free, in conformance with international standards for paper permanency.

MIX
Papier aus verantwortungsvollen Quellen
Paper from responsible sources
FSC® C105338

If you have any concerns about our products,
you can contact us on
ProductSafety@springernature.com

In case Publisher is established outside the EU,
the EU authorized representative is:
Springer Nature Customer Service Center GmbH
Europaplatz 3, 69115 Heidelberg, Germany

Printed by Libri Plureos GmbH
in Hamburg, Germany